1/2014

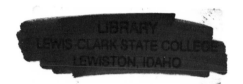

D1443002

GLOBAL HEALTH IN AFRICA

PERSPECTIVES ON GLOBAL HEALTH

Series editor: James L. A. Webb, Jr.

The History of Blood Transfusion in Sub-Saharan Africa,
by William H. Schneider

Global Health in Africa: Historical Perspectives on Disease Control,
edited by Tamara Giles-Vernick and James L. A. Webb, Jr.

GLOBAL HEALTH IN AFRICA

Historical Perspectives on Disease Control

Edited by Tamara Giles-Vernick and
James L. A. Webb, Jr.

Ohio University Press
Athens

Ohio University Press, Athens, Ohio 45701
ohioswallow.com
© 2013 by Ohio University Press

To obtain permission to quote, reprint, or otherwise reproduce or distribute material from
Ohio University Press publications, please contact our rights and permissions department at
(740) 593-1154 or (740) 593-4536 (fax).

Printed in the United States of America
Ohio University Press books are printed on acid-free paper ⊗ ™

COVER PHOTOS: (*top left*) WHO Photo 1991, ARCO 12, PRINT-AFRO-MALARIA. "After the spraying is
completed in any house the foreman records the date of spraying on the wall." Photograph by P. Palmer. WHO Copyright; (*top center*) courtesy Tamara Giles-Vernick; (*top right*) WHO Photo 11761, ARCO 12, PRINT-AFRO-MALARIA.
"Laboratory Technicians Collect Blood Specimens From School Children in a Survey to Determine the Incidence of
Malaria in the Town of Ho." Photographer Unknown. WHO Copyright; (*primary image*) courtesy Tamara Giles-Vernick

23 22 21 20 19 18 17 16 15 14 13   5 4 3 2 1

Library of Congress Cataloging-in-Publication Data
Global health in Africa : historical perspectives on disease control / edited by Tamara Giles-
Vernick and James L. A. Webb, Jr.
     pages cm. — (Perspectives on global health)
"Global Health in Africa had its beginnings in 2008, at a one-day workshop at Princeton
University"—Acknowledgments.
 Includes bibliographical references and index.
 ISBN 978-0-8214-2067-6 (hc : alk. paper) — ISBN 978-0-8214-2068-3 (pb : alk. paper) —
ISBN 978-0-8214-4471-9
 1. Public health—Africa—Congresses. 2. Medical policy—Africa—Congresses. 3. Africa—
Social conditions—Congresses. 4. Public health—International cooperation—Congresses. I.
Giles-Vernick, Tamara, [date]– editor of compilation. II. Webb, James L. A., Jr., [date]– editor of
compilation. III. Series: Perspectives on global health.
 RA545.G56 2013
 614.4096—dc23
                                        2013026979

CONTENTS

ACKNOWLEDGMENTS

Global Health in Africa had its beginnings in 2008, at a one-day workshop at Princeton University. We are grateful to Princeton University's Center for Collaborative History, Center for Health and Wellbeing, Department of History, Shelby Cullom Davis Center for Historical Studies, and Environmental Institute for their financial support for the workshop and to Emmanuel Kreike for his gracious efforts in facilitating it. Emmanuel Akyeampong, Jean-Paul Bado, Barbara Cooper, Susan Craddock, Steve Feierman, Matthieu Fintz, Emmanuel Kreike, Burton Singer, and Helen Tilley made incisive contributions to our workshop discussions and influenced the direction that the resulting volume has taken.

The editors express thanks to their home institutions. Tamara Giles-Vernick conveys her gratitude to Arnaud Fontanet and members of the Institut Pasteur Unit of Emerging Diseases Epidemiology for generously sharing their perspectives on global public health and to Sylvana Thépaut for her superb administrative assistance. Jim Webb thanks colleagues in the Department of History and the Program in Global Studies at Colby College for a congenial work environment and in the administration at Colby College for their support of a National Institutes of Health/National Library of Medicine grant that provided time for research and writing.

The volume has entailed extensive back-and-forth communications between the editors and the contributors, and we are grateful for the spirit of collegiality and goodwill of our contributors. Many of the ideas, interpretations, and data in these essays have been tested in conference presentations in a wide variety of university and research settings, and we are appreciatively aware that the contributions have been strengthened as a result. An earlier version of William Schneider's essay on smallpox appeared in *Medical History* 53, no. 2 (2009), and a slightly modified version of the essay on malaria by Jim Webb was published in the *Journal of the History of Medicine and Allied Sciences* 66, no. 3 (2011).

We thank Patrick Zylberman and Aline Munier for their insights, comments, and suggestions on the various essays in this volume. The external reviewers engaged by the Ohio University Press likewise wrote astute reports that provided helpful guidance for revisions. Gill Berchowitz, director of Ohio

University Press, was continuously supportive of the project and a pleasure to work with.

The editors thank their spouses, Ken Vernick and Alison Jones Webb, for their critical readings, intellectual exchanges, and good humor.

INTRODUCTION

JAMES L. A. WEBB, JR. AND TAMARA GILES-VERNICK

Global health history is a new research field, and to date we know little about the histories of global health initiatives in Africa.[1] In one sense, this is quite surprising. Africa's disease burden is heavy, and international and bilateral agencies, philanthropic organizations, nongovernmental organizations (NGOs), and public-private partnerships in league with African governments have undertaken a broad array of interventions against individual diseases and into health care systems over the past many decades. Most of these interventions were time-limited, ran their courses, and were forgotten. Later iterations of these programs generally took scant advantage of the earlier experiences. There were no specialists charged with understanding the past experiences, and thus there was no systematic effort to analyze the performance of global health programs and to investigate the reasons for failure and partial success. The lessons of the past have thus remained largely unarticulated or misconstrued, unable to inform contemporary global health efforts.

Global Health in Africa is a first exploration of some of the histories of global health initiatives in Africa. The volume is published with the intention of developing the new field of global health history in order to broaden the training of a new generation of public health professionals. Our goal is to promote historical and anthropological research that integrates the social sciences and the biomedical sciences in the service of global public health.[2] This approach owes much to the subdiscipline of historical epidemiology, which evaluates the changing nature of disease over space and time; it integrates social, political, economic, and ecological processes with those of pathogens and with the effects of global health initiatives themselves. In bringing together biomedical and social science approaches, historical epidemiology sharpens our understandings of the biosocial causes of ill health and helps us grasp why some interventions fail.

To date, in the development, implementation, and expansion of public health projects, planners generally have not sensed a first imperative to understand the worlds in which their projects would operate. It has not been their charge to appreciate political constraints and resource scarcities or to explore the ways in which African populations understood the biomedical interventions. They have tended to assume that there was no real need to do so, because the epidemiology and etiology of the diseases were sufficiently well known and the methods and interventions could be universally applied. The biomedical practitioners' lack of training in the social sciences made it difficult for them to appreciate the centrality of nonbiomedical perspectives.

This collection highlights some of the public health consequences of the chasm between the biomedical and social sciences that is an artifact of our system of professional education. It underscores the need to bridge the divide in order to improve the delivery of public health services. The fine-grained analyses of the past illustrate how narrowly conceived technical interventions have failed to account for specific and complex contexts into which they are introduced and how, as a result, these interventions have cast long shadows of unintended consequences. The case studies also show how long-standing policy continuities and unquestioned assumptions still guide some contemporary interventions. We have organized our sampling of global health history in Africa around these linkages between past, present, and emergent to highlight how long-term continuities play a critical, but understudied, role in global health.

Global Health

"Global health" is a term that means different things to different people and suggests different policy choices to different audiences in different geographical locations. It can imply support for rural health systems or primary care centers, individual disease control programs such as the mass distribution of insecticide-treated bed nets to reduce malaria transmission, or an effective ban on health education about contraception and abortion. Its breadth is accommodating. It allows virtually everyone to be in favor of global health. In this respect, it is an analog to the umbrella term "economic development" that likewise has meant very different things to different people at different times.[3]

The term "global health," however, is also frequently used to refer to distinctive configurations of financial, political, and biomedical influence and resources in the post–World War II period. In Africa, although the actors have changed over time, the various configurations have one central element of continuity: all have been characterized by a flow of resources to Africa. Private philanthropies, international health organizations, bilateral health programs, and private-public partnerships based in the North Atlantic have developed the health initiatives and implemented them in Africa with African partner states, nongovernmental organizations, and associations.[4] Recent Chinese investment in large-scale health care infrastructure such as hospitals and clinics, and in health care personnel, has expanded the complement of global health actors in Africa.[5]

In this volume, we use the term "global health" broadly to refer to the health initiatives launched within Africa by actors based outside of the continent. In our usage, global health in Africa has its roots in the colonial period and came into its modern forms in the post-WWII era.[6] This framework accommodates the continuities in external resource flows and the changing groups of actors, institutional configurations, and biomedical, financial, and political priorities.[7]

The contributors to this volume address the history of health interventions into acute and chronic infectious diseases including malaria, cholera, influenza, smallpox, and HIV/AIDS, and chronic, noninfectious conditions such as malnutrition and injection drug use. They explore interventions by European colonial and independent African state institutions, the World Health Organization (WHO), nongovernmental organizations, funding and research institutions such as the Pasteur Institute and its international network, and the US National Institutes of Health; and they explore the responses to these interventions by the Africans whose health the interventions were aimed at improving. They demonstrate that health interventions in Africa have a long history that reflects the changing interests of the intervening institutions, scientific advances in the understanding of disease, the development of new tools for intervention, and the changing nature of the international political and economic order.

The Colonial Antecedents of Global Health in Africa

The antecedents of global health in Africa have their roots in the late nineteenth century, when a new chapter in Africa's relationship with Europe began.[8] During the "Scramble for Africa," competing western European powers used African military conscripts to establish political and economic influence within vast African territories, sometimes in collaboration with local African political authorities; after a transition to formal rule, the Europeans extracted resources and labor to bolster their metropolitan economies. In many of the new colonies, the Europeans forced their African subjects to gather wild rubber or to work on plantations or in mines. These working conditions, as well as African flight from colonial labor demands, heightened colonial subjects' exposure to infectious diseases. In this regard, the imposition of European colonial rule and African responses to it provoked important changes in the disease burdens of African peoples.[9]

Africa's medical history was also profoundly changed by the introduction of Western biomedicine. In one sense, the encounter might be thought of as a collision between African medical knowledge and modes of healing and those of Europe. Specialist healers and midwives in Africa had long traditions of caring for acute and chronic illnesses and knowledge of many other conditions (including pregnancy and childbirth), and European medical authorities challenged these African practices, considering them to be primitive and inefficacious. Yet over time, Western biomedicine made inroads into African approaches to healing and was the most important contribution to a new medical pluralism in Africa. Africans with access to Western biomedicine frequently drew on both African and European medical knowledge. African forms of medical knowledge changed over time, but they largely were not displaced or entirely suppressed.[10]

Early in the colonial period, Europeans found their own medical knowledge inadequate to cope with the major infectious diseases in Africa.[11] In an effort to protect European administrators, soldiers, and merchants, European colonial powers invested resources in biomedical research, seeking new ways to understand and control the major diseases in their colonies. This research gave rise to a new discipline of tropical medicine, which developed in new schools of tropical medicine and hygiene and in research institutes in the metropolitan centers of empire and the colonies.[12] The new knowledge was soon deployed in the African colonies, principally through mobile medical campaigns to treat sleeping sickness, onchocerciasis, yaws, tuberculosis, leprosy, syphilis, yellow fever, and other diseases.[13]

European medical missionaries also launched initiatives to serve the African communities in which they evangelized. Some missionary societies set up clinics that offered rudimentary primary medical care in rural areas, and in some urban areas, missionary societies built hospitals that provided more sophisticated medical services for Africans.[14] The secular colonial authorities developed a system of urban hospitals that provided medical services principally to a European clientele.[15]

The global economic depression of the 1930s constrained the colonial medical systems, and with the outbreak of the Second World War, the colonies adopted even more austere budgets. In the aftermath of the war, the European empires began critical reappraisals of their responsibilities to promote programs of economic and social development in their African colonies. Yet it was notably with the creation of the World Health Organization that African health issues began to be considered from broader international perspectives.

JAMES L. A. WEBB, JR. AND TAMARA GILES-VERNICK

The World Health Organization, one of the original agencies of the United Nations, was founded in 1948. It supplanted the two existing international health organizations—the Office international d'hygiène publique and the League of Nations Health Organization—and it had a new, broader mandate.[16] In the postwar world of shattered economies that were beginning to be reconstructed, massive populations of displaced persons, and the rapid polarization of the Cold War blocs, the WHO embraced the objective of the "attainment by all peoples of the highest possible level of health."[17] New medicines and insecticides were available that portended a range of new possibilities for the improvement of human health.

With limited funding from the UN member states, the WHO attracted talented physicians and public health specialists in an era of high confidence in the power of science to improve the lives of the world's peoples. It acted as a consultative body, and with funding from other UN agencies such as UNICEF, it undertook a range of health initiatives in African colonial territories or independent states, whose histories are largely yet to be explored. With its founding came the beginnings of "global health," which owed much to colonial health, in its adoption of a vertical, "campaign"-style approach to controlling or seeking to eradicate specific diseases.[18]

Conceiving of its scope in "international" terms, the WHO divided the world into six regions (Africa, the Americas, Southeast Asia, Europe, the Eastern Mediterranean, and the Western Pacific).[19] Its earliest, high-profile initiatives sought to eradicate specific diseases—first malaria and then smallpox—and to undertake large-scale campaigns against yaws and tuberculosis. Several historians have commented on how Cold War politics shaped both the rhetoric and the practices of these campaigns. The withdrawal of the Soviet Union and other communist countries from the WHO and the UN system in 1949 left the health institution more open to American influence, and this was notably evident in the World Health Assembly's embrace of a malaria eradication program in 1955.[20] When the Soviet bloc returned to the UN in 1956, the Soviets pushed an initiative to eradicate smallpox that was formally adopted by the World Health Assembly in 1959.[21]

In the 1970s, a movement to reorient health programs in Africa and elsewhere in the developing world challenged this focus on eradication and individual disease campaigns. The "basic health care" or "primary health care" movement gained momentum throughout the decade. In 1978, at the International Conference on Primary Health Care in Alma-Ata (in the Soviet

Republic of Kazakhstan), the WHO adopted a new model of health services for developing countries that promulgated the goal of "Health for All by the Year 2000." Both China and Cuba offered models for the provision of basic health services for the rural poor.[22] Missionary medicine, which had long provided basic health services in Africa and elsewhere, also contributed to this movement, emphasizing the training of village health care workers, the availability of basic supplies, and "appropriate technology."[23]

Yet even as the primary health care movement strengthened, a series of public health disasters, brought about by warfare within and between African states, called forth new externally based humanitarian public health responses. Médecins Sans Frontières, the first of a cohort of late twentieth-century secular humanitarian medical interventionist groups, formed in 1971 and committed its resources to providing frontline medical care in areas where states could not.[24] Other humanitarian organizations formed and followed suit.[25] The massive medical needs of millions of Africans in makeshift, unplanned, burgeoning refugee camps without sanitation infrastructure were framed as "complex emergencies," a concept that proved useful in mobilizing financial resources for broad public health interventions.[26]

Outside of the war zones, primary health care flagged. Although the Alma-Ata Declaration received approvals from many nations, the primary health care approach was dogged by difficulties in translating its ideals into practice.[27] Subsequently, international public health planners modified their ambitious goals and adopted the "selective primary health care" approach by targeting specific problems such as growth monitoring to ensure adequate childhood nutrition, oral rehydration techniques for childhood diarrheal infections, breastfeeding, and immunization.[28] The WHO's Expanded Program in Immunization, created in 1974 prior to both Alma-Ata and "selective primary health care," was one of the few enduring contributions of the broader movement.[29]

The primary health care movement, however, did not attract robust, sustainable political support or funding. The governments of some African states embraced the primary health care movement, but most, despite their rhetoric, did not.[30] Neither the United States nor the Soviet Union offered much support; the United States associated the movement with socialism, and the Soviet Union, although it hosted the Alma-Ata meeting, also expressed misgivings.[31] Moreover, donor support for primary health care entailed funneling monies to African governments, and both multilateral and bilateral donors were reluctant to do so. Their restraint resulted partly because health budgets were already committed, but also because of considerable uncertainty about the costs of training rural health workers, improving water quality, or other

JAMES L. A. WEBB, JR. AND TAMARA GILES-VERNICK

goals.[32] Concerns about the corruption, inefficiency, and instability of African governments also shaped these decisions.

Unwillingness to endorse the primary health care approach also reflected mediocre successes in promoting economic development in Africa. Large-scale agriculture and infrastructure projects generally did not meet their goals, and many development projects, such as those that involved the construction of dams for irrigation, produced a spate of unintended health consequences.[33] Moreover, development monies, whether from grants or loans, typically were disbursed from state coffers, and much was diverted. Billions of dollars made their way into the private accounts of African politicians. Even by the 1970s, it was clear to many observers that the grants and loans would not achieve their development goals, yet the funds continued to flow because they secured political allegiances.[34] A new shift in global health in Africa began during the 1980s, resulting in the contraction of health services on the continent. Structural adjustment policies, economic crisis, and the Soviet Union's dissolution, which brought an end to the Cold War, all reduced external resources for African health care services and contributed to deteriorating health care infrastructures.

Beginning in the late 1970s and bolstered by the elections of Margaret Thatcher as prime minister of the UK in 1979 and Ronald Reagan as US president in 1980, a conservative political discourse gained adherents. It held that bloated public sectors were responsible for slow economic growth, and that "structural adjustment" to reduce the ranks of civil servants, would liberate economic sectors of undue political interference and permit African commodities to compete freely in international markets. The International Monetary Fund imposed structural adjustment programs (SAPs) on most African economies in an effort to shrink the public sector. The public sector strictures, however, did not extend to public health expenditures. In many African countries, public health spending increased, but structural adjustment policies sought to create "economic efficiency" by implementing user fees to recover costs. Some African countries adoped the Bamako Initiative (1987) to improve primary health services through community financing. Both efforts produced mixed results. Most health spending has remained focused on hospitals and clinics in urban areas.[35] Structural adjustment did, however, fan an aversion to health care institution building in Africa, although many public health specialists insisted at the time that the health of African populations could be improved most significantly by expanding basic health services in primary care clinics.[36] This divergence in ideological outlook over the appropriate roles of the private and public sectors remains a fundamental tension into the twenty-first century.

Still another historical development shifted attention from previous decades of large-scale eradication campaigns and subsequently from primary health care investment. As the Cold War waned and the threat of nuclear annihilation diminished, security analysts perceived new threats.[37] The collapse of the Soviet Union led to deteriorating controls on biological weapons and scientists' activities, and security experts and public health planners openly worried that biosecurity threats could emerge from a widening array of sources and that new developments in genomics could facilitate the "weaponization" of new biological threats.[38] One key idea was that the increasing integration of the world economy and the increasing volume of global travel would bring forth new threats to health in the developed world. Scientific researchers and commentators argued that this accelerating globalization enhanced the prospects for "emerging disease" outbreaks, and government funding increased for research on such threats.[39]

During the mid to late 1990s, as the HIV pandemic exploded certain "emerging disease threats" became palpably real. As US policymakers became aware of the extent of the epidemiological disaster in Africa, they judged the HIV pandemic to be a geopolitical threat that could destabilize African states and their economies. This provoked new interest in promoting "development" in order to limit the political and economic disruption that AIDS was projected to cause. Global health became further enmeshed with national security concerns.

Global health, however, was not long to remain principally the domain of governmental actors. During the 1980s, private philanthropic organizations began to insert themselves more publicly into the high-profile arena of global health.[40] Rotary International took on the challenge of the global eradication of polio with the creation of its PolioPlus program in 1985, and in 1988, the WHO, together with Rotary International, UNICEF, and the Centers for Disease Control and Prevention, passed the Global Polio Eradication Initiative.[41] Following the lead of researchers at the Centers for Disease Control who advocated for the eradication of Guinea worm, the Carter Center committed itself to support national eradication projects in 1986, and other international partners signed on to the effort at global Guinea worm eradication.[42]

Within a decade, far larger global health efforts were launched by other philanthropic organizations with far broader aspirations and far deeper pockets. In 1994, with the creation of the Bill and Melinda Gates Foundation, the role of private philanthropy in global health surpassed that of bilateral foreign aid, the WHO, and other philanthropic organizations. This heralded a new world health order.[43] In 2000, Bill and Melinda Gates sparked the creation of

JAMES L. A. WEBB, JR. AND TAMARA GILES-VERNICK

the Global Alliance for Vaccines and Immunizations (GAVI), a private-public partnership whose members included the WHO, UNICEF, the World Bank, and representatives of the pharmaceutical industry. Between 2000 and 2011, GAVI had received donations totaling over US $6.4 billion, of which nearly US $1.5 billion (23 percent) came from the Gates Foundation.[44] In 2002, with seed money from the Gates Foundation, a second, larger, and more massively underwritten private-public partnership formed the Global Fund to Fight AIDS, Tuberculosis, and Malaria. Endorsed by the G-8 countries, the Global Fund, based in Geneva and administered until 2009 by WHO staff, garnered support from the taxpayers of the largest developed nations; the single largest private donor was the Gates Foundation. These partnerships have instigated massive campaigns and programs, including the Global Polio Eradication initiative, the Guinea Worm Eradication program, the provision of antiretroviral drugs to prevent the progression of HIV infections, and the mass distribution of insecticide-treated bednets throughout Africa.

In the late twentieth century and the early decades of the twenty-first century, the financial strength of the global public health organizations was thus of a higher order of magnitude than ever before. There continued to be many bilateral programs of health, such as those of the United Kingdom Department for International Development, the US Agency for International Development, China's various ministries involved in providing aid, and the Cooperation Agencies of France, Germany, Sweden, Norway, the Netherlands, Italy, and other European Union countries. Some agencies joined forces in "multilateral" initiatives. Biomedical research institutions and funding organizations also actively created new public health research initiatives around the world. The US National Institutes of Health, for instance, financed research projects that have brought together American and African university research teams. The French Agence Nationale de la Recherche (ANR) made funds available for innovative, multidisciplinary public health research and intervention in the global South, including in Africa. In France and in its network of institutes, some situated in former French colonies in Africa, the Pasteur Institute continued to carry out biomedical research on numerous infectious diseases, including HIV/AIDS, malaria, tuberculosis meningitis, and cholera. The Wellcome Trust funded ongoing biomedical research in the UK and its research institutes in the former British colonies. More nongovernmental organizations and private charities were involved in African health work than at any time in the past. The funding for global health initiatives was greater than ever before.

The decades since the 1990s have seen an escalation in funding for global health in Africa. The development of African health services, however, has proceeded slowly. Several basic measures—infant and child mortality rates, access to skilled childbirth attendants, vaccination coverage—show that sub-Saharan African health systems have not improved as quickly as in much of the rest of the developing world. Some have even stagnated.[45] A growing number of African health professionals did enter into the ranks of the international health elite, and by the late 1990s, African health professionals enjoyed some success in lobbying donor countries to increase their commitments to global health programs in Africa. In one sense, the older paradigm of the developed countries carrying out health programs in Africa had altered: health professionals in Africa who shared biomedical perspectives in common with health professionals in Europe and North America helped design and implement the programs.

The medical pluralism that combined the biomedical systems of treatment and healing developed in Europe and North America with the manifold cultures of treatment and healing in Africa, however, presented numerous challenges. Medical anthropologists made useful contributions that helped expand definitions of health problems and improve the delivery of global health initiatives. A core challenge, however, was to develop cadres of local health practitioners—such as African nurses—who could translate public health messages into African idioms and bring African perspectives into dialog with Western biomedicine.[46]

Continuity in Global Health Initiatives

Against the background of important changes that have taken place—the inception of the WHO, large-scale campaigns partly inspired by Cold War politics, the "primary health care" movement, structural adjustment policies, fears of the threat of emerging diseases, the massive increase in the participation of private philanthropic organizations, and the Africanization of an international health elite—the history of global health initiatives in Africa demonstrates an important continuity. From the immediate post–World War II period to the present, global health initiatives had been characterized by a commitment to disease-specific programs. These programs target individual diseases—such as malaria, tuberculosis, HIV, measles, whooping cough, tetanus, polio, and smallpox—or indicators of health statuses, such as levels of malnutrition, maternal deaths, or access to clean water, as enshrined in the UN's Millennium Development Goals. Some programs are both conceived and implemented from the "top down," as in the case of polio vaccination in the Global Polio Eradication

JAMES L. A. WEBB, JR. AND TAMARA GILES-VERNICK

initiative. Others have been reshaped by a much broader range of actors: demands for greater access to antiretroviral therapies, for instance, came from African communities and nongovernmental organizations, and subsequently from African states, and multilateral institutions such as UNAIDS and WHO. The activist pressure produced results: multinational pharmaceutical companies, after bearing considerable public criticism, agreed to new dispensations.[47]

Donor engagement with disease-specific programs has consistently reinforced a focus on the biological agents of African diseases, rather than on the social determinants such as poverty, lack of access to resources, and income inequalities. Global public health policy in Africa has sought to increase survival rates through biomedical interventions, rather than improve the health of the poor by increasing access to primary health care. The disease-specific approach has had numerous successes. Childhood vaccinations, in particular, have proved to be highly effective in reducing deaths among younger generations, but "catch-up" programs to vaccinate older generations against preventable diseases have sometimes lagged. Other interventions, such as the provision of antiretroviral drugs to Africans with HIV, have enjoyed good success, although expansion of the programs has been constrained by the unwillingness of donors to make robust contributions during the recent global financial crisis.

To donors, the best investments in global health in Africa have consistently appeared to be disease-specific programs. They offered several key advantages. Disease-specific programs, based primarily in the biomedical sciences, offered technical solutions to achieve measurable outcomes. The implementation of such programs appeared not to require social sciences training, basic linguistic or cultural competency, or familiarity with the societies for which the interventions were planned. In principle, these technical interventions were neutral, able to be applied without entanglement in African struggles over political and economic priorities. They were also expected to produce results promptly.

The disease-specific approach had important implications for how global health projects have been conceived and implemented in Africa. Because public health specialists conceptualized diseases as primarily biological in nature, abstracted from their social, political, and economic contexts, they assumed that therapies and tools proven effective elsewhere could be applied in Africa with minimal adjustment. The disease-specific model thus considered global health interventions as a portable universal good. Experts who had proved their mettle in other world regions could consult and provide useful guidance. The social, political, and economic contexts of the delivery of health interventions were scarcely taken into account. The fact that the interventionists generally did not speak the languages of the people who were intended to profit from the interventions ensured that the gulf in understanding was large.

Organization and Central Themes of the Volume

The essays in this collection are organized in three parts. Part I, "Looking Back," contains four chapters that analyze colonial era interventions and reflect on their implications for contemporary interventions. The first essay, by William Schneider, focuses on the colonial-era smallpox vaccination campaigns in West Africa, in an era before the global smallpox eradication campaign. He calls these campaigns "partial successes," and his essay sheds new light on the success of smallpox eradication by illuminating the colonial programs' constraints, piecemeal efforts, and limited goals. What made colonial efforts only "partial successes," Schneider argues, was a lack of international coordination and "global" framework for these vaccination campaigns. He uses lessons from this analysis to comment on recent efforts to eradicate polio.

James Webb's essay on the first large-scale use of synthetic insecticide to control malaria brings to light the constraints faced by the pilot malaria eradication programs in tropical Africa during the era of the first global malaria eradication program. The repeated application of synthetic insecticides produced resistance in the vector mosquitoes; and the flow of people across political boundaries between Guinea and Liberia pointed up the fact that regional collaborations were essential to effective antimalarial interventions. Webb also reveals the epidemic malaria that was unleashed among the Liberian communities in the protected zones when control efforts ended. His essay demonstrates that the history of malaria eradication efforts offers important lessons for present-day malaria control efforts, in particular that the failure to sustain malaria control can lead to epidemic malaria among populations whose acquired immunities have degraded during the period of effective malaria control.

Guillaume Lachenal explores the colonial antecedents of the therapeutic approach known as "treatment as prevention" (TasP) and its relation to contemporary efforts to reduce HIV transmission. He traces a genealogy of TasP, from its beginnings in colonial mass treatments for malaria control, to the sleeping sickness and yaws campaigns of the 1920s and 1930s, through disastrous sleeping sickness treatment and prophylaxis measures in French and Belgian colonies in the 1950s. He explores how mass pentamidine use as both treatment and prophylaxis against sleeping sickness in Cameroon resulted in significant medical accidents. His essay provides an essential historical context for understanding the contemporary global health campaign for HIV.

Jennifer Tappan investigates the tangled scientific understandings of severe childhood malnutrition from the 1950s to the 1970s. Her essay explores how prevailing definitions of severe malnutrition, based on "protein deficiency," led medical nutritional researchers to prescribe dried skim milk. This was the beginning of a global program to introduce powdered skim milk into the diets of malnourished infants and young children. Physicians did not recognize that the therapy of adding dried skim milk to food unwittingly promoted bottle-feeding with skim milk that in turn caused disastrous health consequences. Tappan's research underlines how narrow biomedical understandings of nutrition that did not take account of the production, reception, interpretation, and long-term impact of the intervention produced entirely unanticipated outcomes. Her essay points to the need to have a broader social and cultural analysis of the reception and potential impacts of the contemporary ready-to-use therapeutic food (RUTF) such as the Nutriset product, Plumpy'nut.

Part II of this collection, "The Past in the Present," contains essays exploring the historical dimensions and unexamined assumptions of contemporary disease control programs. Tamara Giles-Vernick and Stephanie Rupp develop new insights into the deep history of human–great ape encounters in the tropical forest. They draw on the oral evidence of Africans in the forests whose stories demonstrate that their "contact" with great apes has been fluid and multifaceted, and not always pathogenic. The authors show that the northern equatorial forests, where great apes live and where some notable host shifts have occurred, have had a long, complex, and nonlinear history of human mobility, settlement, trade, and forest exploitation. Their essay offers a historical corrective to the frequently invoked trope that early twentieth-century human incursions into the forest have provoked the emergence of new infectious diseases. It also sheds light on the difficulties of surveillance in and the "biosecuring" of ecological zones in which human–great ape contact can facilitate cross-species transmission.

Anne Marie Moulin's contribution explores the history and broader public health significance of Egypt's hepatitis C (HCV) epidemic. It constitutes one of the most massive iatrogenic infections of modern history, a consequence of the coercive population-level campaigns of schistosomiasis treatment from the late 1950s to the early 1980s. The infections were so widespread that HCV has become naturalized as an endemic condition. Moulin traces the processes by which Egyptian and other researchers identified the relationship between the mass treatment campaigns, what they recognized as jaundice, and what they later characterized as the world's most serious epidemic of hepatitis C. The coercive schistosomiasis treatment campaigns and the Egyptian government's subsequent denial of the HCV epidemic have fostered a deep popular mistrust of state public health. Moulin suggests that this mistrust has played a significant role in the ongoing political revolution that has shaken Egypt in 2011–12.

Myron Echenberg's essay investigates the seventh global pandemic of cholera that developed in Africa late in the second half of the twentieth century. He explores the multifaceted processes through which an exotic bacterium became an endemic "African" disease. Echenberg homes in on a fundamental paradox. Cholera no longer constitutes the threat that it once was in much of the world. Yet since 1995, over 95 percent of the world's cases have occurred in Africa. His essay makes clear that both biological and social explanations are necessary to explain why *Vibrio cholera* has become more widespread and lethal. He identifies political chaos, economic crises, climatic and anthropogenic environmental changes, and policy choices of governing African elites as critical factors in these outbreaks. His essay suggests that some of the most effective measures to counter the infections will be rooted in social and political choices.

Part III, "The Past in the Future," examines two fields of public health intervention in which efforts to reduce disease transmission and future harm are premised on an understanding of the past. In their chapter on medical male circumcision (MMC), Michel Garenne, Alain Giami, and Christophe Perrey offer a critique of the controversial 2007 WHO/UNAIDS recommendation to promote male circumcision as an effective measure to control female-to-male HIV transmission. They trace the history of male circumcision practices in Africa and explore past assumptions about male circumcision and its putative medical contributions. In this light they evaluate the past decade's epidemiological studies that have concluded that this intervention is efficacious. They compare the demographic evidence drawn from direct observation of HIV prevalence and incidence among circumcised and intact populations in Africa with the epidemiological evidence derived from clinical trials. They find that these two disciplinary approaches yield apparently disconsonant results. The authors subsequently analyze the decision-making processes that led to the WHO/UNAIDS recommendation for male circumcision.

Sheryl McCurdy and Haruka Maruyama's chapter examines the contemporary history of heroin trafficking and use in Africa, and pays particular attention to experiences of the drug trade and its fallout in Tanzania. The authors explore the causes and consequences of different responses to heroin trafficking and use in Africa, focusing first on the US-led "War on Drugs" and then on the "harm-reduction" approach. McCurdy and Maruyama's essay offers a potent critique of the inability of the "War on Drugs" to eliminate drug trafficking and injection drug use. In 2006–7, the Tanzanian state, recognizing that this approach had failed to reduce either trafficking or drug use, adopted a grassroots "harm-reduction" approach to minimize the harms to drug users and to those within their social networks. The authors illuminate the broader political and social contexts that have shaped the contours of this approach in Dar-es-Salaam and determined its efficacy.

Africa has long served as a laboratory for human research and experimentation.[48] Its disease environments and public health challenges have called forth a succession of interventions that are increasingly the focus of a new generation of scholarship in the field of historical epidemiology. The essays in this collection address some of the most important interventions in disease control: mass vaccination, large-scale treatment and/or prophylaxis campaigns, harm-reduction efforts, and nutritional and virological research. Despite the technological promise offered by both research and intervention, the enthusiasm of their proponents, and the successes of some of the interventions, many of these efforts have had far-reaching, unanticipated social and medical consequences for African populations. The essays illustrate vividly the need for a fuller integration of social science and biomedical perspectives, in order to translate global health initiatives to local needs, capacities, and constraints and to better anticipate the social consequences of these interventions. This will require the multidisciplinary training of public health specialists. Global health practitioners need to understand African conceptions of disease etiology, African therapeutic practices, and the various political, economic, and resource constraints that affect African access to medical care. The study of past efforts, part of the emerging field of global health history, is a powerful tool to allow us to grasp more fully the nature of the contemporary challenges.

Notes

1. Some recent works in historical epidemiology have explored the histories of individual diseases. For exemplary studies of HIV/AIDS and cholera, see John Iliffe, *The African AIDS Epidemic: A History* (Athens: Ohio University Press, 2006), and Myron Echenberg, *Africa in the Time of Cholera* (New York: Cambridge University Press, 2011). For an overview of African historical epidemiology, see James L. A. Webb, Jr.,

"Historical Epidemiology and Infectious Disease Processes in Africa," *Journal of African History* 54, no. 1 (2013): 3–10.

2. Medical anthropologists recently have called for the development of a new field of global health diplomacy to bring health care professionals into dialog with foreign-policy professionals and medical anthropologists to address the problems of failed public health initiatives. See Vincanne Adams, Thomas E. Novotny, and Hannah Leslie, "Global Health Diplomacy," *Medical Anthropology* 27, no. 4 (2008): 315–23. For a survey of the discipline of anthropology's engagement with global health, see Craig R. James and Kitty K. Corbett, "Anthropology and Global Health," *Annual Review of Anthropology* 38 (2009): 167–83. For essays that explore the narratives of international epidemics, see Sarah Dry and Melissa Leach, eds., *Epidemics: Science, Governance and Social Justice* (London: Earthscan/Routledge, 2011).

For a reflection on the role of history in health policy making with special reference to the UK, see Virginia Berridge, "History Matters? History's Role in Health Policy Making," *Medical History* 52, no. 3 (2008): 311–26.

3. H. W. Arndt, *Economic Development: The History of an Idea* (Chicago: University of Chicago Press, 1989).

4. For an example of African NGOs and association activities, see Vinh-Kim Nguyen, *The Republic of Therapy: Triage and Sovereignty in West Africa's Time of AIDS* (Durham, NC: Duke University Press, 2010).

5. Barry Sautman and Yan Hairong, "Friends and Interests: China's Distinctive Links with Africa," *African Studies Review* 50, no. 3 (2007): 75–114.

6. Some scholars have interpreted the broadening effectiveness of the twenty-first-century WHO disease surveillance networks as marking a fundamental transformation under way in the aftermath of the 2003 SARS (severe acute respiratory syndrome) epidemic. See, for example, David P. Fidler, "Germs, Governance, and Global Public Health in the Wake of SARS," *Journal of Clinical Investigation* 113, no. 6 (2004): 799–804, and Lorna Weir and Eric Mykhalovskiy, *Global Public Health Vigilance: Creating a World on Alert* (New York: Routledge, 2010).

Recently, George Dehner has examined the WHO influenza surveillance system that operated in earlier decades, bringing to light continuities over time. He notes that there were other expert groups within the WHO that developed policies to counter threats to global health, including for other diseases such as influenza that were not required to be reported to health authorities (George Dehner, *Influenza: A Century of Science and Public Health Response* [Pittsburgh: University of Pittsburgh Press, 2012], 15).

7. Oliver-James Dyer and Ayesha de Costa, "What Is Global Health?" *Journal of Global Health* 1, no. 1 (Spring 2011), accessed online at http://www.ghjournal.org /spring-2011-issue; Andy Haines, Antoine Flahault, and Richard Horton, "European Academic Institutions for Global Health," *Lancet* 377 (January 2011): 363–65; Ilona Kickbush, "Mapping the Future of Public Health: Action on Global Health," *Revue canadienne de santé publique* 97, no. 1 (2006): 6.

8. H. L. Wesseling, *Divide and Rule: The Partition of Africa, 1880–1914,* trans. Arnold J. Pomerans (New York: Praeger, 1996); Thomas Pakenham, *The Scramble for Africa: The White Man's Conquest of the Dark Continent from 1876 to 1912* (New York: Avon, 1992);

A. Adu Boahen, *African Perspectives on Colonialism* (Baltimore: Johns Hopkins University Press, 1989).

9. The most extensive disease problem appeared to be trypanosomiasis, also known as sleeping sickness. It became epidemic among African populations in several territories. The colonial medical campaigns to control trypanosomiasis involved forced relocation and medical coercion, and the early drugs used produced devastating consequences for many of the survivors. The medical campaigns are best documented in northern Zaire and French Equatorial Africa. See Maryinez Lyons, *The Colonial Disease: A Social History of Sleeping Sickness in Northern Zaire, 1900–1940* (Cambridge: Cambridge University Press, 2002); Rita Headrick, *Colonialism, Health, and Illness in Equatorial Africa, 1885–1935,* ed. Daniel Headrick (Atlanta: African Studies Association, 1994); Jean-Paul Bado, *Eugène Jamot, 1879–1937* (Paris: Karthala, 2011); Kirk Arden Hoppe, *Lords of the Fly: Sleeping Sickness Control in British East Africa, 1900–1960* (Westport, CT: Praeger, 2003). For the broader history of trypanosomiasis, see John Ford, *The Role of the Trypanosomiases in African Ecology: A Study of the Tsetse Fly Problem* (London: Oxford University Press, 1971).

Africans who labored in mines ran a major risk of disease from tuberculosis and silicosis, and the sufferers were sent away from the mines to die elsewhere. See Randall M. Packard, *White Plague, Black Labor: Tuberculosis and the Political Economy of Health and Disease in South Africa* (Berkeley: University of California Press, 1989); Elaine N. Katz, *The White Death: Silicosis on the Witwatersrand Gold Mines, 1886–1910* (Johannesburg: University of Witwatersrand Press, 1994).

10. See Steven Feierman and John Janzen, eds., *Health and Healing in Africa* (Berkeley: University of California Press, 1992); John Janzen, *The Quest for Therapy: Medical Pluralism in Lower Zaire* (Berkeley: University of California Press, 1978); Julie Livingston, *Debility and the Moral Imagination in Botswana* (Bloomington: Indiana University Press, 2005).

11. Europeans had, however, achieved major reductions in the mortality and morbidity among European troops in Africa and elsewhere in the tropics, beginning in the 1850s. See Philip D. Curtin, *Death by Migration: Europe's Encounter with the Tropical World in the Nineteenth Century* (New York: Cambridge University Press, 1989). On the disease problems of the Europeans involved in the military conquest of the continent, see Philip D. Curtin, *Disease and Empire: The Health of European Troops in the Conquest of Africa* (Cambridge: Cambridge University Press, 1998).

12. The literature on the emergence of tropical medicine is extensive. For some representative approaches, see Michael Worboys, "The Emergence of Tropical Medicine: A Study in the Establishment of a Scientific Specialty," Gerard Lemaine et al., eds., *Perspectives on the Emergence of Scientific Disciplines* (The Hague: Mouton, 1976), 75–98; Michael Worboys, "Tropical Diseases," in *Companion Encyclopedia of the History of Medicine,* ed. W. F. Bynum and R. Porter (London: Routledge, 1993), 1:512–36; Warwick Anderson, "Immunities of Empire: Race, Disease, and the New Tropical Medicine," *Bulletin of the History of Medicine* 70, no. 1 (1996), 94–118; John Farley, *Bilharzia: A History of Imperial Tropical Medicine* (Cambridge: Cambridge University Press, 2003); David Arnold, ed., *Warm Climates and Western Medicine: The Emergence of Tropical Medicine* (Amsterdam: Rodopi, 1996); Anne Marie Moulin, "The Pasteur Institutes between the

Two World Wars: The Transformation of the International Sanitary Order," in *International Health Organizations and Movements, 1918–1939,* ed. Paul Weindling (Cambridge: Cambridge University Press, 1995).

13. Jean-Paul Bado, *Médecine coloniale et grandes endémies en Afrique, 1900–1960: Lèpre, trypanosomiase humaine et onchocercose* (Karthala: Paris, 1996); Headrick, *Colonialism, Health, and Illness in Equatorial Africa*; Heather Bell, *The Frontiers of Medicine in Anglo-Egyptian Sudan, 1889–1940* (New York: Clarendon Press, 1999).

14. Ralph Schram, *The History of the Nigerian Health Services* (Ibadan: Ibadan University Press, 1971), 59–180. This book covers a far broader field of historical study than indicated by its title.

On the social history of missionary medicine, see David Hardiman, ed., *Healing Bodies, Saving Souls* (Amsterdam: Rodopi, 2006); Nancy Rose Hunt, *A Colonial Lexicon of Birth Ritual, Medicalization, and Mobility in the Congo* (Durham, NC: Duke University Press, 1999); Megan Vaughan, *Curing Their Ills: Colonial Power and African Illness* (Stanford, CA: Stanford University Press, 1991), chap. 3; John Comaroff and Jean Comaroff, *Of Revelation and Revolution,* vol. 2, *The Dialectics of Modernity on a Southern African Frontier* (Chicago: University of Chicago Press, 1997); Terence Ranger, "The Influenza Pandemic in Southern Rhodesia: A Crisis of Comprehension," in *Imperial Medicine and Indigenous Societies,* ed. David Arnold (Manchester: Manchester University Press, 1988), 172–88; John Manton, "Making Modernity with Medicine: Mission, State, and Community in Leprosy Control, Ogoja, Nigeria, 1945–50," in *The Development of Modern Medicine beyond the West: Historical Perspectives,* ed. Hormoz Ebrahimnejad (New York: Routledge, 2009), 160–83; David Simmons, "Religion and Medicine at the Crossroads: A Reexamination of the Southern Rhodesian Influenza Epidemic of 1918," *Journal of Southern African Studies* 35, no. 1 (2009): 29–44.

15. William H. Schneider and Ernest Drucker, "Blood Transfusions in the Early Years of AIDS in Sub-Saharan Africa," *American Journal of Public Health* 96, no. 6 (2006): 984–94. On urban hospitals in colonial Zimbabwe, see Tamara Giles-Vernick, Susan Craddock, and Jennifer Gunn, "Mobility Restrictions, Isolation, and Quarantine: Historical Perspectives on Contemporary Debates," in *Influenza and Public Health: Learning from Past Pandemics,* ed. Tamara Giles-Vernick and Susan Craddock (London: Earthscan/Routledge, 2010), 201–2, 205.

16. The Office international d'hygiène publique, formed in 1907, was largely concerned with overseeing international rules for quarantining ships to prevent the spread of plague and cholera. The League of Nations Health Organization, in principle, had a broad mandate, but it was an underfunded organization with a small staff that depended fundamentally on the pro bono advice of European and US public health experts. On the League of Nations Health Organization, see Iris Borowy, *Coming to Terms with World Health: The League of Nations Health Organization, 1921–1946* (New York: Peter Lang, 2009).

17. "The Constitution of the World Health Organization," Article 1 in *Basic Documents of the World Health Organization,* supplement 2006 (Geneva: World Health Organization, 2006), 2.

18. On the imperial roots of eradication in the Americas, see Nancy Leys Stepan, *Eradication: Ridding the World of Diseases Forever?* (London: Reaktion Books, 2011), 35–64.

JAMES L. A. WEBB, JR. AND TAMARA GILES-VERNICK

19. Theodore M. Brown, Marcos Cueto, and Elizabeth Fee, "The World Health Organization and the Transition from 'International' to 'Global' Public Health," *American Journal of Public Health* 96, no. 1 (2006): 64.

20. J. A. Gillespie, "Europe, America, and the Space of International Health," in *Shifting Boundaries of Public Health: Europe in the Twentieth Century,* ed. Susan Gross Solomon, Lion Murard and Patrick Zylberman, Rochester Studies in Medical History, vol. 12 (Rochester, NY: University of Rochester Press, 2008), 114–37, esp. 124–32; Socrates Litsios, "Malaria Control, the Cold War, and the Postwar Reorganization of International Assistance," *Medical Anthropology* 17 (1997): 255–78; J. Siddiqi, *World Health and World Politics: The World Health Organization and the U.N. System* (London: Hurst and Company, 1995).

21. Erez Manela, "Smallpox Eradication and the Rise of Global Governance," in *The Shock of the Global: The 1970s in Perspective,* ed. Niall Ferguson et al. (Cambridge, MA: Harvard University Press, 2010), 251–62; Stepan, *Eradication,* 120–23; Brown, Cueto, and Fee, "World Health Organization," 64–65.

22. Stepan, *Eradication,* 227.

23. Marcos Cueto, "The Origins of Primary Health Care and Selective Primary Care," *American Journal of Public Health* 94, no. 11 (2004): 1865.

24. Humanitarian medicine owed its beginnings to colonial medical and Christian missionary activities, the International Red Cross, Second World War relief organizations such as Catholic Relief Services and CARE, and to the UN High Commission on Refugees, created in the aftermath of World War II (Michael Barnett and Thomas G. Weiss, eds., *Humanitarianism in Question: Politics, Power, Ethics* [Ithaca: Cornell University Press, 2008]; Guillaume Lachenal and Bertrand Taithe, "Une généalogie missionnaire et coloniale de la médecine humanitaire: Le cas Aujoulat au Cameroun, 1935–1973," *Le mouvement social,* no. 227 [2009]: 45–63; Patrick Aeberhard, "A Historical Survey of Humanitarian Action," *Health and Human Rights* 2, no. 1 [1993]: 30–44). During the Nigerian civil war (1967–70), humanitarian groups offered basic medical and nutritional services to those targeted by or caught in violent conflict. This emergency led to the development of Médecins Sans Frontières (Doctors without Borders), and the proliferation of interventions that expanded beyond efforts to secure "basic survival" (Peter Redfield, "Doctors, Borders, and Life in Crisis," *Cultural Anthropology* 20, no. 3 [2005]: 331); Michael Barnett, *Empire of Humanity: A History of Humanitarianism* [Ithaca: Cornell University Press, 2011]).

25. Over subsequent decades, new humanitarian medical organizations proliferated, including Action contre la faim (1979), Oxfam (1995), and the UAE-financed, France-based Women and Health Alliance International (2009), as well as centers within academic institutions, such as Harvard University's François-Xavier Bagnoud Center for Health and Human Rights in the School of Public Health, founded by the AIDS researcher/activist Jonathan Mann. Since the 1970s, humanitarian medical interventions have taken place in Sudan, Somalia, Rwanda, the Democratic Republic of Congo, Mozambique, and elsewhere in Africa (Neil Middleton and Phil O'Keefe, "History and Problems of Humanitarian Assistance in Sudan," *Review of African Political Economy* 33, no. 109 [2008]: 543–59; Johan Pottier, "Roadblock Ethnography: Negotiating Humanitarian Access in Ituri, Eastern DR Congo, 1999–2004," *Africa* 76, no.

2 [2006]: 151–79; Steven Robins, "Humanitarian Aid beyond 'Bare Survival': Social Movement Responses to Xenophobic Violence in South Africa," *American Ethnologist* 36, no. 4 [2009]: 648).

26. Jennifer Leaning, Susan M. Briggs, and Lincoln C. Chen, eds., *Humanitarian Crises: The Medical and Public Health Response* (Cambridge, MA: Harvard University Press, 1999); Ezekiel Kalipeni and Joseph Oppong, "The Refugee Crisis in Africa and Implications for Health and Disease: A Political Ecology Approach," *Social Science and Medicine* 46, no. 12 (1998): 1637–53.

27. Stepan, *Eradication*, 228–29.

28. Marcus Cueto notes that some planners contended that selective primary health care complemented the Alma-Ata Declaration, while others believed that it contradicted the 1978 measure. Cueto, "Origins of Primary Health Care," 1868–69.

29. Ibid., 1870. In the 1980s, "Child Survival Programs" were the core focus of the selective primary health care programs; by the mid-1990s the focus had shifted to the "Integrated Management of Childhood Diseases."

30. Kwesi Dugbatey, "National Health Policies: Sub-Saharan African Case Studies (1980–1990)," *Social Science and Medicine* 49, no. 2 (1999): 223–39.

31. Cueto, "Origins of Primary Health Care," 1867.

32. Ibid., 1871. The WHO's recent assessment of primary health care appears in *World Health Report 2008 (Now More Than Ever)*, http://www.who.int/whr/2008/en /index.html.

33. William R. Jobin, *Dams and Disease: Ecological Design and Health Impacts of Large Dams, Canals, and Irrigation Systems* (London: E & FN Spon Press, 1999).

34. George B. N. Ayittey, *Africa Betrayed* (New York: Palgrave Macmillan, 1993).

35. David Sahn and Rene Bernier, "Have Structural Adjustments Led to Health Sector Reform in Africa?" *Health Policy* 32, nos. 1–3 (1995): 193–214; Lucy Gilson and Anne Mills, "Health Sector Reforms in Sub-Saharan Africa: Lessons of the Last 10 Years," *Health Policy* 32, nos. 1–3 (1995): 215–43.

36. Hilary Standing, "An Overview of Changing Agendas in Health Sector Reforms," *Reproductive Health Matters* 10, no. 20 (2002): 19–28.

37. Andrew Lakoff and Stephen J. Collier, eds., *Biosecurity Interventions: Global Health and Security in Question* (New York: Columbia University Press, 2008), and Andrew Lakoff, "Preparing for the Next Emergency," *Public Culture* 19, no. 2 (2007): 256–58.

38. Joshua Lederberg, ed., *Biological Weapons: Limiting the Threat,* BCSIA Studies in International Security (Cambridge, MA: MIT Press, 1999); Jonathan B. Tucker, *Scourge: The Once and Future Threat of Smallpox* (New York: Atlantic Monthly Press, 2001).

39. Nicholas King traced how an "emerging diseases worldview" captured American scientific, media, and public attention during the 1990s (Nicholas B. King, "Security, Disease, Commerce: Ideologies of Postcolonial Global Health," *Social Studies of Science* 32, nos. 5–6 [2002]: 763–89).

40. Private philanthropic engagement, of course, was not new. The Rockefeller Foundation, created in 1913, had carried out medical initiatives in the southern states of the USA, the Caribbean, Central America, and South America, although it had ratcheted back its public health activities after the Second World War (John Farley, *To*

JAMES L. A. WEBB, JR. AND TAMARA GILES-VERNICK

Cast Out Disease: A History of the International Health Division of the Rockefeller Foundation [1913–1951] [New York: Oxford University Press, 2003]). In the United Kingdom, the Wellcome Trust, founded in 1936, became the largest philanthropic funder of biomedical research in Europe.

On international health organizations and movements after the First World War, see Paul Weindling, ed., *International Health Organizations and Movements, 1918–1939* (Cambridge: Cambridge University Press, 1995).

41. David Heymann, "Global Polio Eradication Initiative," *Bulletin of the World Health Organization* 84, no. 8 (2006): 595.

42. Sandy Cairncross, Ralph Muller, and Nevio Zagaria, "Dracunculiasis (Guinea Worm Disease) and the Eradication Initiative," *Clinical Microbiology Reviews* 15, no. 2 (2002): 223–46.

43. In the late 1990s, the WHO adopted the term "global health" in preference to the term "international health," in an effort to shore up its position in the changing configuration of global health actors. See Brown, Cueto, and Fee, "World Health Organization."

44. GAVI Alliance, *Progress Report 2011*, downloaded March 26, 2012, at http://www.gavialliance.org/.

45. World Health Organization, *World Health Report 2008*.

46. See, for instance, Rachel R. Chapman, *Family Secrets: Risking Reproduction in Central Mozambique* (Nashville: Vanderbilt University Press, 2010); Barry L. Hewlett and Bonnie S. Hewlett, *Ebola, Culture, and Politics: The Anthropology of an Emerging Disease* (Belmont, CA: Thomson Wadsworth, 2008).

47. David Barnard, "In the High Court of South Africa, Case No. 4138/98: The Global Politics of Access to Low-Cost AIDS Drugs in Poor Countries," *Kennedy Institute of Ethics Journal* 12, no. 2 (2002): 159–74; Michael Zisuh Ngoasong, "The Emergence of Global Health Partnerships as Facilitators of Access to Medications in Africa: A Narrative Policy Analysis," *Social Science and Medicine* 68 (2009): 953–54.

48. The history of science in Africa during the colonial period has been more thoroughly explored for the British colonies than for other European imperial powers. On science in British Africa, see Helen Tilley, *Africa as a Living Laboratory: Empire, Development, and the Problem of Scientific Knowledge, 1870–1950* (Chicago: University of Chicago Press, 2011), and Joseph M. Hodge, *The Triumph of the Expert: Agrarian Doctrines of Development and the Legacy of British Colonialism* (Athens: Ohio University Press, 2007).

PART I

❖

Looking Back

1

THE LONG HISTORY
OF SMALLPOX ERADICATION
Lessons for Global Health in Africa

WILLIAM H. SCHNEIDER

One of the longest held and most ambitious goals of global health has been disease eradication. Yet support for this idea over the years has waxed and waned, as efforts have achieved mixed results. The malaria eradication campaign in the 1950s by the World Health Organization (WHO) was a highly publicized failure, but it was not the first. The Rockefeller Foundation sponsored an ambitious program to eradicate yellow fever in the 1920s that ended in disappointment after much initial success.[1] Likewise, at the same time as the malaria campaign the WHO launched an effort against yaws that similarly achieved initially encouraging results only to be followed by recognition of the persistence of the disease in isolated pockets. But these discouragements were soon followed by success against smallpox that in turn prompted the decision to target polio (initiated by Rotary International).

The difficulties encountered since the 1980s and, even more seriously, the new emerging diseases have greatly sobered even the most ardent supporters of this goal of global health.[2] Currently, the only diseases endorsed by the World Health Assembly for eradication are Guinea worm and polio. The sixth Millennium Development Goal uses the following language to describe efforts against disease, "halt and begin to reverse the incidence."

In the debate about eradication, there are frequent references to history, with the smallpox success figuring quite prominently. Although the studies of smallpox are numerous, they are uneven. They typically follow one of two approaches. First, and most common, are accounts of the campaign proposed by WHO beginning in the 1950s, which was finally funded and implemented in the late 1960s with support and leadership by the United States and the Soviet Union. The magisterial volume by the principal leaders of that effort, Frank Fenner and his coauthors, has been taken as more or less the last word on the subject, and this is appropriate, to a large extent. The volume is thoroughly documented, based on a large amount of evidence, and certainly the starting point for anyone wishing to revisit the subject.[3] But these authors have a particular point of view, given their involvement in the campaign, which minimizes earlier efforts. Hence the chapters on colonial rule focus primarily on the epidemiology of smallpox, with little about attempts to prevent or respond to epidemics when they occurred.[4] Variations on this approach usually share the similarity of having been written by participants, who minimize earlier efforts.

The second approach is a broad sweeping history of smallpox, generally focusing on the toll it has taken on humans since the earliest times and efforts to discover and implement a means to combat it. These studies are broad and hence not particularly in depth.[5] They focus on discovery and comparisons of approaches in different countries over long periods of time.

The interest in the recent success against smallpox is certainly justified because of the uniqueness and impact of the campaign. The lessons to be learned from successes are numerous, as long as one can distinguish similar and different features and the broader context of smallpox in comparison to other diseases under consideration for eradication. But lessons can also be learned from failures and partial successes, which have more often been the case in campaigns against infectious diseases.[6]

This essay looks at the campaigns against smallpox in Africa during European colonial rule that can be considered partial successes.[7] As such, they are valuable in two important respects. The first is for comparison to the successful efforts that followed. This examination will, thus, help complement the official WHO history of smallpox eradication and similar accounts that have only a passing treatment of efforts immediately preceding the successful campaign of the 1960s and '70s, especially in the areas such as Africa and Asia where the disease persisted. In fact, there were long and extensive campaigns against smallpox in these regions, which succeeded at least in controlling the disease.

These colonial smallpox campaigns are important for a second and perhaps more important reason. They resemble the more numerous campaigns against infectious diseases in the past century that can also be characterized as having been partially successful. They therefore may offer even more lessons for contemporary global health efforts.

The campaigns against smallpox were the earliest, most extensive and effective health measures undertaken by African colonial authorities in the first half of the twentieth century. Yet they have been largely characterized by their failure at eradication, in contrast to the subsequent success of the WHO campaign that occurred after the independence of African and Asian countries. To the extent they succeeded, even though not completely, these efforts at smallpox control and prevention from the 1920s to the end of colonial rule in

WILLIAM H. SCHNEIDER

West, Central, and East Africa were a model for further public health efforts, including the WHO eradication campaign. To the extent that they failed, the campaigns offer a lesson for contemporary efforts to reduce, let alone eradicate, diseases in tropical settings.

This essay will review that history and examine in that light the discussions and efforts at eradication of other diseases that, with the exception of smallpox, so far have met a similar fate: much effort and progress but falling frustratingly short of their ultimate goal.

Smallpox in 1900

Just as the WHO eradication program of the 1960s–1970s did not start from scratch, the new European colonial rulers did not confront an unknown disease when they arrived in Africa at the end of the nineteenth century. Although the cause was unknown, Africans had a means of diagnosis, at least to the extent that they recognized those who were struck with smallpox, because of its distinctive symptoms, especially the pustules and eventual pock markings on the skin. This facilitated prevention by instinctive avoidance of the sick, although there is little evidence of systematic quarantine in traditional society.

More noteworthy was knowledge of prevention through inoculation by variolation. This practice of using the material in pustules (liquid or dried) from an infected person to give a mild case of smallpox to individuals in order to make them immune to the disease was reported in China by the tenth century, and it spread to Ottoman lands and Africa. Europe and its colonies in the Americas adopted the practice in the seventeenth and eighteenth centuries, although they learned of it by different means. Lady Montagu was the most highly visible proponent in England after she returned from Constantinople in 1715, and Cotton Mather's inoculations in a Boston smallpox epidemic shortly thereafter (1721) were learned from slaves.[8] The practice of variolation was most common in African societies with Muslim populations or those in contact with the Muslim world, that is, the east coast and sahel regions just south of the Sahara.[9]

Colonial rulers used some of these same tools, but also some new ones, to fight smallpox in their new African colonies. They still had no treatment for smallpox and no new diagnosis tools, although the early symptoms were pretty readily apparent and well known. More important, by 1900 Europeans understood the cause and means by which the disease spread, something that gave additional reason for applying a tool of prevention long practiced in European medicine: isolation and quarantine.

Both the practice of diagnosis and isolation depended on the machinery of colonial government administration that underlay a number of features of colonial rule and was crucially important to other measures taken in the campaigns against smallpox. Most obvious and extensive were the mass vaccination campaigns that began in Africa well before the First World War. They had been developed during the nineteenth century in European home countries, following Edward Jenner's discovery of the cowpox method of inoculation. This vaccination, as he called it, was superior to the use of smallpox material because there was no risk of smallpox infection, as was the case with variolation.[10] Moreover, animals could be used as the source for the production of vaccine. Typically, pustules were scraped from the flanks of infected calves, a process that could be conducted on the scale needed for the mass campaigns. There were problems of loss of potency in the heat of Africa that was an ongoing concern, not to mention training a sufficient number of people to undertake the systematic campaigns. By and large, however, the colonial authorities were successful in establishing vaccination campaigns in every African colony, which, even if it did not eliminate the disease, greatly reduced and contained the cases of smallpox.

A final feature of the new colonial administrative structure was its ability to provide surveillance that identified and reported cases, especially once the mass campaigns brought smallpox under control. As will be seen, the effectiveness in obtaining this information varied greatly from colony to colony, just as the ability to carry out systematic and effective vaccination campaigns varied. In the end, surveillance was one of the most important reasons why the WHO campaign was able to achieve its goal of eradicating the disease.

The Record of Colonial Smallpox Campaigns

Campaigns against infectious diseases in Africa began shortly after the European "scramble for Africa." A method of preventing smallpox had been known for hundreds of years, and when Europeans moved in to occupy Africa, they had almost a century of experience back home with Jenner's much-improved method of vaccination. By 1900, smallpox had dramatically declined in a number of European countries, including all those with colonies in Africa, thanks largely to systematic vaccinations and revaccination programs with glycerated calf-derived vaccine.[11] It is, therefore, not surprising that smallpox vaccination quickly became one of the first and most widely practiced medical interventions in African colonies.

Even before the turn of the twentieth century, the French reported inoculation campaigns in Senegal and what later came to be called the French

Soudan (present-day Mali).[12] In 1902, France passed a mandatory smallpox vaccination law, which two years later was also applied to the colonies, and in 1905 systematic vaccinations began in French West Africa. In the Belgian Congo smallpox vaccination was required for all urban residents as early as 1894, and in 1920 vaccinations were made mandatory in the British colony of the Gold Coast.[13]

As colonial medical services expanded between the wars and especially after 1945, smallpox campaigns grew along with them. Other efforts of care and prevention also grew but were still overshadowed in terms of numbers reached. For example, a 1954 health service report for French West Africa listed over 3.6 million mixed smallpox–yellow fever vaccinations and another 1.6 million for smallpox alone, while there were 87,529 inoculations for yellow fever separately, and 53,994 BCG (Bacillus Calmette-Guérin) vaccinations for tuberculosis.[14]

The smallpox vaccinations were extensive and began early. Systematic statistics for African colonies are difficult to find before the 1920s, but there are a number of reports from enough colonies that indicate colonial rulers introduced vaccination quickly, following the experience back in the home country. Moreover, since variolation (arm to arm) was widespread in traditional African societies, especially in the west, east and south, Africans were familiar with the disease and the idea of prevention.

Statistics for French African colonies began to be kept shortly after the mandatory French vaccination law was extended to the colonies in 1904, and over a million vaccinations were reported annually by 1911 in French West Africa.[15] Like the overall report of cases, however, it is difficult to assess the effect of the vaccinations. Annual colonial medical reports indicate that increased vaccinations were an important response to an outbreak of smallpox; but so too was a call for stepped-up regular vaccination.

In French West Africa the variations in number of cases and vaccinations were too great to draw any conclusions about the overall effectiveness of vaccination. Data for specific colonies are more helpful in discerning the relationship. In some there were years when no cases of smallpox were reported, hence authorities could argue that the disease was eliminated. Elsewhere, some of the spikes in cases (sharp rise and quick decline) are likely explained by outbreaks of smallpox that prompted a rise in vaccinations during and after.[16]

There are less complete statistics for French Equatorial Africa, but the order of magnitude, except for Chad, was much smaller than in French West Africa. For example, the number of smallpox cases reported in Gabon, French Congo, and Ubangi-Shari (Central African Republic) was never more than a few dozen between the 1920s and 1940s, figures that were far overshadowed when epidemics of thousands of cases hit Chad. It is not surprising that vaccinations in Gabon only exceeded 100,000 in 1947, although Ubangi, which bordered Chad, had closer to 200,000 or more vaccinations beginning during the Second World War. More complete figures for cases and vaccinations are available for Chad, as well as the large mandate territory of Cameroon.[17] In both colonies, the epidemics were infrequent and presumably managed well by vaccination and isolation (figures 1 and 2).

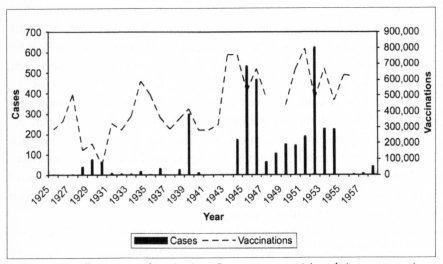

FIGURE 1.1. Smallpox cases and vaccinations, Cameroon, 1925–58 (population: 2,230,000 in 1926; 5,246,00 in 1957)

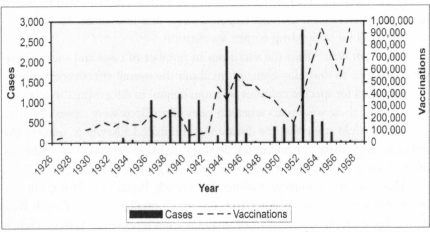

FIGURE 1.2. Smallpox cases and vaccinations, Chad, 1929–58 (population: 1,073,120 in 1931; 2,579,600 in 1958)

In the British colonies, the data are uneven, but some pattern of correlation can be discerned between cases and vaccinations. For example, vaccinations in Sierra Leone, Uganda, and Tanganyika appear to have followed closely the rise and fall of smallpox cases, suggesting that vaccinations were a response to epidemics. The Gold Coast is of interest because data are good, but the pattern is not clear. Data for vaccinations in Kenya are incomplete, whereas, the numbers for Nigeria are so large that regional analysis is necessary.[18]

In Nigeria cases reported during the mid-1930s indicate a much higher prevalence of smallpox in the northern provinces. Figures from the early 1950s, however, show that the south and east were not spared during the most serious epidemic of smallpox in any African colony during the twentieth century. Part of the reason is that even though the number of vaccinations in Nigeria was large, the population of the colony was even larger, hence the rate of vaccinations was lower overall compared to French West Africa. In 1937, for example, the rate in the French colonies was over 3.5 times that of Northern Nigeria, and by 1951, although both colonies increased, the French rate was still almost 2.5 times higher. Both smallpox cases and vaccinations reported in the Belgian Congo rose during colonial rule. The colony was so large and the numbers so big, however, that, like Nigeria, it would require analysis at a smaller regional level to understand the relationship between vaccinations and prevalence (figure 3).[19]

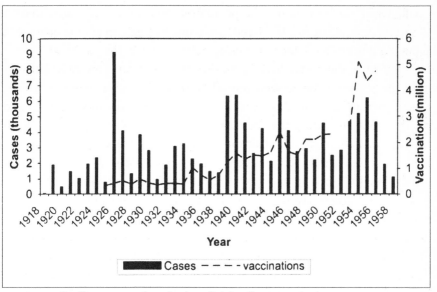

FIGURE 1.3. Smallpox cases and vaccinations, Belgian Congo, 1918–58

In assessing the effectiveness of colonial campaigns against smallpox, the most dramatic measurement would be against the successful eradication program of the 1960s and '70s. In other words, how close did the colonial campaigns come to eradicating smallpox? And what did the WHO program do differently that explains its success?

There are usually two main reasons given for the success of the eradication campaign. First is the nature of the disease, its rapid appearance, obvious symptoms, and lack of an animal reservoir. Of course, this had been the case before, during, and after colonial rule but was fully appreciated only in hindsight. The other reasons cited for the success have more to do with the specific strategies and techniques of the WHO campaign, such as improvement in vaccination techniques, systematic and effective vaccination procedures, surveillance and containment of new cases, and global coordination of efforts.[20]

Of these reasons, the ones that have received the most attention are the new technologies developed and used. These included a more effective vaccine, especially the use of freeze-dried vaccine that was not affected by the heat of tropical countries. Another innovation was the development of a procedure for mass vaccinations using a pump and jet injection of vaccine. Initially the pump ran on electricity, but then was modified to be foot-powered to solve the problem of lack of electricity. Eventually this was simplified by the development of a bifurcated needle, which was easier to use, cheaper to make, and which used a small amount of vaccine very efficiently. The health personnel had only to jab the upper arm about ten times to break the skin and leave the vaccine in the subsurface.

Helpful as these may have been, they were not fundamentally different from the Jennerian vaccination procedure that was implemented on a mass scale in Europe and elsewhere after 1800. Most knowledgeable observers and participants acknowledge that the earlier mass campaigns in Europe and North America had eliminated most of the smallpox cases, but even with the new refinements of effective sera and vaccination, it would have been very costly, if possible at all, to eradicate smallpox in Africa and Asia by mass campaigns alone. In addition, a crucial last step of surveillance and containment was needed to eliminate the last areas of endemic smallpox.

In hindsight, the technique was remarkably simple and effective, but it was initially attempted almost by accident, first in Africa then subsequently in Bangladesh, Indonesia, and Afghanistan. "In retrospect it seems clear—we didn't know how to eradicate smallpox when we started," according to William Foege who is given credit for first practicing it, in an account that was a reconsideration of the

West African success thirty years later.[21] There was a shortage of vaccine when an outbreak of smallpox occurred in Eastern Nigeria in the late 1960s. Unable to implement the usual mass vaccination, he carefully identified exactly who was infected and using local knowledge and a network of missionary medical personnel, they anticipated who had been and who were likely to be exposed to those in contact. This population was then isolated, and they were the only ones vaccinated as a preventive measure.[22] The result was just as effective as a mass campaign and much cheaper. From November 1966 through May 1967 the total number of vaccinations that Foege and his team performed using surveillance and containment was only 750,000 in a region whose population was 12 million. On May 30, 1967, Eastern Nigeria proclaimed itself smallpox free.[23]

How close were the colonial health authorities to eradication, and how conscious of this were their assessments? The main effort of authorities was regular and massive vaccination. As mentioned above, this was no surprise, since it had been the method used in their home countries with effective results. It was recognized that the process would take more time in the colonies, but after the Second World War, as more money was put into more disease campaigns, there was a growing impatience with the continuing existence of smallpox. Much was written about this failure, but the reasons most frequently mentioned were shortcomings of the vaccination campaigns. For example, some authorities blamed Africans for resistance to vaccination. This was more common in the early years, when racist stereotypes were stronger. Later references were vague and usually blamed failure on low numbers of vaccinations for a given year.[24] In fact, reports more often indicated how well and eager Africans were for vaccines. For example, following an outbreak of smallpox in the Gold Coast in 1929, the colonial medical report stated, "A feature of the outbreak was the extraordinary manner in which the chiefs and people cried out for vaccination. This demand did not cease on the cessation of the epidemic and many areas are still demanding vaccination."[25]

The most frequent subject of concern was the effectiveness of vaccines. As in the WHO campaign, this was easy to identify and offered the promise of a quick fix. The problems were technical in nature and almost always focused on two recurring difficulties: the potency of vaccines and the thoroughness of administration both in following procedures and reaching enough of the population. Vaccine was produced locally in French West Africa before 1900, and a large-scale vaccine production facility was established at the Pasteur Institute in Kindia, Guinea, in 1905 shortly after the French law of April 14, 1904, was passed requiring vaccination. This permitted 18,392 vaccinations in the colony that year. In 1909 Kindia also began producing a more stable dried vaccine with positive results reported in 71–89 percent of vaccinations.[26] By the 1930s, the following facilities existed for smallpox vaccine production in French colonial Africa.

TABLE 1.1. French West and Equatorial Africa smallpox vaccine production, 1931

Colony	Locations	Notes
Senegal	St. Louis	For all of Senegal and Mauretania
French Sudan	Bamako + 4 centers	
Upper Volta	2 centers	
Niger	7 centers	All closed in March 1931; replaced by dry vaccine
Guinea	Kindia (Pasteur Inst)	Also produced dry vaccine
Ivory Coast	Bouaké	Closed end of 1931 and replaced by dry vaccine from Paris and fresh vaccine from Upper Volta
Dahomey	Abomey + 2 centers	More dry vaccine used (78%) than fresh
Cameroon	N'Gaoundéré	Replaced center at Douala in July 1931
French Equatorial		Only dry vaccine from Paris used

Source: Lucien Camus, "Rapport général annuel sur les vaccinations et revaccinations pratiquées en France pendant l'année 1931," Bulletin de l'Académie de médicine 110 (1933): 561–66.

Production facilities were also established in Sudan, Nigeria, and Kenya in Anglophone Africa.[27] There was continuing testing and retesting of efficacy of the vaccines, especially the problem of weakening potency due to the heat.

A related concern was proper use and administration of the existing vaccines. Most colonies required vaccination in the first year of life and periodic vaccinations thereafter, usually every ten years. An alternative and supplemental approach was the campaign in a targeted area where all were vaccinated if there was fear of an outbreak. The other question that was often debated concerned the training and thoroughness in following procedures by the personnel doing vaccinations. These continued to be discussed and debated up until the time that the WHO campaign began.

Despite the shortcomings, and although not appreciated at the time, the vaccination techniques were good enough to greatly reduce and even eliminate smallpox in a number of locations by the time the WHO program began in the 1950s. This was true in Europe and in many countries of the Americas; and despite the characterization by Fenner et al. ("in most developing countries, few people were successfully vaccinated and smallpox was essentially uncontrolled")[28] it was also true in parts of Africa.

WILLIAM H. SCHNEIDER

TABLE 1.2. Colonial control of smallpox in Africa

Colony	Years with no cases of smallpox reported	Years when less than 100 cases of smallpox were reported
Dahomey		1936–37
		1939
		1932
		1944
		1955–56
French Soudan		1934
		1940–41
		1948–49
Gold Coast	1935	1927–28
		1932–37
		1940
		1949
		1954–55
Guinea		1927
		1939–41
		1948–51
Ivory Coast		1928–35
		1941–42
Kenya	1931–33	1935–36
	1938–42	1949
	1952–53	1951–55
N. Rhodesia		1932
		1934–42
		1947
		1949–51
Senegal		1934–35
		1941–42
		1947–51
		1956
Sierra Leone		1931
		1938–43
		1950–55
Uganda	1931–34	1931–42
	1937–39	1949–51

Source: Annual reports of African colonial health departments, 1927–55.

As these figures show, a few colonies reported no cases of smallpox for a number of years, and even more colonies (ten) reported several years with fewer than one hundred cases. Moreover, the list was likely longer, because not all African colonial reports were examined, and in many years reports were not made. It is, therefore, not too far of a stretch to say that in most African colonies smallpox was under control and surveillance was such that when outbreaks occurred, they were quickly brought under control.

Evidence of the effectiveness of eliminating or controlling smallpox as well as monitoring new cases can be found in the reports of colonies whose efforts had the greatest success in reducing smallpox, such as Kenya and Uganda in the 1930s. As the 1934 annual report of the Kenya Medical Department noted, after three years of no incidents and sixteen years since anything like an epidemic (as occurred at the end of the First World War), a smallpox epidemic broke out "among certain Somalis in the northern frontier district," herders crossing the border. In all there were 1,781 cases and 645 deaths that year. "Hospitalization was out of the question," the report went on, and vaccinations were given so as to establish "a barrier of vaccinated people between the infected areas and the closely populated highland and lake districts." These began, according to the report, within three days and eventually totaled over 408,000 vaccinations, which successfully confined the outbreak. Some vaccine was sent by air, taking hours as opposed to weeks by surface transport. The report boasted, "Fortunately in 1934 it was possible, as it was not in 1916–18, to ensure that the disease did not spread into any of the densely populated areas."[29] By 1938 (and continuing through 1942) there were again no cases of smallpox reported in the colony.

In 1935 when smallpox appeared in Uganda for the first time in many years, the annual report attributed it to visitors from India and a pilgrim returning from Mecca.[30] The cases were quickly contained, and by 1937 no cases were reported. Earlier, authorities in Tanganyika attributed an outbreak in 1930 to a passenger from Bombay, and a later report of a smallpox epidemic in 1943 concluded that it was introduced from the northern border.[31]

In French colonial Africa the best success was achieved in Equatorial Africa (Gabon, Congo, Ubangi-Shari, and Chad). From 1931 to 1938 a total of 1,201 smallpox cases were reported in these colonies, all but 134 of which were in Chad, and 842 of them occurred in the epidemic of 1938.[32] A special report by the new Vichy government on "Health efforts in French Equatorial Africa" in March of 1941, described in great detail the source and response to the 1938 epidemic in Chad.

WILLIAM H. SCHNEIDER

According to this report, the origin of the smallpox epidemic was in the region of Bol, on Lake Chad, on the southern edge of the Sahara and in the northwest of the inhabited part of Chad. It was described as "a region very difficult to monitor and where the inhabitants, generally nomadic, avoid vaccination and thus represent a veritable danger for neighboring populations." In addition to the pastoral Fulani who ignored the Nigerian border to the west, there were Hausa merchants and pilgrims who moved from Nigeria to Mecca and regions to the east.[33] Once colonial health authorities recognized the outbreak, they reacted like authorities in Kenya during the epidemic in the early 1930s, by setting up a quarantine line at Abeché, the largest regional center east of the capital which was on the route to the Anglo-Egyptian Sudan. In the words of the report, "Vaccinations numbering 8,441 for a resident population of 6,500 inhabitants stopped any further spread of the epidemic." Reports for the following years, however, show even more cases (1,206), and the epidemic did not subside until after the Second World War.[34]

These efforts were strikingly similar to the surveillance and containment strategy of the WHO smallpox eradication program. That means all of the most frequently mentioned elements of the successful program existed during the colonial period, with one exception. Not mentioned in the assessments of problems in colonial health reports on campaigns against smallpox, or at least not discussed in any depth, were questions of regional cooperation and cross-border surveillance. It is a truism, often ignored because it is so obvious, that as Fenner et al. stated as the first of their principles and lessons, "For a world-wide programme against a disease to be successfully undertaken, all countries must agree to it and there must be a mechanism for coordinating and monitoring the work."[35]

A detailed comparison of colonial efforts in Africa to the WHO global eradication campaign makes this crucial difference very apparent. Despite the success of the mass vaccination campaigns in reducing cases of smallpox to few or none, and where surveillance and rapid response such as in Kenya or Chad contained new outbreaks, smallpox would continue to occur as long as neighbors in Somalia or Nigeria failed to achieve similar success in reduction and control. Even though Fenner et al. did not think it applied to Africa, where they stated there was "continued endemicity of smallpox in all countries,"[36] their conclusion about the limited success in the rest of the world also applied in sub-Saharan Africa as this essay has shown.

Through the 1950s, most national governments and colonial administrations had conducted smallpox control programmes, some of which were very effective. . . . However, the interest of national authorities in smallpox control waxed and waned with the varying incidence of the disease and as they became temporarily free of it or, on the contrary, were reinfected from abroad. A concerted and sustained initiative, supported by one or more bilateral assistance agencies, might have succeeded in eliminating smallpox from many countries but it is unlikely that it could have achieved world-wide eradication.[37]

This was the most novel feature of the WHO campaign: international cooperation and a global approach to the campaign against smallpox that was the feature most lacking in colonial efforts to eliminate smallpox in Africa.

Lessons Learned

Lessons learned from comparing colonial campaigns against smallpox with the successful eradication effort after the 1960s can be summarized as follows. Most important is to recognize the significant work of reduction and control that was achieved during the colonial period. This has been underappreciated partly because of ignorance about how much was done but also because of frustration among colonial authorities themselves from the fact that outbreaks continued despite decades of effort, including effective elimination in some colonies and regions. The success of the eradication campaign that followed only made the shortcomings of earlier efforts stand out even more.

Second, as admitted by leaders of the eradication campaign, success was not simply the result of new vaccination techniques. To be sure, higher quality vaccines and more efficient needles helped, but procedures used during the colonial campaign were sufficiently effective to reduce and control smallpox. New techniques alone were not sufficient to eliminate the disease.

Systematic monitoring, isolation, and response to outbreaks have been correctly identified as the keys to eradication. This was not entirely new, however, since some colonial campaigns adopted some of these same measures in addition to the mass periodic vaccinations done everywhere. Especially in colonies where smallpox was eliminated or greatly reduced, such as Kenya, the response to new outbreaks was very similar to the strategy Foege developed in Eastern Nigeria that became the model for the rest of the eradication campaign.

A final lesson is that international cooperation, which is taken for granted today, was perhaps the most novel element in the successful eradication effort that was lacking during the colonial period. Besides sharing resources, expertise, and pooling vaccine development efforts, cooperation was crucial to prevention of cross-border and imported spread of smallpox. This was especially the case where colonial authorities succeeded in eliminating or greatly reducing smallpox only to see outbreaks from those entering the country from places it was still endemic.

WILLIAM H. SCHNEIDER

Reinforcing the validity of these lessons is the experience of the most extensive eradication effort since the elimination of smallpox: the campaign against polio (currently called "Global Polio Eradication Initiative").[38] It has benefited from effective vaccines, international cooperation, and the funding necessary to be on the brink of success. Most assessments, however, find shortcomings in the monitoring, isolation, and targeted vaccination that have prevented the final goal of eradication. It is hardly an accident, therefore, that the same places that harbored the last pockets of smallpox (Nigeria, Pakistan, and India) are the same places (along with Afghanistan) that the last polio cases are found. The underlying difficulties of population density, isolation, and resistance to following the program are further proof that any plans for additional efforts at eradication need to study these historical experiences before developing new strategies.

Notes

1. Fred L. Soper, "Rehabilitation of the Eradication Concept in Prevention of Communicable Diseases," *Public Health Reports* 80 (October 1965), 855–69.

2. For examples of the debate, see R. Aguas et al., "Prospects for Malaria Eradication in Sub-Saharan Africa," *PLoS One* 3 (3): e1767, March 12, 2008; S. Taylor, "Political Epidemiology: Strengthening Socio-Political Analysis for Mass Immunisation—Lessons from the Smallpox and Polio Programmes," *Global Public Health* 4, no. 6 (2009): 546–60; and Walter R. Dowdle and Donald R. Hopkins, eds., *The Eradication of Infectious Diseases: Report of the Dahlem Workshop on Eradication of Infectious Diseases,* Berlin, 16–22 March 1997 (New York: John Wiley and Sons, 1997).

3. For the official WHO history of the smallpox eradication campaign, see F. Fenner et al., *Smallpox and Its Eradication* (Geneva: World Health Organization, 1988). Henderson, who directed the campaign, wrote a separate account, D. A. Henderson, *Smallpox: The Death of a Disease: The Inside Story of Eradicating a Worldwide Killer* (Amherst, NY: Prometheus Books, 2009).

4. The sources used by Fenner et al. and others for the period before the WHO campaign were mainly secondary, which, in turn, relied on data collected by the League of Nations and WHO or accounts by doctors in the field at the time. They did not use archival reports and colonial government records.

5. Donald R. Hopkins, *Princes and Peasants: Smallpox in History* (Chicago: University of Chicago Press, 1983), reissued as *The Greatest Killer: Smallpox in History* (Chicago: University of Chicago Press, 2002). See also Gareth Williams, MD, *Angel of Death: The Story of Smallpox* (New York: Palgrave Macmillan, 2010).

6. Some studies attempt historical perspective, but focus mostly, if not entirely, on the period since the WHO smallpox campaign in the 1960s. See, for example, Iso Arita, John Wickett, and Miyuki Nakane, "Eradication of Infectious Diseases: Its Concept, Then and Now," *Japanese Journal of Infectious Diseases* 57 (2004), 1–6; or Bruce Aylward et al., "When Is a Disease Eradicable? 100 Years of Lessons Learned," *American Journal of Public Health* 90, no. 10 (2000): 1515–20.

7. Much of the material is drawn from a more extensive study that can be found in William H. Schneider, "Smallpox in Africa during Colonial Rule," *Medical History* 53, no. 2 (2009): 193–228.

8. Laurence Farmer, "When Cotton Mather Fought the Smallpox," *American Heritage* 8, no. 5 (1957); O.T. Beall, Jr., "Cotton Mather, the First Significant Figure in American Medicine," *Bulletin of the History of Medicine* 26, no. 2 (1952): 103–16; G. Miller, "Putting Lady Mary in Her Place: A Discussion of Historical Causation," *Bulletin of the History of Medicine* 55, no. 1 (1981): 2–16.

9. Eugenia W. Herbert, "Smallpox Inoculation in Africa," *Journal of African History* 16, no. 4 (1975): 539–59.

10. Fenner et al., *Smallpox and Its Eradication*, 261–73.

11. The last epidemic of smallpox in Europe (1870–71) which prompted most compulsory vaccination laws, coincided with the beginning of the Scramble for African colonies. See Fenner et al., *Smallpox and Its Eradication,* 232; 271–73; and J. D. Rolleston, "The Smallpox Pandemic of 1870–74," *Proceedings of the Royal Society of Medicine, Section of Epidemiology and State Medicine* 27, no. 2 (1933): 177–92. The last cases of endemic smallpox were recorded in France, Belgium, and Britain in the 1920s and '30s.

12. For a good but not exhaustive survey of these efforts, see Hopkins, *Greatest Killer,* 194–97. For the broader context of health in Senegal, see Angélique Diop, "Les débuts de l'action sanitaire de la France en AOF, 1895–1920: Le cas de Sénégal," in *AOF: Réalités et héritages,* ed. Charles Becker, Saliou Mbaye, and Ibrahima Thioub (Dakar: Direction des Archives du Sénégal, 1997), 2:1212–27.

13. AOF, "Rapport, 1953," op. cit., note 8 above, pp. 36, 42–44; Maryinez Lyons, "Public Health in Colonial Africa: The Belgian Congo," in *The History of Public Health in the Modern State,* ed. Dorothy Porter (Amsterdam: Rudopi, 1994): 365; Gold Coast Colony, *Report on the Medical Department, 1933–34* (Accra, Gold Coast: Government Press, 1934), 5 (hereafter Gold Coast, *Report,* with relevant date).

14. IMTSSA Box 84, AOF Directeur général de la Santé publique, "Rapport sur le fonctionnement du Service de Santé, 1954, pt. 1," 28.

15. AOF, "Rapport, 1953," 42.

16. See Schneider, "Smallpox in Africa," 222–26.

17. The estimated population of Chad for 1958 was 2,579,600. In Cameroon the estimated population was 2,230,000 in 1926 and 5,426,000 in 1957, from http://www .populstat.info (accessed 4 November 2008).

18. See Schneider, "Smallpox in Africa," 219–22.

19. Unfortunately, those figures were not available for this study.

20. The best summary remains the closing chapter of Fenner et al., *Smallpox and Its Eradication,* available online at http://whqlibdoc.who.int/smallpox/.

21. W. H. Foege, "Commentary: Smallpox Eradication in West and Central Africa Revisited," *Bulletin of the World Health Organization* 76, no. 3 (1998): 233–35.

22. In addition to Foege, see Jonathan B. Tucker, *Scourge: The Once and Future Threat of Smallpox* (New York: Atlantic Monthly Press, 2001), 76–80.

23. Henderson, *Smallpox: The Death of a Disease,* 137.

24. For an example from Sierra Leone, see Sierra Leone, *Annual Report of the Medical and Sanitary Department, 1933* (Freetown, Sierra Leone, 1933), 37; *1934,* 33. For

a Francophone example, see Lucien Camus, "Rapport général annuel sur les vaccinations et revaccinations pratiquées en France pendant l'année 1931," *Bulletin de l'Académie de médicine* 110 (1933): 564.

25. Gold Coast *Report, 1929–30*, 28.

26. J. G. Breman, A. B. Alécaut, and J. M. Lane, "Smallpox in the Republic of Guinea, West Africa, Part 1, History and Epidemiology," *American Journal of Tropical Medicine and Hygiene*, 1977, 26, no. 4 (1977): 757; R. Fasquelle and A. Fasquelle, "A propos de l'histoire de la lutte contre la variole dans les pays d'Afrique francophone," *Bulletin de la Société de pathologie exotique* 64, no. 5 (1971): 741.

27. A. Bayoumi, "Smallpox in the Sudan, 1925–1964," *East African Medical Journal* 51, no. 1 (1974): 135. Other facilities are reported in Kenya Medical Department, *Annual Medical Report 1950* (Nairobi, Medical Department, 1950), 20; Tanganyika Territory, *Annual Medical and Sanitary Report, 1951* (Dar es Salaam, 1951), 46; Nigeria, *Annual Report on the Medical Services for the Year 1937* (Lagos: Government Press, 1937), 15; ibid., *1941*, 7; ibid, *1956*, 28. The first production reports from Yaba appear in the 1941 Nigerian medical report.

28. Fenner et al., *Smallpox and Its Eradication*, 1345. On the elimination of smallpox in Europe and the Americas, see Fenner, 317–33.

29. Kenya Medical Department, *Annual Medical Report 1934* (Nairobi, Medical Department, 1934), 11–12. In 1935 the number of cases of smallpox reported dropped back to fifteen for the year.

30. Uganda Protectorate Medical Department, *Annual Medical and Sanitary Report 1935* (Entebbe: Government Printer, 1935), 39–40.

31. Tanganyika Territory, *Annual Medical and Sanitary Report, 1930* (Dar es Salaam, 1930), 8; ibid., *1943*, 9–10; Kenya, *Annual Medical Report, 1943*, 4. D. G. Conacher, "Smallpox in Tanganyika, 1918–1954," *East African Medical Journal* 34, no. 5 (1957): 157–81, compiled a list of "extra-territorial sources of infection" in Tanganyika with seven incidents reported from 1925 to 1944.

32. IMTSSA Box 81, État français, Secretariat d'état aux colonies, Direction du Service de santé des colonies, "L'oeuvre sanitaire de la France en Afrique Equatoriale," 8 March 1941, partie médicale, "lutte contre variole," pp. 19–20.

33. Ibid., 29.

34. Ibid. There were 1,670 cases in 1945; 243 in 1946; and 41 in 1947.

35. Fenner et al., *Smallpox and Its Eradication*, 1349.

36. Ibid.

37. Ibid., 1349–50.

38. For the last two reports, see "Every Missed Child: Independent Monitoring Board of the Global Polio Eradication Initiative " (June 2012), http://www.polioeradication .org/Portals/0/Document/Aboutus/Governance/IMB/6IMBMeeting/IMB6 _Report.pdf, and "Ten Months and Counting: Report of the Independent Monitoring Board of the Global Polio Eradication Initiative " (January 2012), http://www .polioeradication.org/portals/0/document/aboutus/governance/imb/5imbmeeting /imbreport_january2012.pdf.

2 THE FIRST LARGE-SCALE USE OF SYNTHETIC INSECTICIDE FOR MALARIA CONTROL IN TROPICAL AFRICA

Lessons from Liberia, 1945–62

JAMES L. A. WEBB, JR.

Apparently no Administration of any African territory has, so far, shown the willingness of setting up a project of this kind. Certainly some campaigns have given good results, but as far as I am aware, no endeavor has been made to find out in rural west or East Africa, the method which is the most effective and the least expensive at the same time. If WHO can help to determine it, it will have rendered a great service to all Health Administrations of African countries and territories.

—Dr. E. J. Pampana, 2 January 1952

Prior to the widespread use of DDT and free distribution of anti-malarial drug, most of Liberia appeared to be under the false sense of hyperendemic malaria protection. The colossal slaughter of the young was not as carefully recognized as malaria death and the relative freedom from serious clinical attacks gave the impression of an immuned population. This was false security as analysis will show because economic inefficiency and retardation of mind and body is associated with high malaria incidences. Nevertheless, the introduction of DDT and free distribution of anti-malarial drugs have disturbed that immunity and whenever defects occur now in the effective use of these control measures, the clinical manifestations are more frequent and more severe in the adults. These manifestations assume epidemic proportion at times.

— Hildrus A. Poindexter, 5 August 1952

In the immediate aftermath of the Second World War, the prospects for the global control of malaria—and perhaps even global eradication—appeared promising.[1] The older approaches to malaria control in tropical Africa, based on environmental management techniques such as the drainage and larviciding of anopheline mosquito breeding grounds, had been used with success before the war in some urban areas and in some plantation and mining sites,[2] and during the war in some of the important coastal ports, including Freetown and Accra. These techniques, however, were relatively expensive and could not be "scaled up" to provide protection to most African communities. The wartime successes in vector-borne disease control using dichloro-diphenyl-trichloroethane (DDT) in southern Europe and within the United States, however, suggested another path to disease control that could be replicated in other malarious regions, including tropical Africa.[3]

At the first World Health Organization Conference on African Malaria, held in Kampala, Uganda, in 1950, a major schism had emerged between malariologists who believed that DDT and other synthetic insecticides should be used to reduce malaria transmission in rural Africa and those who believed that such efforts, if unsuccessful, would compromise the acquired immunity of those who had survived malarial infections in childhood. Those in favor of interventions with synthetic insecticides won the day, and concerns over the potential loss of acquired immunity did not figure into the considerations of those who planned the Liberian interventions, in part because they were invigorated by the prospect for full success—the eradication of malaria—and chose not to plan for the potential consequences of partial success.[4]

In Monrovia, the capital of the Republic of Liberia, the Americans launched the first initiative to bring powerful synthetic chemical insecticides to bear on the tropical African malaria problem. Several years later, the program expanded to the areas surrounding the capital, and in 1953 the WHO developed a pilot project in Central Province to explore the feasibility of malaria eradication. These projects uncovered a spate of difficult issues that challenged the pretensions of the global malaria eradication campaign.

Prelude to the American Initiatives at Mosquito Control (1941–44)

In March 1941, the government of the United States of America passed the Lend-Lease Act that facilitated the US provision of essential war matériel to the United Kingdom and other Allied powers.[5] In July 1941, the US government requested that Pan American World Airways build an airfield in Liberia. Pan American turned to the Firestone Tire and Rubber Company—which had established a rubber plantation in Liberia in 1926[6]—to undertake the project, and for its part Pan American agreed to fly US-made aircraft from the United States to Brazil, then across the South Atlantic to Liberia, and then on to British forces in the Mediterranean. A runway at the newly constructed

Use of Synthetic Insecticide to Control Malaria in Liberia

Roberts Field airbase opened in January 1942.[7] The US Army Air Force took over the airfield and extended it to accommodate giant B-29 Flying Fortress bombers. By late 1942, an estimated five thousand US troops were garrisoned at the airbase in Liberia.[8]

The further development and protection of strategic wartime assets in Liberia appeared vital. In early 1942, the Japanese seizure of the British colonial rubber plantations in Malaya cut off the supply of the Allies' principal source of natural rubber—a critically important resource. The Firestone rubber plantation in Liberia—by far the largest in the Atlantic basin—thus took on greater significance, even as a new technology of synthetic rubber production, legal restrictions on civilian use of rubber tires, and an active "reclaim" program for used tires allowed the United States to meet its essential wartime needs.[9]

President Franklin Delano Roosevelt, the first US head of state to visit Africa, touched down at Roberts Field in January 1943, signaling a new era in US-Liberian relations.[10] In conversations with the Liberian president Edwin J. Barclay, Roosevelt reached an agreement for the United States to construct a deepwater port at Monrovia.[11] The US strategic goal was to provide maritime protection for the Allies in the South Atlantic. Barclay took the decision, effective 31 December 1943, to adopt the US dollar—instead of the pound sterling—as the sole legal tender in Liberia. The arrangements drew Liberia and the United States into a closer embrace.

William Tubman assumed the presidency of Liberia in January 1944, and within weeks of his accession, the government of Liberia had declared war on the Axis powers. Tubman then took steps to restructure the internal politics of Liberia. He announced a "Unification Policy" that, in principle, would diminish the cultural division between the Americo-Liberians, who were the descendants of US freed slaves and who controlled the Liberian state along the Atlantic coast, and the "upcountry" native Africans. In 1944, a joint US and Liberian force began the first continuous road into the Liberian interior, from Monrovia to Ganta, near the border with French Guinea, and on to Saniquellie to the northeast.[12]

In October 1944 the United States signed a Lend-Lease agreement with Liberia and arranged to send a Foreign Economic Administration mission to Liberia with a broad general portfolio.[13] Tubman sought assistance from the United States in planning for improvements in the sanitation of Monrovia and other coastal towns. His request was folded into the military program in Liberia. The United States approved a United States Public Health Service (USPHS) mission to Liberia to provide additional military sanitation, in cooperation with the government of Liberia, to protect US military personnel; to render the environs of the airport free of mosquito species that would be dangerous if introduced to the United States; to assist the government of Liberia in planning for the sanitation of coastal towns; and to render aid to the government of Liberia in the event of a request to enlarge its public health program.[14]

Mosquito Control Arrives in Liberia (1945–47)

In 1945, an "all-Negro" team of eleven US physicians, engineers, entomologists, and nurses from the United States Public Health Service, headed by Dr. John B. West, arrived in Monrovia to create a five-year development plan in public health.[15] One of their principal charges was to bring malaria under control, and in March 1945 they launched a malaria control program in the greater Monrovia area. The efforts were largely makeshift. DDT solution insecticides (10 percent DDT in kerosene) were used for indoor residual spraying (IRS). Intensive larviciding (with 5 percent DDT in kerosene), as well as some drainage operations, were carried out over an area about twelve miles long and three miles wide.[16]

In the greater Monrovia area, much of the insecticide use was inefficient because more than 50 percent of the interior house walls had sorptive surfaces of laterite soils that were high in iron and aluminum through which the solvent carried the insecticide into the wall, rendering it ineffectual. At the time there was no entomologist or chemist in Liberia who understood the issue. Work proceeded on an ad hoc basis. When the DDT seemed no longer to do the job—that is, to kill the mosquitoes inside the dwelling—the sprayers were called back in. The result was roughly a once-a-month spraying cycle with exceedingly high per capita costs.[17]

The larvicidal and drainage operations also faced daunting logistical problems. There were an estimated 90,000 acres of mangrove swamps in the greater Monrovia area in which mosquito breeding could not be controlled with routine ground methods of larviciding. Airplane spraying was costly, and it was estimated that only 5 percent of the mangrove swamps would produce mosquitoes at any one time. Moreover, the heavy rainfalls would dilute the larvicide and make it almost impossible to reduce anopheline vector populations to a level at which transmission of malaria would not occur.[18]

Yet, the mosquito control program, although very expensive, at least by one measure produced positive public health results: Malaria admissions to the public health hospital in Monrovia decreased by almost 95 percent from 383 in 1945 to 21 in 1947. This decline may have been in part a result of the

Use of Synthetic Insecticide to Control Malaria in Liberia

local community's access to antimalarial drugs that reduced the severity of the malarial attacks, as well as a result of the vector control program.[19]

The initial mosquito control efforts in Monrovia were well received by the local population, once it was appreciated that the spraying resulted in the near disappearance of flies, bed bugs, and other insects, in addition to mosquitoes. Another benefit flowed from the drainage operations that dried out some swamp areas that were then planted in food crops.[20] According to Dr. J. N. Togba, the sole Western-trained Liberian physician—who in October 1950 became director of the newly formed Bureau of Public Health and Sanitation and from October 1952 the director of the newly formed National Public Health Service (NPHS) of Liberia—interest in public health further intensified following a successful effort to counter an outbreak of smallpox in 1947 that involved the vaccination of roughly 95 percent of the total population. Requests for hospitals and clinics poured in from the counties and provinces.[21]

Retraction (1948–52)

By 1947, the malaria control program had thus achieved some positive results in reducing hospital admissions and in reducing nuisance insect and mosquito densities. But for the Americans the expense of the program argued against its continuation. The US mission withdrew the malaria control officer from Liberia and replaced him with a "sanitary engineer" who had no expertise in malaria control and who was given a wider scope of work. By 1948, the malaria control efforts had been cut back by 80 percent. And from 1947, the population of Monrovia surged, nearly doubling in the next five years, as the restrictions against the immigration of "upcountry" Africans were relaxed. The immigrants were highly parasitized, and they lived in close proximity to Monrovians whose acquired immunity—maintained by recurrent inoculations by malaria-carrying mosquitoes—had deteriorated as a result of the vector control program and their access to antimalarial drugs. The result was a sharp increase in malarial infections and a surge of resentment against the US mission.[22]

From 1948 to 1950, the control efforts deteriorated as a result of inexpert direction and restricted resources. From an epidemiological point of view, the malaria control program had spiraled into ineffectiveness. Mosquito densities had declined markedly, but an analysis of blood smears in 1950 indicated that the control program had no impact whatsoever on rates of infection.[23] The Americo-Liberians' view of the malaria control program, however, had gained traction. Americo-Liberians considered the program to be a powerful good, because it reduced the problem of nuisance mosquitoes and house vermin.

They enthusiastically seized the opportunities to have their houses sprayed. As Professor C. W. Kruse, a World Health Organization (WHO) consultant from the Johns Hopkins University, noted in his 1950 report: "One gets the impression that almost everybody in the town is supervising the operation and issuing instructions. . . . This control program, inspected from the standpoint of apparent effectiveness, cost, and permanence does not appear favorable."[24] At the time of Professor Kruse's survey, there were only about four thousand buildings (including homes and huts) that were sprayed in the Monrovia region, and the average cost was $2.25 per house per year. This made it one of the most expensive spraying operations in the world. The larvicidal program in principle followed a set routine: the control zone had been divided into five sectors and the crews went from one to another during the five days of the workweek. But the zone had been established without any reference to mosquito flight ranges. Some of the zones extended five miles to the east or five miles to the west of Monrovia, far beyond the flight ranges of the mosquitoes.[25]

As the mosquito control efforts waned, mosquito densities increased, and vermin returned in large numbers. The reduced malaria control efforts soon appeared to be nearly futile, and Dr. Togba added his voice to those of others who stridently criticized the US program. Dr. Poindexter, the director of the USPHS mission in Monrovia, recommended to his superiors in Washington that the program be scrapped, arguing that a holding pattern would damage the prestige of the United States. Dr. Togba put additional pressure on the United States by threatening to ask the World Health Organization to send a malaria control team to Liberia, and in 1951, the medical officer in charge of the Division of International Health Relations of the USPHS visited Monrovia and promised a US team, composed of a malariologist, a sanitary engineer, and a sanitarian, to reinvigorate the malaria control efforts.

The WHO sent Dr. Ragnar Huss, a specialist in public health, to visit Liberia in 1951. His recommendation was for a scale-up of operations: the US malaria control program should be extended "to cover the important malarial regions outside Monrovia." He suggested that, if the USPHS was not prepared to extend the control program, Liberia should request assistance from the WHO. The fundamental rationale for the scale-up was the extent of the economic loss due to malaria that was imposed on the laboring population of the country.[26]

The US team arrived later in 1951. They recommended the establishment of a control zone of twenty-five square miles around Monrovia in which drainage and larvicidal operations would be carried out. The Liberian Institute of Tropical Medicine in October of 1951 countered with a recommendation that residual spraying with a DDT emulsion should take place at four- to five-week intervals in all the houses in the Monrovia area, in what was essentially a resumption of the earlier IRS program.[27] By November 1951, the program had stabilized to include limited larviciding in a main part of Monrovia; the abandonment of the project of large-scale drainage of the mangrove swamps; and a concentration on IRS using insecticides other than DDT, because of concerns over its effectiveness in coastal Liberia, or benzene hexachloride (BHC), because of its objectionable odor.[28]

In 1951, following on the scaling down of mosquito control efforts in the immediately preceding years, mosquito populations "exploded" in the Monrovia region. As a stopgap measure, the USPHS sent a "Fog Generator" to blanket the large breeding areas near the coastal settlements with insecticide. It caused quite a stir. Its first trial suggested smoke from a conflagration, and the local fire brigade mobilized to stamp it out.[29] The fog generator achieved limited success, owing to the difficulty of getting proper wind direction and movement and the need to release the fog before the sun's heat became intense after 9 A.M.[30] A technology that had worked reasonably well in the United States did not transfer well to coastal Liberia.

Toward the end of the same year, Dr. Togba submitted a malaria control proposal for inland areas to UNICEF. It was forwarded to T. A. Austen, the Public Health Officer to General F. Daubenton, the acting director of the WHO Regional Office for Africa, who considered the request to be unrealistic: The road system into the interior was rudimentary; there were no maps showing where villages were located; there was no rural medical network; and all supplies of insecticide would have to be carried by porters into the interior. In testy conversations with Togba, Austen was frustrated in his efforts to get the most basic information about the public health prospects for a Liberian malaria control program; he was unable even to confirm the number of administrative districts in Liberia.[31]

Austen followed up by making inquiries about the prospects for collaboration between UNICEF and the WHO. Austen learned that UNICEF was already operating a small malaria control program about forty miles from Monrovia in a group of thirty villages with a population of about fifteen hundred. When he tried to learn more about the program, he waded into troubled political waters. The local head of UNICEF was unforthcoming and refused to confirm his own estimate of population. The project workers were hesitant to count the villagers for fear that they would be accused of helping the government seize the villagers' food and livestock and that they would lose the confidence of the villagers.[32]

In Monrovia proper, the malaria control program was struggling to cope with an ongoing economic boom. By 1952, the population of the capital was estimated at somewhere between 10,000 and 15,000, with a considerable fluctuation of migrants. With Monrovia burgeoning, government officials began to push for an extension of the malaria control program into the rest of the country. The motivation was straightforwardly economic: to attract foreign enterprise to Liberia and to be able to offer an environment for investment that was free from malaria. This was a variation on the theme "malaria blocks development" that had earlier focused on the biophysical burden borne by malaria sufferers.[33] Healthy workers would now attract investments. In Liberia, the "antimalaria" program was at the vanguard of development ideology.[34]

In 1952, Dr. E. J. Pampana, chief of the Malaria Section of the WHO, assessed the Liberian situation. In his view, a new IRS model of malaria control would be required:

> Monrovia, in spite of seven years of control activities, does not teach us anything as regards the solution of the problem of Liberia. There is no doubt that malaria is hyper-endemic all over the country, that it causes a very severe death rate amongst children and is certainly responsible for some deterioration in the physique of young people and perhaps for the apathy of the indigenous population. On the other hand there is no reason why, once a simple, efficient and economical method of insecticide application is found, Liberia could not try to control malaria with its own personnel in the areas of greatest developmental importance.[35]

In 1952, the USPHS personnel in Monrovia made the decision to switch from DDT to dieldrin, known as DLD. (It was not appreciated at the time that DLD was a more toxic pesticide with potentially more serious effects on human health.) The major advantages seemed to be that the chemical was stable and remained toxic even in contact with iron and aluminum and that it appeared to have a longer residual effect. It thus promised the possibility of a once-per-year spraying regime that would drastically reduce the labor and materials costs of the malaria control program.

The Dieldrin Campaign in Monrovia (1953–57)

The DLD campaign in the greater Monrovia area was launched in September 1953, and the initial results were highly positive. The United States International Cooperation Administration (ICA) malariologist noted that, after spraying the houses in Monrovia, Bushrod Island, and Sinkor, the anopheline mosquito populations dropped dramatically and that both the adult and the larval populations remained at low levels. Moreover, whenever adults and larvae were found, they were always associated with a significant number of unsprayed houses. Treating the unsprayed houses immediately brought about dramatic reductions in the breeding pools.[36]

Progress was rapid. By August of 1954, the spraying program had been so successful that the malaria control teams could find no vector larvae in Monrovia. Then DLD resistance began to emerge, and by 1955, the control program had shifted back to the use of DDT in Monrovia on a twice-yearly basis. The NPHS of Liberia began to take part in the operations, and the Americans drew down their staff, and by 1956, there was only one American participant.[37] And from March 1956 until 1957, the vector absence was regularly monitored. The teams appeared to have achieved the local eradication of the malaria vectors. This was deemed highly significant. As the final report noted: "The main thing we have accomplished is to prove that malaria control can be effective in the hyperendemic tropics and have created an organization which can expand to cover the whole country as more people are available."[38] The accomplishment was limited to Monrovia, but nonetheless the success was real. It had been achieved despite the loss of trained men who quit their jobs to go to the diamond fields and the time-consuming necessity to train the replacements.[39]

Beyond Monrovia: Mosquito Control in Kpain, Central Province (1953–58)

In 1953, the WHO in collaboration with UNICEF, launched an antimalaria program in the upcountry of Central Province as one of the first pilot projects to investigate the feasibility of malaria eradication in tropical Africa.[40] The extension of malaria control into the interior of Liberia posed new challenges. One was architectural. The upcountry houses were not like the houses in the greater Monrovia area. They were built from timber, rather than clay, and the roofs were not close fitting. The weight of the house structure was borne by heavy-uprights and joists, rather than by mud walls. Mosquitoes flew unimpeded through the wide gaps at the eaves.[41]

A more intractable problem arose from the rhythms of the rural agricultural economy. In the towns of the interior—that were accessible by a motorable road and had one or more Lebanese trading stores—only a quarter to half of the houses were occupied during the daytime. Nighttime occupation rose to 80 or 90 percent. In the villages—that typically could be approached only on foot and sometimes required up to twenty miles of rough walking from a motorable road—the daytime residents were mainly the sick, aged, or the disabled. Nighttime occupation in the villages, as in the towns, was around 80 or 90 percent. Spraying could only take place during the daytime hours and during the dry season, from November through April. During the wet season, many farmers stayed near their fields and slept in their open shelters.

During the dry season, most adults and children worked their fields and were gone during the daylight hours. In their fields they built other structures—usually a "rice kitchen," which was a sizable structure with an open ground floor and a substantial ceiling with an upper-storey storage granary, and a "farm kitchen," which had the same open architecture without the storage granary. The storage granary was a suitable resting place for the vector mosquitoes, but it was kept locked, and thus was inaccessible to the spray teams who found their way into the fields. In practice, this happened infrequently, because the farmers refused to tell the spray teams where their rice kitchens were located because they sensed that sharing this information would leave them vulnerable to predation by Liberian government workers.[42] As one observer noted bluntly: "No villagers will direct the spraying squads and they will never say where the rice-kitchens are located."[43] The farm kitchens were accessible only by discontinuous forest paths, and only the local people knew the traces.

By contrast, the enthusiasm for the extension of the antimalaria campaign into the upcountry on the part of the international community was great. It bubbled up from the success in Monrovia and from the support that was building for the idea of a WHO-led global malaria eradication campaign. Although Dr. Pampana of the WHO had stressed the need for experiments to determine the best means of control, within Liberia the antimalaria program went forward without much in the way of planning. For this reason, from its beginnings the upcountry spraying campaign evolved as a cavalcade of errors. As in the greater Monrovia area, there was no malariological survey before the IRS campaign began, and thus no baseline data of infection against which to measure progress. Nor was there an entomological survey. The project directors simply assumed that the same vector that was principally responsible for malaria transmission in Monrovia—*Anopheles gambiae*—had the same epidemiological significance in the upcountry. This, alas, was not the case.

In haste to protect the largest number of people in the shortest possible time, the campaign began along the northern terminus of the Monrovia–French Guinea road and its spurs. The approach was to spray along the ribbons of the road network. The logistics were daunting. The spraying could take place only during the dry season; materials had to be brought 180 miles by road from Monrovia to the project headquarters at Kpain; and soon a shortage of transport vehicles brought the project to a near standstill. Moreover, the spraying along the ribbons of roadway was uneven. At frequent intervals, strips of unsprayed areas were left as "check areas." These would normally have been at considerable distance from a sprayed area, to prevent the easy infiltration of mosquitoes.[44]

On top of this confusion was layered a poorly considered effort to try out a variety of different insecticides at various dosages. Some areas were sprayed with DLD, others with BHC, and yet others with DDT. The result was that a practical evaluation of the differential effectiveness of the insecticides was impossible.

The logistics of the project were further complicated by the fact that during the wet season, the local roads were barely negotiable. The team leader, Dr. W. Möllhausen, paid visits to the local authorities in Voinjama and Kolahun in the nearby Western Province in May of 1957. The distance between the two towns was twenty-six miles, but the trip took nine hours and involved crossing sixty-two "bad" bridges, "reconstructing" twenty bridges by adding planks, and frequent unloading the heavily packed cars because the bridges would not bear their weight.[45]

During the rainy season, the inundations also caused damage to the walls of the upcountry houses and huts. Rural Liberians seasonally replastered their walls to repair the damage. When the malaria team members became aware of replastering, they realized that the newly applied wall surfaces would likely diminish the utility of the residual spray, and that the replastered buildings might have to be resprayed. This possibility challenged the pretension to full coverage; and there was no surveillance network to alert the sprayers to the instances of replastering.

In 1955 the enthusiasm generated by the formal commitment of the WHO to the global eradication of malaria raced through the malaria control projects. Yet by 1956 at least one prescient specialist had realized that the eradication project in Liberia could not meets its goal. The larger significance of the replastering problem was apparent to the consulting entomologist M. T. Gillies. He noted:

> If . . . effective coverage with the insecticide of all inhabited shelters is
> not possible, then the only rational policy left open would be the aban-
> donment of the attempt at country wide spraying and its replacement by
> an intensification of treatment centres. Such a suggestion, in the heady
> atmosphere of eradication schemes, may sound retrogressive and hereti-
> cal. But to this outside observer at least, it appears that the problems of
> Liberia (which in some ways are unique) may ultimately force the in-
> ternational organization concerned to adopt this unpopular policy.[46]

In 1956, the upcountry malaria control program opened a new portfolio. The WHO/UNICEF project received a supply of antimalarial drugs as a supplement to the indoor residual spraying campaign.[47] The drugs were dispensed initially in a haphazard manner: the health propagandist at Kpain, on the orders of Dr. Möllhausen, the team leader, handed out the pills freely to children that he encountered in the villages, and Möllhausen himself reportedly gave to each child from whom he took blood a Nivaquin pill.[48] Möllhausen was worried about the impact of the indoor residual spraying program on the immunological status of the children. As he wrote to the WHO Regional Director: "If the houses are sprayed, they will not get infection during this time and they might loose [sic] some immunity, so that the children get probably worse attacks by re-infection while staying in the farms for the other months."[49]

How effective was the spraying? Had the rates of malarial infection declined as a result of the interventions? Here—as with the issue of the differential effectiveness of insecticides—it was necessary to have baseline data, and the best measure was the parasite rate in human blood samples. (The less expensive, but less telling diagnostic test was palpation of the spleen. The percentage of patients found to have distended spleens was expressed as a "spleen rate.") The rural townspeople, however, were uncooperative. The default was to examine schoolchildren; but because the students' homes were often far away from the schools, their parasite rates did not reflect the local parasite rates in towns where the schools were located. Some medical officers secured the support of the local chiefs and district commissioners and arrived with an escorting soldier and forced the townspeople to comply.[50]

The project's activities were concentrated on the inhabited areas along the main roads. Although the team claimed that they covered a depth of twenty miles on either side of the roads, large areas were never explored and uncounted hamlets and rice kitchens went unsprayed. Moreover, the work of the spraying squads was impossible to supervise fully. In principle, teams of six spraymen went into villages with two supervisors, and in the best-case scenario, two of every six houses were checked for quality. Many supervisors, however, stayed in town taking care of private business rather than accompanying their teams into the bush.[51]

The WHO retrospective assessment held that even in the easily accessible villages the insecticide coverage was incomplete. Some houses were left unsprayed. The DLD spray cycle was on an annual basis, but no consideration was given to the importance of completing the spray cycle before the peak mosquito-breeding season. Moreover, the rural villagers replastered

Use of Synthetic Insecticide to Control Malaria in Liberia

their houses frequently and rebuilt houses and even entire villages in the course of the year. The result left "a great percentage" of houses unsprayed in most areas.[52]

One consequence of the uneven rate of coverage was that the parasite rates of infants varied widely. One important variable was whether the infants slept inside or outside the sprayed houses. Yet even in the heavily sprayed areas, the infant parasite rate was never suppressed below 29 percent.[53]

There was a spate of other difficult issues. The team suffered interpersonal conflicts among the expatriate staff, and the lines of authority over the Liberian staff members were blurred. When Dr. M. E. C. Giglioli, the WHO entomologist, discovered that one of the chief insect collectors had been submitting false reports to him for three continuous months, he demanded that the collector be fired. The Liberian administrator intervened to save the man's job.[54] Giglioli resigned in July 1957, amid charges from Möllhausen that he had not done his job.[55]

By 1957, resistance to DLD was confirmed and cross-resistance to BHC was reported. In the WHO project area, *A. gambiae* had become highly resistant.[56] By the second half of 1957, resistance to DLD had become widespread, and spraying operations were suspended in February of 1958.[57]

Toward the end of the project, in 1957, Möllhausen asserted that an epidemic of malaria was exacting an extraordinary toll in morbidity and mortality—on the order of 25 percent—from infants and children. An emergency treatment program with chloroquine was launched, but a WHO report disparaged the effort on the grounds that it would have little effect on future malaria control. "Such a rather ill-planned and unmethodical drugging may have some propagandistic value and may be prompted by humanitarian consideration, but their value as an effective means of malaria control is more than doubtful, especially in view of the fact that according to inquiries made only a small proportion of sick children could be treated as at this time of year the majority of the people live in rather inaccessible shelters on their farms."[58]

The impact of the indoor residual spraying program on the immunological status of the adult villagers was also marked. The initial use of DLD had been highly effective in interrupting malaria transmission, until the emergence of resistance. During this period of interrupted transmission, the acquired immunities of the adult villagers began to degrade. After the emergence of resistance to DLD and the reestablishment of transmission, a malaria epidemic surged through the adult villagers. The project staff measured spleen rates and had no doubts. As a quarterly project report concluded, "Vector resistance to DLD [dieldrin] has been followed by a malaria epidemic of which the adult spleen rate obtained in the Project Area is ample proof."[59]

The WHO program that began in 1953 lasted for five years. The "protected" population was sizable and increased over the life of the project.

TABLE 2.1. Estimated population protected by the Kpain Malaria Project, 1953–57

Year	Population
1953	54,000
1955	142,000
1956	200,000
1957	300,000

Source: WHO, AFR/MAL/61/43, Dr. C. Guttuso, "The Kpain (Liberia) Malaria Project," 30 May 1962, 1.

Was the Kpain project worth following up? What lessons were to be drawn from it? The WHO position was that the Kpain program had been so poorly led and executed that it would have been highly improbable if it had achieved the interruption of malaria transmission. The WHO decided to fund a new project at Kpain, staffed by a malariologist, an entomologist, and a sanitarian. The expectation was that it could achieve the interruption of malaria transmission and thereby pave the way toward eradication.[60]

The ICA/UNICEF/GOL Pilot Project in Montserrado (1958–62)

In 1958, the government of Liberia in collaboration with the ICA of the US State Department decided to open a new field of antimalaria operations immediately inland from the greater Monrovia area, to build on the success of their earlier program. The insecticide of choice was DDT, and in 1958, the spray campaign in the Montserrado region began. As early as 1959, however, major difficulties loomed. Some 6 percent of rural Liberians refused to open their houses to the spray teams, and the buzzing nuisance culicine mosquitoes, rather than the silent anophelines, had become resistant to DDT.[61] The two issues were directly linked—because one of the immediate benefits of the IRS program was that it eliminated nuisance mosquitoes, and when this benefit was lost, the percentage of "spraying refusals" would climb. The UNICEF/ICA project assessment was blunt: "The general conclusion to be drawn from these and similar surveys in Liberia is that in rural areas residual house spraying is not sufficient for interruption of transmission. It is expected that more efficient control will be achieved by insecticides supplemented with mass-drug treatment."[62]

Use of Synthetic Insecticide to Control Malaria in Liberia

Round Two: The Kpain Project, 1958–62

At the WHO Technical Meeting on Malaria convened in Brazzaville in December 1957, specialists agreed that the pilot projects to date throughout West Africa had failed to achieve the interruption of transmission, and that new projects should include large-scale experiments in mass drug administration. Because the cost of training special health teams to record the dispensation of drugs was very costly, mass drug administration typically meant that the spray teams would leave behind tablets with heads of family who, in principle, would hand them out to family members who were away in the fields or give the tablets to the village chiefs who would then hand them out to the villagers.[63] In theory, this would ensure a low-cost chain of supply that would extend to the hard-to-reach villagers. The issue of actual usage—who took the antimalarials, in what doses, and how this would be measured—was not broached.

The new Kpain project, far smaller in scale than the first, would thus attack both the vector *and* the reservoir of parasites within the human population—what was termed "the human factor." It was planned for the upcountry towns of Bahn and Saniquellie, which were readily accessible from the Kpain headquarters and had a combined population of about 45,000–50,000. The initial malaria eradication operations had started in this region, and even after four continuous years of IRS, the malaria indices had stayed very high.

By design, half the population would be treated with indoor residual spraying and mass drug treatment and the other half with only indoor residual spraying. The Bahn sector (population 24,000) would receive IRS and drug treatment with chloroquine and pyrimethamine. To accomplish this, the Bahn sector was to be divided into four subsectors as treating units, and a total of sixteen "treaters" would be employed. The Saniquellie sector would receive IRS alone.[64]

The "human factor," however, was a lot more complicated—and mobile—than the project designers appreciated. Residents of the Bahn sector, in particular, frequently traveled to French Guinea where malaria was also hyperendemic, and residents of French Guinea frequented the Bahn sector. This regional epidemiological integration was not factored into the program, despite the fact that the problem had been laid out clearly by the Haematological Malaria Survey reports in earlier years: "The movement of the [Bahn] population is variable,—many of them like to stay for a long time in the adjacent French colonies, where no spraying is carried out. On the other hand many visitors and traders from other African countries can be found here regularly, which results in a complete mixture of all West African strains of malaria (and other) parasites."[65]

In September 1958, the first DDT spraying cycle began. The entomological realities had shifted enormously. *Anopheles funestus* had been all but eliminated from the upcountry regions that had been sprayed, and into its ecological niche flitted the *Anopheles gambiae,* formerly a minor upcountry vector.

In this second round of the Kpain malaria project, the Liberian government took steps to neutralize the resistance of the villagers. It issued signed letters of authority to headmen, and pressured chiefs and local authorities to facilitate the work of the malaria teams. The "plan-ops" called for twice yearly spraying with DDT, and the first two spray cycles met with grand success. Indoor residual spraying with DDT caused *A. gambiae* to disappear from the larger settlements. Emboldened by this achievement, the project managers took the next logical step. They shifted the focus of the spraying teams to the rice kitchens, farms, hamlets, and the small settlements.

Here the rate of progress of the teams was slower—and the field of operations was larger—than had been anticipated. The number of rice kitchens was found to equal or exceed the number of permanent houses. The spray teams fanned out into the remote countryside. This was extremely time-intensive work. Dr. Guttuso, the project director, insisted on thoroughness—the spraying of the entire interior of all of the village houses and of all the isolated farm shelters.[66] The expanded field of work was beyond the means of the spray teams, and in their efforts to cover more ground, the insecticide spraying cycle lapsed from twice to once per year.

The shift to DDT also necessitated some logistical adjustments. DDT was packaged in unwieldy 200 lb. drums. The initial plan was for "specially selected" porters who could handle heavy loads, organized in four-man teams, to carry the drums using a hammock. This proved impractical when winding down narrow trails in the bush and in fording streams. Because the rice kitchens were often at great distance from one another and each required only a small amount of insecticide, the porters transferred the DDT into the small DLD drums of 40 lbs. each. And as the malaria work expanded, the labor arrangements also had to be revamped. The men who initially had been "selected" as unpaid insecticide porters had labored under compulsion from the village chiefs. During the following year (1959), the system of forced labor was reformed to one of compensated labor.[67]

As the work advanced, the scientific surveys from a few fully sprayed areas turned up good news. The laboratories at Kpain reported that both the mosquito dissections and the human blood surveys were negative for parasites.

Yet at the same time, diamonds were discovered in the project region, and migrants began to flood in. They built houses that went undiscovered and thus unsprayed. The parasite rates of infants who had been born in and had remained in the sprayed areas were nil. Yet there was still malaria in the project region. The positive cases had been introduced—in what was known as "malaria without anophelism"; the increase in mining activity had drawn in parasitized workers from afar.[68] Soon thereafter, *A. gambiae* built up its numbers in the unsprayed houses, and the transmission of malaria was reestablished.

By 1959, other serious problems were emerging. The old DLD and BHC zones had been re-sprayed with DDT, and there were reports of an increasing tolerance of *Anopheles gambiae* to DDT, although laboratory tests did not corroborate the reports. At the project headquarters at Kpain, visitors in mid-1959 described critical lapses. Only one of the two zones had been sprayed; the laboratory technicians had no blood slides to analyze; and the distribution of antimalarial drugs had ground to a halt. A major constraint was transport. Only three vehicles were in working condition, and there was no mechanic who knew how to fix the vehicles that were out of repair.[69]

Could the problems be addressed through economies of scale? One possibility was to fold the smaller ICA/UNICEF/GOL pilot project into the WHO project. The smaller project involved a program of spot spraying in Monrovia and the Montserrado region, just inland from Monrovia. Yet the execution of the ICA/UNICEF/GOL program was haphazard at best. The former Rockefeller Foundation malariologist Fred L. Soper—who had led a successful species eradication campaign in Brazil and was a former director of the Pan American Sanitary Bureau—was highly critical of the organization of the spraying campaign. As he noted in his diary, "There are no maps, the houses are not numbered, the only number in use is the numerical order of the house in the day's work of a squad in a certain district of the city; there is no way in which the past work of individual squads can be evaluated; no-one knows how many houses nor in what districts the service is responsible for; men doing work get different pay scales according to the circumstances of their employment; range for spraymen [is] from $17.50 to $35.00 monthly." The larvicidal operations were judged no better.[70]

In addition to the deficient management, other sticking points made collaboration difficult. By US law, the ICA could hire only Americans and Liberian nationals. And if there were to be institutional cooperation, on what basis would it take place? Soper pushed for an integration of the antimalaria programs and for the participation of all institutions on the same projects on a percentage basis.[71] This was not to be.

The WHO funding for the Kpain project ended in 1961.[72] As the guiding hand of WHO sponsorship was lifted, the professional antimalaria project staff in Kpain arranged to be transferred back to Monrovia; the NPHS withdrew five UNICEF vehicles from Kpain; administrative oversight procedures were jettisoned.[73] Malaria control unraveled.

Assessments

The malariological lessons were many, complex, and difficult to assimilate. On the technical side, the most striking lesson was that DDT's impact was both immediate and long-lasting. In some areas that had been left unsprayed during the second cycle, the DDT residue was still active as long as twenty-six months after spraying, even though full coverage had not been achieved. On the conceptual side, at least for those who had carried out the malaria projects, the notion of a static rural malaria problem in tropical Africa was overturned. By the end of the project, the project staff recognized that the malaria problem was a dynamic one. The large number of migrants who flowed in and out of the "industrial" zones and the movement of people between the Liberian upcountry into Sierra Leone and French Guinea portended a complicated program that would have to extend across political borders: In the upcountry of Liberia, the boundaries of the tropical African state clearly did not constitute a workable unit of epidemiological intervention. Effective malaria control or eradication in Liberia—and by extension elsewhere in West Africa—would require close collaboration between neighboring states.

In financial terms, the costs of the WHO antimalaria project were higher than had been anticipated. The IRS program far exceeded estimates. This was principally a function of the average surface per capita that had to be sprayed. Originally estimated at 44 square meters, in practice the figure was at least 100 square meters per capita. This was owing to the large number of crop huts and to the fact that the houses were frequently built over 6 meters in height, and *A. gambiae* could be found resting in the apexes. This greater surface area, in addition to the time necessary to locate and travel to the rice kitchens and to spray the houses' high ceilings, drove the cost "through the roof."[74] The 1959 monthly program of mass drug administration also proved administratively complex and expensive, and it was abandoned. Mass drug administration had reached only six thousand recipients, a smaller number than anticipated.[75]

The DDT spraying operations by themselves proved remarkably effective in reducing mosquito density. *Anopheles funestus* had been the most important malaria vector in the Liberian countryside, and it had proved highly vulnerable to DLD. As *Anopheles funestus* died off, however, *Anopheles gambiae* had moved into its ecological niche. Some specialists suspected that the initial susceptibility of *Anopheles gambiae* to DDT was the result of its imperfect adaptation to the new environment. The implication was that as its adaptation improved, *Anopheles gambiae* would become less susceptible to spraying operations.[76]

Faced with these divergent, complex, and incomplete results, the WHO crafted an interpretation of the Liberian antimalaria campaign as troubled but ultimately successful. The main constraints were identified as the high costs of the project and the lack of the administrative capacity to manage the project. The WHO characterized the participation of the government of Liberia as "exemplary."[77]

The WHO claimed that the interruption of malaria transmission had been achieved with IRS alone, although some specialists did not support this claim because it implied a *sustainable* interruption of transmission. The movement of parasitized in-migrants and the migrants' construction of new buildings in the project zone had facilitated the rapid reestablishment of transmission.[78]

The WHO did not give any retrospective consideration to the medical consequences of reinfection in populations that had had their acquired immunities to malaria compromised by the antimalaria programs, even though those who were directly involved with the projects had observed the onset of epidemic malaria in the adult population. The WHO assessment was also silent on the issue of post-project epidemic malaria among children.

Dénouement

By 1962, following on a series of early pilot projects across tropical Africa, WHO malaria specialists had come to the view that, while technically feasible, the logistical and financial problems of eradicating malaria in tropical Africa were insurmountable at the present time. The best approach was thought to be to encourage the establishment of a "pre-eradication" program in the newly emerging independent African states. In addition to the training of technical personnel, a key component of the "pre-eradication program" was to be the development of a rural health infrastructure that could serve as the basis for the program. In principle, this would allow for the efficient treatment and cure of severe malaria.

In July 1962, at Yaoundé, the WHO convened a conference on African malaria, and a meeting took place there that included the WHO, NPHS of Liberia, and USAID. All were agreed on the WHO pre-eradication program for Liberia. Definitive decisions, however, were being taken elsewhere. In Monrovia, USAID had signed a new program agreement with the Liberian government that lacked a rural health infrastructure component.[79] The program goal was simply to expand the residual spraying program into the interior, from Montserrado County into the Central Province, as quickly as possible.

A new malaria control project began in Monrovia in 1962, aimed at protecting an urban population that had grown to 100,000. The WHO appointed a public health advisor who served for five years, from 1963 to 1968. The Liberian government never appointed a counterpart.[80] The Malaria Pre-Eradication Project was folded into the Department of Basic Health Services in January 1968, and the project headquarters shifted from Kpain to Monrovia.[81]

By 1970, when Dr. Arnaldo Gabaldón, an eminent malariologist who had chaired several of the malaria expert committees of the WHO, visited Liberia, the antimalaria projects outside of Monrovia had collapsed. In Monrovia, the efforts were directed at nuisance, rather than vector, mosquito control. Gabaldón was unable to get any cooperation, data, or even an expression of interest about the malaria problem.[82]

Before the antimalaria projects in Liberia, mosquito control efforts in West Africa had been concentrated in urban areas and on plantation or mining sites. Before World War II, drainage and larvicidal interventions had been effective in reducing the density of anopheline mosquitoes and the intensity of local malaria transmission. The projects had evolved on an ad hoc basis, taking account of local microenvironments.

In the immediate postwar period, the Americans introduced malaria control with synthetic insecticides to Monrovia. The early successes of the mosquito control programs in the Liberian capital created a demand for "scaled-up" projects in the surrounding areas and in the "upcountry" of Central Province that dovetailed with the government of Liberia's political program of "unification." A spate of difficulties troubled the early efforts at malaria eradication in upcountry Liberia and foreshadowed the general retreat from malaria eradication efforts across tropical Africa by the mid-1960s.

The WHO assessment of the Liberian experience highlighted the institutional, logistical, and financial difficulties encountered by the pilot projects and claimed that the goal of the interruption of malaria transmission through the use of IRS alone had been achieved. This underplayed some of the core challenges that the malaria eradication pilot project had encountered, and it did not address the issues of the medical consequences of the epidemic malarial reinfection of adults after the partial loss of acquired immunity or of the epidemic malarial infection of children.

❖

The malaria eradication pilot projects of the 1950s and 1960s have direct relevance for the malaria "elimination" campaigns of the early twenty-first century. The contemporary campaigns rely on two of the same approaches to malaria control: synthetic insecticides for indoor residual spraying to reduce vector density and chemical therapy to treat severe cases of malaria. The major difference is the contemporary mass distribution of insecticide-treated bed nets.

The early twenty-first-century campaigns are encountering mosquito resistance to the insecticides used for indoor residual spraying and treating bed nets. The use of synthetic insecticides today, as in the past, is changing the species composition of the mosquito fauna and thus the epidemiology of malaria transmission. The emergence of parasite resistance to the new chemical therapies is forecast. To date, the development of an effective malaria vaccine that could be deployed widely or the engineering of a transgenic mosquito that is unable to transmit the parasite and could be released in African environments are not close at hand. The weakening financial commitment to malaria control raises the specter of a lapse in malaria control and a resurgence of epidemic malaria.

Notes

Complete information for the epigraphs is as follows. For the first epigraph: World Health Organization (WHO)7.0022, Liberia. JKT I. SJ 4, "Report on my Visit to Liberia." Dr. E. J. Pampana to General F. Daubenton, 2 January 1952. For the second epigraph: National Archives and Records Administration (NARA), RG469, Liberia Subject Files, Box 3, Liberia Program Reports, Biennial Reports Folder. "Annual Report Fiscal Year 1952," Hildrus A. Poindexter, Chief, Public Health Staff, TCA, to Acting Country Director, 5 August 1952, 26.

1. For recent surveys of malaria history that discuss the global malaria eradication program, see James L. A. Webb, Jr., *Humanity's Burden: A Global History of Malaria* (New York: Cambridge University Press, 2009), and Randall M. Packard, *The Making of a Tropical Disease: A Short History of Malaria* (Baltimore: Johns Hopkins University Press, 2007). On the history of biomedical research on malaria, see Leo B. Slater, *War and Disease: Biomedical Research on Malaria in the Twentieth Century* (New Brunswick, NJ: Rutgers University Press, 2009).

2. For the environmental management techniques in the Zambian copper belt, see Jürg Utzinger et al., "The Economic Payoffs of Integrated Malaria Control in the

Zambian Copperbelt between 1930 and 1950," *Tropical Medicine and International Health* 7, no. 8 (2002): 657–77.

3. For wartime Europe, see Edmund Russell, *War and Nature* (New York: Cambridge University Press, 2001), 119–44; Darwin H. Stapleton, "The Short-Lived Miracle of DDT," *Invention and Technology* 15, no. 3 (2000): 34–41; Frank M. Snowden, *The Conquest of Malaria: Italy, 1900–1962* (New Haven:Yale University Press, 2006), 198–212.

In the United States, during the 1940s DDT played a role in the decline of malarial infections in the southern states, and enthusiasm for vector control with the newly deployed synthetic insecticide was high. In the United States, the decline was measured in clinical cases of malaria. Retrospective analysis indicates that malarial infections were in marked decline before the use of DDT. This decline was principally owing to the widespread destruction of mosquito habitat brought about by the environmental transformations of the 1930s that included the drainage and impoundment programs of the Tennessee Valley Authority and the out-migration of the once-vulnerable populations to cities and towns. See Margaret Humphreys, "Kicking a Dying Dog: DDT and the Demise of Malaria in the American South, 1942–1950," *Isis* 87, no. 1 (1996): 1–17; Margaret Humphreys, *Malaria: Poverty, Race, and Public Health in the United States* (Baltimore: Johns Hopkins University Press, 2001).

In Liberia, by contrast, there were virtually no baseline data. No malariological studies had been carried out beyond the Firestone plantations since 1936. Ludwik Anigstein, "Medical Exploration in Liberia," *Bulletin of the Health Organisation of the League of Nations* 6, no. 1 (1937): 93–127.

4. Webb, *Humanity's Burden*, 160–66; Socrates Litsios, *The Tomorrow of Malaria* (Karori, NZ: Pacific Press, 1996), 106–23.

5. The United States had previously extended naval assistance to the United Kingdom through the 1940 "Destroyers for Bases Agreement," and before the Lend Lease Act of 1941, the UK had been obliged to pay in gold for other war matériel.

6. For the early history of Firestone in Liberia, see Arthur J. Knoll, "Firestone's Labor Policy, 1924–1939," *Liberian Studies Journal* 16, no. 2 (1991): 49–75.

7. Alfred Lief, *The Firestone Story: A History of the Firestone Tire and Rubber Company* (New York: Whittlesey House, 1951), 321–23.

8. Harrison Akingbade, "U.S. Liberian Relations during World War II," *Phylon* 46, no. 1 (1985): 30.

The US troops suffered high rates of malarial infection, owing in part to fluctuating policies in the administration of antimalarial prophylaxis. See John W. H. Rehn, "Africa-Middle East Theater," in Medical Department, US Army, *Preventive Medicine in World War II*, vol. 6, *Communicable Diseases: Malaria* (Washington, DC: Office of the Surgeon General, Department of the Army, 1963), 303–46.

9. Lief, *Firestone Story*, 271–81; for general background on Firestone in Liberia, see Ibrahim Sundiata, *Brothers and Strangers: Black Zion, Black Slavery, 1914–1940* (Durham, NC: Duke University Press, 2003), 107–26.

10. US-Liberian relations had been seriously strained by the government of Liberia's involvement with forced labor practices that came under investigation by the League of Nations. On the labor abuses and the League of Nations investigation, see Sundiata, *Brothers and Strangers*, 79–139.

11. As part of an agreement with the government of Liberia in 1926, the Firestone Tire and Rubber Company committed to building a harbor at Monrovia at a cost not to exceed $300,000. The Liberian government was to repay the expense of construction to Firestone. Harvey J. Firestone, president of the Firestone Tire and Rubber Company, spent $115,000 toward this end, before engineers determined that the project was impracticable; Firestone absorbed the financial loss. Lief, *Firestone Story,* 164.

12. Wayne Chatfield Taylor, *The Firestone Operations in Liberia* (Washington, DC: National Planning Association, 1956), 14–15; Akingbade, "U.S. Liberian Relations during World War II," 25–36; David McBride, *Missions for Science: US Technology and Medicine in America's African World* (New Brunswick, NJ: Rutgers University Press, 2002), 169.

13. J. H. Mower, "The Republic of Liberia," *Journal of Negro History* 32, no. 3 (1947): 299.

14. National Archives and Records Administration (NARA), RG469, UD504, Liberia Subject Files, Box 4, Liberia-Reports-Travels, Misc. Unfiled Materials Folder, Interdepartmental Advisory Council on Technical Cooperation, Country Study on Liberia, 17 January 1951, 66.

On the political culture of Liberia and the corruption of the Tubman era, see Tuan Wreh, *The Love of Liberty . . . The Rule of President William V. S. Tubman in Liberia, 1944–1971* (London: C. Hurst, 1976).

15. "US Will Help Liberia in 5-Year Health Work," *New York Times,* 22 November 1944; Lawrence A. Marinelli, *The New Liberia: A Historical and Political Survey* (New York: Frederick A. Praeger, 1964), 80.

The surgeon Dr. John B. West was stationed in Liberia with the US Army medical corps. McBride, *Missions for Science,* 178.

16. NARA, RG469, UD754, Liberia-Personnel 1951–1958, Box 2, Liberia-Reports Folder 3/3, Roy F. Smits, "Historical Review of the Malaria Control Program in Liberia, 1944–1955," 23 August 1955, 1; WHO7.0022, Liberia 1932–1951, JKT I. SJ 4, "Report on my Visit to Liberia," E. J. Pampana to General F. Daubenton, 2 January 1952; WHO7.0022, Liberia 1953–1956, JKT II. SJ 3; Charles E. Kohler, Malariologist [ICA], "A Five Year Malaria Eradication Plan for the Republic of Liberia," 1–2.

17. Kohler, "Five Year Malaria Eradication Plan," 2.

18. NARA, RG469, UD504, Liberia Subject Files, Box 2, Liberia-Health, Annual Report, Public Health Activity Joint Commission, 1953, 4–6.

19. NARA, RG469, UD504, Liberia Subject Files, Box 4, Liberia-Reports-Travels, Misc. Unfiled Materials Folder, Interdepartmental Advisory Council on Technical Cooperation, Country Study on Liberia, 17 January 1951, 68–70; NARA, RG469, Subject Files-Liberia, 1947–1952, Box 16, Hildrus A. Poindexter to Dr. Louis L. Williams, Jr., Chief, Division of International Health, USPHS, 20 July 1952.

20. NARA, RG469, E-530, Liberian Branch-Subject Files, 1948–1955, Box 20, Dr. Estabrook to Mr. Eason, "Resume of Accomplishments in Public Health Mission to Liberia," 23 August 1951, 3.

21. WHO7.0022, Liberia 1932–1951, JKT 1. SJ3, J. N. Togba, "Official Report of the Bureau of Public Health and Sanitation: For the Fiscal Year October 1, 1950–September 31, 1951," 7–8.

JAMES L. A. WEBB, JR.

Dr. J. N. Togba trained in the United States and received his medical degree in 1946. He returned to Liberia for one year, and then went to the United States for two years of public health training at Harvard University (NARA, RG469, E-529, General Correspondence-Liberia, 1948–1955, Box 1, Memorandum from Haldore Hanson, "Notes on My Liberian Visit—February 23 to March 2, 1951," 7). For the broader West African context of Western-trained African physicians, see Adell Patton, Jr., *Physicians, Colonial Racism, and Diaspora in West Africa* (Gainesville: University Press of Florida, 1996).

22. NARA, RG469, E-1313, Subject Files-Liberia, 1947–1952, Box 16, Hildrus A. Poindexter to Dr Louis J. Williams, Jr., Division of International Health, USPHS, 20 July 1952.

23. WHO7.0022, Liberia, 1932–1951, JKT 1, SJ 2, C. W. Kruse, Associate Professor of Sanitary Engineering, The Johns Hopkins University, School of Hygiene and Public Health, "Sanitary Survey of the Republic of Liberia," [1950], 36.

24. Ibid., 33–34.

25. Ibid.

26. WHO7.0022, Liberia, JKT 1, SJ 3, WHO/PHA/5, Ragnar Huss, "Public Health Medical Services in Liberia," 10 April 1951, 22.

27. The Liberian Institute of the American Foundation for Tropical Medicine, known as the Liberian Institute of Tropical Medicine, was endowed by a gift from Harvey J. Firestone, Jr., as a memorial to his late father, in 1947. Its research mission was to investigate both human and animal diseases. See [Anon.], "Liberia, Scene of New International Institute for Tropical Medicine," *American Journal of Tropical Medicine*, s-1-27 (July 1947): 517–19. Its work was supported by the Liberian Foundation. For details on the Liberian Foundation, see Stanley J. Leland, "The Liberian Foundation: Aims and Methods," *Milbank Memorial Fund Quarterly* 28, no. 1 (1950): 43–51. The Americans withdrew their support of the Institute in the late 1960s. In 1975, a Liberian Institute for Biomedical Research came into existence, "somewhat in succession to the Liberian Institute for Tropical Medicine" (D. Elwood Dunn, Amos J. Beyan, and Carl Patrick Burrowes, *Historical Dictionary of Liberia* [Lanham, MD: Scarecrow Press, 2001], 209).

28. WHO7.0022, Liberia, 1957–1967, JKT 3, SJZ, C. E. Kohler, "Malaria Control Terminal Report 1957," 4.

29. WHO7.0022, Liberia, JKT 1, SJ 3, T. A. Austen to General F. Daubenton, Acting Director, Regional Office for Africa, dated 3 December 1951, from Monrovia, para. 6.

30. NARA, RG469, Liberia Subject Files, Box 3, Liberia Program Reports, Biennial Reports Folder, Annual Report Fiscal Year 1952, Hildrus A. Poindexter, Chief, Public Health Staff, TCA, to Acting Country Director, 5 August 1952, 6–7.

31. WHO7.0022, Liberia, JKT 1, SJ 3, T. A. Austen to General F. Daubenton, Acting Director, Regional Office for Africa, dated 3 December 1951, from Monrovia, para. 6.

32. Ibid., para. 12. For an overview of Americo-Liberians' exploitation of the peoples of the interior, see M. B. Akpan, "Black Imperialism: Americo-Liberian Rule Over the African Peoples of Liberia, 1841–1964," *Canadian Journal of African Studies* 7, no. 2 (1973): 217–36.

For economic evidence of the government's "requisitioning" crops and livestock without compensation and forced labor recruitment, see Robert W. Clower et al., *Growth without Development: An Economic Survey of Liberia* (Evanston, IL: Northwestern University Press, 1966), 17–20.

33. On the transition between an older literature that stressed the economic costs of malaria and an emerging postwar literature that held that malaria control would produce economic development, see Randall M. Packard, "'Roll Back Malaria, Roll in Development?': Reassessing the Economic Burden of Malaria," *Population and Development Review* 35, no. 1 (2009): 53–87.

34. WHO7.0022, Liberia, JKT 2, SJ3, A. Avery-Jones, "General Summary of the Situation of Malaria Project Liberia-5," [1956], 1.

35. Pampana, "Report on my Visit to Liberia."

36. Kohler, "Five Year Malaria Eradication Plan," 2.

The spraying program also covered Tchien in the Eastern Province and Harper in Maryland County. In 1954, 8,493 houses had been treated and 52,716 people had been "protected." NARA, RG469, UD504, Liberia Subject Files, Box 3, Liberia Programs Reports, The Cooperative Liberia–United States Public Health Program (1954), 5.

37. National Library of Medicine, History of Medicine Division, MS C 359, Fred L. Soper Papers, 1919–1975, Visit to Africa [23 November 1959], 32.

38. WHO7.0022, Liberia, JKT 3, SJ 1, "Malaria Control Activities, National Public Health Service—R.L. February 1957. Monthly Report," 1; Kohler, "Malaria Control Terminal Report 1957," 9–10.

39. WHO7.0022, Liberia, JKT 3, SJ 1, "Malaria Control Activities, National Public Health Service—R.L. March 1957, Monthly Report," 2.

40. James L. A. Webb, Jr., "The WHO Pilot Projects in Tropical Africa and the Global Malaria Eradication Program," in *The Global Challenge of Malaria: Past Lessons and Future Prospects,* ed. Frank M. Snowden and Richard Bucala (New York: World Scientific, forthcoming); Matthieu Fintz, "Moustiques et gouvernement du paludisme en Afrique: De la conservation de la nature à l'organisation du marché des biens de lutte," doctoral thesis, Université Robert Schuman—Strasbourg III, 2004.

41. WHO AFR/MAL/17, R. Elliott, "Report on a Consultant Appointment to Project Liberia 16" (1958), 5.

42. Ibid., 6–7, 33.

43. WHO7.0022, Liberia, Dr. P. C. Issaris, "Report on the Joint UNICEF/WHO Malaria Project, Kpain (Liberia) [25 March to 10 May 1957]," 7.

44. WHO AFR/MAL/4, M. E. C. Giglioli, "Report of the Entomologist 1955–1957," 4.

45. WHO7.0022, Liberia, JKT 3, SJ 1, WHO/UNICEF Joint Malaria Project. Kpain, Liberia, Dr. W. Möllhausen to the Regional Director, AFRO, Monthly Report, May 1957, 1.

46. WHO7.0200, JKT 4, SJ 2, M. T. Gillies, "Report on a Travelling Fellowship to Study Malaria Control Problems in West Africa (June–September 1956)," 3.

47. WHO. E/ICEF/309/add.2, 18 February 1956, General Progress Report of Executive Director: Programme Developments in Africa, para. 35.

48. WHO7.0022, Liberia, JKT 3, SJ 1, Dr. K. W. C. Sinclair-Loutit, WHO Medical Advisor, UNICEF-AERO, "Report on a Visit to West Africa [4–11 April 1957]," 3.

49. WHO7.0022, Liberia, JKT 3, SJ 1, Dr. W. Möllhausen, "The Activities of the Malaria Team for the Quarter Jan.–March 1957 (Quarterly Report)," 2.

50. WHO7.0022, Liberia, JKT 3, SJ 1, "Reports on the Haematological Malaria Survey 1956 [2 May 1957]," 1.

51. WHO7.0022, Liberia, JKT 3, SJ 1, Dr. P. C. Issaris, "Brief Report on the Joint UNICEF/WHO Malaria Project. Kpain (Liberia)," 1–2. Dated 22 May 1957.

52. AFR/Mal/8, O. Mastbaum, "Report on the Joint UNICEF/WHO Malaria Project, Kpain (Liberia) [1957]," 3; Guttuso, "Kpain (Liberia) Malaria Project," 4.

53. WHO7.0022, Liberia. Dr. P. C. Issaris, "Report on the Joint UNICEF/WHO Malaria Project, Kpain (Liberia) [25 March to 10 May 1957]," 5.

54. WHO7.0022, Liberia, JKT 3, SJ 1, Dr. P. C. Issaris, "Brief Report on the Joint UNICEF/WHO Malaria Project. Kpain (Liberia) [22 May 1957]," 3.

55. WHO7.0022, Liberia, JKT 3, SJ 1, Liberia-5, TA (LIR-16) UNICEF ICA, Malaria Control Project 2.1.4, 1.

Giglioli got in the last word. As he observed in an official WHO report after he had been posted to Nigeria, "This debacle of the Project is an excellent example of the results of planning scientific work on a basis of political expediency." WHO AFR/MAL/4, M. E. C. Giglioli, "Report of the Entomologist 1955–1957," 4.

56. WHO/MAL/198, C. D. Ramsdale, "Report on a Visit to Liberia for the Testing of Dieldrin-Susceptibility in A. Gambiae (18 October–4 December 1957)," 14.

57. WHO AFR/MAL/61/43, Dr. C. Guttuso, "The Kpain (Liberia) Malaria Project," 30 May 1962, 1.

58. WHO7.0022, Liberia, JKT 3, SJ 2. [n.a.], "Report on the Joint UNICEF/WHO Malaria Project, Kpain (Liberia)," 2.

59. WHO7.0022, Liberia, JKT 3, SJ 4, Republic of Liberia, UNICEF-WHO Malaria Project, Kpain (LIB 16), Second Quarterly Report (July–September 1959), 22.

60. WHO. M2/87/13 + Annex, Report of Meeting of Regional Malaria Advisors from 29 July to 9 August 1959, 56.

61. National Library of Medicine, History of Medicine Division, MS C 359, Fred L. Soper Papers, 1919–1975, Visit to Africa [23 November 1959], 32.

62. WHO7.0022, Liberia, JKT 3, SJ 1, Liberia-5, TA (LIR-16) UNICEF ICA, Malaria Control Project, 3.

63. WHO7.0202, JKT 7, SJ 2, M. A. C. Dowling, "The Use of Mass Drug Administration in Malaria Projects in the African Region [1960]," Technical Meeting on Chemotherapy of Malaria, Working Paper No. 44, 2.

64. WHO7.0022, Liberia, Dr. P. C. Issaris, "Report on the Joint UNICEF/WHO Malaria Project, Kpain (Liberia) [25 March to 10 May 1957]," 9–10.

65. WHO7.0022, Liberia, JKT 3, SJ 1, "Reports on the Haematological Malaria Survey 1956. [2 May 1957]," 2.

66. National Library of Medicine, History of Medicine Division, MS C 359, Fred L. Soper Papers, 1919–1975, Memorandum on Trip to Africa and Geneva, 31 October to 10 December 1959, 2.

Use of Synthetic Insecticide to Control Malaria in Liberia

67. WHO7.0022, Liberia, JKT 3, SJ 4, Dr. L. J. Bruce-Chwatt, "Report on a Visit to Ghana, Liberia, and Gambia (7–23 January 1959)," 12. (Bruce-Chwatt was a leading malariologist who had worked extensively in Nigeria. He was one of the foremost advocates for IRS spraying in tropical Africa to explore the prospects for malaria eradication.)

68. WHO, AFRO/MAL/7, Afro Malaria Year Book No. 2, December 1960, 141.

69. WHO7.0022, Liberia, JKT 3, SJ 4, Dr. R. Marti and Dr. R. Lavoipierre, "Visit to Liberia (18–26 May 1959)," 7.

70. Dr. Fred L. Soper, a physician and epidemiologist who became the director of the Pan-American Sanitary Bureau in 1947, was a leading authority on malaria control as a result of his successful work for the Rockefeller Foundation in Brazil in eradicating an introduced African anopheline species. National Library of Medicine, History of Medicine Division, MS C 359, Fred L. Soper Papers, 1919–1975, Visit to Africa [2 December 1959], 37, 40–41.

By 1959, Dr. Togba had invested many of his energies in business opportunities: a taxi business, trucking business, rubber plantation, mining, and lumbering. Soper judged Togba to be in the millionaire class and to spend more time on his private businesses than on the department (National Library of Medicine, History of Medicine Division, MS C 359, Fred L. Soper Papers, 1919–1975, Visit to Africa [26 November 1959], 33). In 1960, Togba was arrested and imprisoned on charges of embezzling $209,000 in government funds (*Jet,* 17 March 1960, 50).

71. National Library of Medicine, History of Medicine Division, MS C 359, Fred L. Soper Papers, 1919–1975, Visit to Africa [7 November 1959], 15.

72. Guttuso, "Kpain (Liberia) Malaria Project," 5.

73. WHO7.0022, Liberia 1957–1967, JKT III, SJ 5, Dr. C. Guttuso, "Report on a Visit to Liberia, July 1962," 7.

74. WHO, AFRO/MAL/7, Afro Malaria Year Book No. 2 [December 1960], 141.

75. Ibid.

76. Guttuso, "Kpain (Liberia) Malaria Project," 5–9.

77. WHO, AFRO/MAL/7, Afro Malaria Year Book No. 2 [December 1960], 142.

In late 1959, President Tubman allocated $100,000 for the suppression of annoyance mosquitoes in Monrovia during his 1960 presidential inauguration. He went over the heads of his health officials to do so. National Library of Medicine, History of Medicine Division, MS C359, Fred L. Soper Papers, 1919–1975, Visit to Africa, 7 November 1959, 13.

78. In a pilot project in South Cameroon, the WHO did achieve the interruption of malaria transmission in the sprayed zone around Yaoundé; the WHO position was that the interruption of transmission had been "virtually obtained" in the western highlands of Uganda (WHO, AFR/MAL/67, "The Malaria Eradication Programme in the African Region, January 1965, 1–2). For a general overview of the pilot projects, see Webb, "WHO Pilot Projects in Tropical Africa"

79. WHO7.0022, Liberia 1957–1967, JKT III, SJ 5, Dr. C. Guttuso, "Report on a Visit to Liberia, July 1962," 2.

80. WHO7.0022, Liberia, JKT 4, SJ 1. [n.a.], "Assignment Report," Liberia 0033 (Ex-Liberia 20), AFR/Mal/96, AFR/PHA/44, 20 September 1969.

81. WHO7.0022, Liberia, JKT 4, SJ 2, Dr. P. G. Lopez-Tello, "Assignment Report: Basic Health Services (Monrovia)," 1.

82. Small-scale malaria control projects in and around Monrovia flickered on and off for the next decade and a half. See AFR/Mal/152, Dr. Le Du and Mr. V. Ramakrishna, "Malaria Control in Liberia: Report of Missions Carried Out in 1974–1976 by a WHO Consultant Team," and WHO7.0022, Liberia, JKT 4, SJ 3, AFRO-memorandum from Dr. Wilfred S. Boayue to Dr. Comland A. A. Quenum, 29 April 1983.

3 A GENEALOGY OF TREATMENT AS PREVENTION (TASP)

Prevention, Therapy, and the Tensions of Public Health in African History

GUILLAUME LACHENAL

This essay seeks to bring together global health's past and present in Africa. It situates current debates over AIDS "treatment as prevention" in historical perspective, comparing them with previous programs that undertook collective prevention by treating individual carriers of infectious diseases. The chapter traces linkages between distant episodes in Africa's medical history to reinvigorate both historical inquiry into and current critiques of contemporary health policies in Africa.

In the field of HIV-AIDS, "treatment as prevention" (TasP) has been a big story in the past two years. Today a familiar acronym in global health circles, TasP began as an exercise in epidemiological modeling. The question was: Knowing that antiretroviral therapy (ART) drastically reduces HIV transmission, what population-level effect would result from screening and immediately treating *all* HIV-infected individuals? The answer, published in 2009 by WHO expert Reuben Granich in the *Lancet*,[1] was that universal "test and treat" would eliminate HIV by the year 2050; it would prevent new infections and disrupt the epidemic's current dynamics.[2] In other words, *treatment* made universal and extended to newly infected and nonprogressive individuals could serve as collective *prevention*. TasP promised to overcome unending hesitations about whether to prioritize treatment or prevention in resource-limited settings: it would do both. Based on a simulation, the idea immediately inspired "real" studies to test it, including large-scale randomized trials in Africa. TasP became the key feature of all major AIDS conferences in 2009 and 2010.[3] In the context of donor fatigue and general "boredom"[4]—as the French AIDS activist Didier Lestrade put it—TasP reinvigorated hope and excitement. It also marked the return of controversy to the AIDS academy.[5]

Skeptics doubted the model's assumptions, not to mention the ethics and feasibility of implementing TasP in Africa.[6] Some critics observed that HIV carriers in the early phase of infection could escape detection by serological testing, and thus constitute an unknown and contagious population. Others suggested that the very high coverage needed for efficient prevention would require compulsory adherence to treatment, or incite health workers to promote it. Many worried about ART's toxicity, particularly when such drugs were given to healthy, immunocompetent individuals who did not otherwise require treatment. And finally, some critics noted that seeking the "elimination" of HIV would likely distract resources from other preventive approaches, or that this "new" prevention strategy would discredit other preventive measures as "inefficient."[7]

TasP enthusiasts, in contrast, called for a paradigm shift in the fight against AIDS, especially in Africa. This shift would include more aggressive and massive screening policies, new treatment guidelines to include HIV-positive patients with no signs of disease progression, and exceptional efforts from donors, governments, and health workers. With such investment, according to Reuben Granich, it would thus be possible to realize the goal "of relegating HIV to the history books."[8]

What does history have to do with TasP? Strikingly enough, both the promoters and the critics of the TasP strategy invoked references to the history of public health. This is an original feature of these debates. One might have expected the contrary: health experts speaking of the immediate present and future, and historians lamenting their amnesia. But in this case, scientists were not indifferent to history. Among the dozen authors participating in the first debates on TasP, certainly a few resembled AIDS luminary Harold Jaffe,[9] arguing that there was "little precedent for the approach of 'treating for the common good' " or of the ethical dilemmas that TasP posed.[10] Most participants, however, knew the historical classics of public health. At the International AIDS Society (IAS) Conference in July 2010, Reuben Granich began his plenary lecture on "HAART[11] as Prevention" with a slide show about smallpox eradication, showing pictures of Edward Jenner, CDC heroes, WHO posters, and African children lining up for vaccines. Although Granich was careful about using the "e word" (eradication), he evoked specific memories: past predictions of future public health victories. He then compared his own forecast of HIV's future with Thomas Jefferson' prophecy about smallpox: Jefferson "wrote to Jenner

A Genealogy of Treatment as Prevention

in 1806 that 'future generations will know by history only that this loathsome disease has existed.'"[12]

By contrast, TasP critics recalled episodes of public health authoritarianism and hubris. In the *Lancet,* Geoffrey Garnett, for instance, worried that TasP would be an "extremely radical" strategy, "with medical intervention for public health benefits rather than individual patient's benefits." Referring to a magisterial article by the medical historians Dorothy Porter and Roy Porter,[13] he added that "the history of the control of sexually transmitted infections documents several examples of compulsory screening and treatment of stigmatized populations, and there is a danger of a well-meaning paternalistic medical model following such a route."[14] Less polite, but with similar examples in mind, was Georges Sideris from the Parisian gay health group "the Warning." Exasperated by the collectivist and coercive implications of TasP, he queried, "What have we learned from examples of the past about public health policies of STI control?"[15]

History thus served both camps in the "treatment as prevention" controversy. This omnipresence of the past contrasts starkly with AIDS specialists' traditional disregard for the "burden of history," which has shaped the uneven epidemiology of AIDS in African societies and the interpretative framework through which it has been (poorly) understood. Social scientists have rightly criticized the repetitive culturalist, if not racist, reflexes in analyses and control of the African AIDS epidemic, often inherited from colonial medicine. They have lamented the dearth of historical political-economic perspectives that undergird the spread of and response to AIDS.[16] Yet in the case of TasP, history is not absent, but everywhere. It has not been silenced, but instead strategically used.

The chapter thus proposes a *genealogy* of treatment as prevention, reconstructing its contingent trajectory and analyzing critically the ambiguities around treatment as prevention and its historical precursors in Africa's public health history. It engages with contradictory uses of the past, emphasizing that the novel, critical feature of TasP debates is *precisely* the presence of the past—the ambiguous remains (successes, excesses, unfulfilled promises) of twentieth-century public health in Africa. Rather than positioning itself "above" the controversy, offering historical lessons for the present, or using historical insight to resolve ethical dilemmas, the chapter demonstrates that TasP debates evoke unstable categories (prevention versus treatment; individual risks and rights versus population health), whose meanings and relations have been complicated or inversed in African history. In short, it is a historical inquiry into the basic categories and values through which we describe and assess public health in the past and present. In so doing, I follow Mitchell

GUILLAUME LACHENAL

Dean's Foucauldian definition of genealogy as a "a history of the present . . . concerned with that which is taken for granted, assumed to be given, or natural with contemporary social existence, a givenness or naturalness questioned in the course of contemporary struggles"[17] and as a "form of criticism, able to induce critical effects and new insights without grounding itself in a system of values exterior to the domain and object under analysis."[18]

To my knowledge, the expression "treatment as prevention" has never been used before now, and yet many colonial struggles to control infectious diseases in Africa were explicitly framed by this "test and treat" paradigm. Colonial health authorities referred to it as "collective medicine" or "social prophylaxis," but no one thought to explain the dialectic between two contradictory terms—treatment and prevention—because it was so omnipresent and self-evident. This historical analysis reveals constant indecision over what constituted (individual) treatment and (collective) prevention. With few exceptions, these terms were interchangeable in the racialized context of colonial medicine. Although many historians now see a classic tension between the individual and the "common good" as foundational to the history of public health,[19] this opposition and the dilemma between individual interests and public health were far from obvious in colonial Africa. The historical equivalents of "treatment as prevention" were neither problems nor promises, but rather routine methods.

The chapter begins with a brief description of Robert Koch's and his followers' early twentieth-century experimentation with the idea of mass treatment as a prevention in colonial malaria control. It emphasizes several neglected aspects of this intervention, including the role of racial visions and tensions in the "treatment as prevention" paradigm. A second section analyzes the well-known history of sleeping sickness and yaws control in Africa during the interwar period, when health authorities promulgated collective treatment, yet simultaneously theorized and practiced it as "social prophylaxis."

The third part of this essay reveals how a forgotten chapter in the history of sleeping sickness control illustrates further complications in the relationship between treatment and prevention. In the 1950s, French and Belgian colonial health authorities used a new method to control sleeping sickness: prophylactic pentamidine injections to protect healthy individuals against infection. But the chemoprophylactic strategy posed numerous practical and theoretical issues, leading doctors to insist increasingly on its collective, rather than individual, efficacy. In the end, individual prevention functioned as collective treatment. The episode reveals the racial thinking inherent in the social prophylaxis paradigm.

The Colonial Invention of Treatment as Prevention

In the 1920s, mass screening and treatment of carriers of infectious diseases became the favored medical strategy of colonial medical services in their struggles against most infectious diseases, including sleeping sickness, yaws, and syphilis and other venereal diseases. The strategy aimed to reduce the "virus reservoir" collectively constituted by germ carriers, and thus to protect the entire population. For this reason medical services systematically presented it as a preventive, or prophylactic, method.

Medical experts and officials termed this strategy the "Koch method," referring to the epidemiological work of German bacteriologist Robert Koch, who contended that mass screening and treatment of germ carriers, including "healthy carriers," was the key to controlling and eradicating infectious diseases.[20] Classic accounts of the bacteriological revolution single out Koch's 1902 screening campaign against typhoid in Germany as the first experiment of this approach. Koch thus demonstrated that infected but healthy individuals sustained epidemic outbreaks and set mass identification of "healthy carriers" as the new priority for public health.[21] Koch's experiments, first against malaria and then against sleeping sickness in New Guinea and German East Africa illustrate the complex genealogy and internal contradictions of colonial treatment as prevention strategies, and the racial logics underpinning key concepts of "virus reservoir" and "germ carriers."[22]

Robert Koch's work on malaria began in German East Africa in 1897–98, when he showed that therapeutic quinine destroyed the plasmodium parasite found in the blood of individuals with malaria fevers. At a moment when the role of *Anopheles* mosquitoes in malaria transmission was not yet established, this finding led Koch to devise a systematic approach to malaria control, based on a strict bacteriological model: first, to expand microscopic diagnosis of malaria infection in both sick and healthy individuals; second, to treat all plasmodium-infected individuals with repeated doses of quinine; third, to repeat screening and treatment until the entire population was malaria-free. Koch tested his approach in 1900 on seven hundred New Guinea plantation workers and summarized his successful results in a famous address to the British Medical Congress of Eastbourne in 1901.[23] He argued that screening and treating the entire population with quinine was materially and financially feasible; it would wipe out malaria in New Guinea. Koch also mentioned that German colonial doctors in Dar es Salaam (the German East African capital) had begun in 1901 to use his experimental method to fight malaria, having set up laboratories and dispensaries to test and treat the city's entire population.

Historians have documented how quickly the Dar es Salaam scheme failed. Not only was it costly and undesirable to submit a population to repeated blood screening and treatment, but "mobile" germ carriers such as migrant workers also undermined complete coverage of treatment. Historians have also described how the failure of quinine distribution (called "quininisation"[24]) set the foundations for a segregationist approach to malaria control, separating the "native virus reservoir" from European settlements.[25] But they have been less attentive to the fundamental ambiguity of these initial attempts to control malaria in Africa, because some have confused Koch's test-and-treat approach with "chemoprophylaxis."[26]

Although Koch did not explicitly discuss the preventive use of quinine, notably because he aimed to treat *visible* germs, medical practitioners had used "quininisation" as a preventive method even before the emergence of the germ theory of disease. The use of cinchona bark and quinine to "preserve" healthy individuals against malaria predates the understanding of malaria and of quinine's action within the framework of parasitological models established after 1897. Hence Koch's method drew on a well-established use of quinine that was indiscriminately preventive and therapeutic, individual and collective, and not specific to malaria.[27] His work thus simultaneously clarified and complicated understandings and approaches to malaria control. Reinterpreting malaria's decline in Europe as collective consequence of widespread individual quinine use,[28] Koch introduced a crucial displacement: he stated that the *screening and treatment of infected individuals* functioned as *prophylaxis* at the scale of the population. *Treatment was prevention,* for two reasons: because treating individual germ carriers amounted to protecting the whole collective body and because in colonial Africa, reducing the "native reservoir of virus" protected Europeans.

Koch's formulation was complicated by two facts that blurred distinctions between therapy and prevention: first, many assumed a priori that all native populations were chronically infected (which often proved true); and second, prophylactic quinine remained officially recommended for European settlers in Africa, although they rarely followed guidelines. "Quininisation" was a key aspect of malaria control in French Algeria and Indochina during the interwar period, although for French colonial doctors, quininization simultaneously meant preventive quinine use by healthy Europeans, and indiscriminate treatment of supposedly infected natives to "sterilize the virus reservoir."[29] Preventive quinine remained exceptional among colonial subjects, restricted to such groups as soldiers, plantation workers, and schoolchildren. For French doctors, then, the meaning of "la quininisation" was defined along racial lines.

A Genealogy of Treatment as Prevention

The definition of the "test and treat" approach in Koch's malaria studies left a paradoxical legacy. Although malaria specialists remained unconvinced by Koch's grand project, its rationale (and perhaps arrogance) permeated most programs of colonial medicine targeting other diseases. Rarely has a failure been so successful in public health history.[30]

The Test-and-Treat Paradigm in Colonial Africa

Despite its impracticability for malaria, "Koch's method" became the foundation for early twentieth-century French and Belgian programs against sleeping sickness (Human African trypanosomiasis). Koch extended his method to sleeping sickness in German East Africa and Uganda in 1906−7,[31] believing that the German drug atoxyl would simultaneously cure and prevent sleeping sickness.[32] Testing the drug, he proposed a plan to fight the epidemic, attacking the human "reservoir of virus" by screening cases, treating them with atoxyl, and isolating incurable cases. Here again, Koch's master plan never materialized: German East Africa and neighboring British colonies would opt for vector control and mass population resettlements. German colonies Togo and Kamerun implemented his method briefly before Allied nations assumed control in World War I.[33]

Historians have extensively studied interwar initiatives to fight sleeping sickness, an illness perceived as the major threat to colonial demographic and economic development.[34] The French, Belgian, Portuguese, and to a lesser extent British[35] programs were organized as "test-and-treat" schemes, based explicitly on Koch's method. One of most renowned examples was Eugene Jamot's "Mission Permanente de Prophylaxie de la Maladie du Sommeil" in Cameroun.[36] The "Mission Jamot," although described as a "prophylaxis" mission, consisted of screening and treating local populations and segregating incurable cases, in the absence of what we would now call proper "preventive" or "chemoprophylactic" measures. As Jamot himself put it, "The medical prophylaxis of sleeping sickness . . . is closely linked to its treatment."[37] Screening more than 1 million persons per year, Jamot's semiautonomous service became famous for its efficient "mobile teams," which went on rounds to villages with microscopes and syringes to diagnose and treat trypanosome carriers. It inspired equivalents in other French colonies and became the model for French colonial health service reorganization after the Second World War. In 1944, the Brazzaville Conference (a major conference on postwar economic planning and political reforms in French Africa)[38] created the "Services d'hygiène mobile et de prophylaxie" (SHMP). The SHMPs extended the test-and-treat strategy to additional endemic diseases, including leprosy, tuberculosis, syphilis, and yaws, and took charge of smallpox, yellow fever, and tuberculosis (BCG) vaccination. The SHMPs received considerable funding, mobilized most of the colonial medical staff, and exemplified the primacy of "prevention," other individual care, and mobile teams over "fixed" networks of dispensaries and hospitals. For tens of millions of African subjects, then, "prophylaxis" meant compulsory treatment.[39]

Belgian and British colonies implemented similar programs emphasizing "social prophylaxis" in the interwar period. In addition to sleeping sickness programs, authorities in Kenya, Uganda, Ruanda-Urundi, and the Belgian Congo launched intensive campaigns against yaws (a nonvenereal treponematose) to screen cases and treat with bismuth and arsenical salts injections.[40] This yaws test-and-treat approach, largely influenced by the sleeping sickness programs, expanded after 1945 with penicillin use and became the one of the first major WHO eradication programs.[41] Colonial test-and-treat programs also targeted tuberculosis, syphilis, and leprosy, although they rarely opted for active screening and treatment.[42]

Colonial test-and-treat programs had no equivalent in Europe, where the approach was limited to controllable and disciplined communities. Even large-scale international health programs, including the hookworm campaigns in America and Asia,[43] could not match the scale and influence of colonial African schemes against sleeping sickness or yaws.

Although colonial test-and-treat programs differed in scale and goal, they shared several principles and problems inherent in colonial "treatment as prevention." First, they were *exceptional* operations, largely independent of "normal" health services. Focusing on a single disease, they functioned with special funds and staff. They relied on specific "wonder drugs," such as atoxyl, tryparsamide, and Bayer 205 (Germanin) for sleeping sickness, and neo-salvarsan and stovarsol, Novarsénobillon (NAB) for yaws and syphilis.[44] Charismatic leaders—Eugène Jamot in French Central Africa, Vittorio Pratti in Ruanda-Urundi, John Gilks in Kenya, for instance—embodied the programs and made prophecies of eradication that appealed to a metropolitan public. The programs also inspired specific professional cultures and ethos.[45] They gained exceptional status, with ad hoc laws that enabled coercive measures to assemble and treat colonial populations. Interwar period French and Belgian programs against sleeping sickness offered spectacular examples of "exceptionalism," for their administrative and financial autonomy enhanced their efficacy but provoked conflict with other health services, other colonial state agencies, and such actors as missionaries and traders. Such conflicts accelerated their dismantlement or reintegration in the general health care system.[46]

Second, these programs exemplified "collective medicine," not simply because they relied on standard, "taylorized" procedures to simultaneously screen and treat hundreds of patients, but also because authorities conceived and evaluated them at the level of the "collective body." They organized the campaigns to treat "populations"—termed "races," "tribes," or "ethnies"—understood as geographic, biological, and social entities. In keeping with colonial administration from the early twentieth century, health authorities confounded people with places, using toponyms/ethnonyms to name both the population and epidemic "focus." Their main objective, moreover, was demographic progress, to be achieved through eradication. What mattered was, as Eugène Jamot put it, to "save the black race" for humanitarian and economic reasons.[47] Authorities thus evaluated the programs' costs and successes at the population scale: total numbers had to rise, and "contamination indexes" had to fall.

Third, because the first, crucial step of these programs was to screen for carriers, they were caught in endless discussions about complete population coverage and diagnostic reliability.[48] Finding and treating *all* carriers necessitated the use of force and the development of elaborate diagnostic procedures. These were the heaviest aspects of the campaign—quite literally, since "mobile laboratories" had to be transported by porters. They routinely involved such invasive procedures as lumbar punctures to detect sleeping sickness infection of the nervous system, or systematic genital examination of women for yaws control.[49] The need to treat the entire "human reservoir" and to produce a "preventive effect" at the level of the population justified these costs and risks of diagnosis.

The low reliability of diagnostic procedures and insistence on complete coverage frequently meant that some individuals were over-treated. Medical workers considered certain patients to be "trypanosomés" based solely on their clinical presentation and subjected them to years of repeated injections, exposing them to iatrogenic infections and problems related to drug toxicity. Some presumed cases were confined to closed camps without evidence of actual infection or of response to treatment.[50] Colonial doctors zealously justified treating every suspected case on the presumption that untreated infection led to death, although a rare few noted the existence of mild forms of sleeping sickness and that systematic treatment of suspect cases would never be acceptable to European patients.[51] They considered terrible therapeutic accidents to be "side effects" of the "noble aim" of eradication. Among the worst cases included the 1930 Bafia accident, when a medical team of the Mission Jamot experimented with a new dosage of the drug tryparsamide, provoking permanent blindness in hundreds of patients, and the anti-yaws campaigns in Ruanda-Urundi (1931–33) that resulted in 113 deaths.[52] The massive scale of the campaigns prompted drastic cost-saving measures (including staff cuts and cheaper, more toxic drugs) and clearly aggravated death tolls.[53]

Conversely, low sensitivity of certain diagnostic procedures enabled many infected persons to escape early detection; only later were such individuals found to be infected, which complicated collective prevention and individual cure. As early as 1930, some observers thought that sleeping sickness screening missed 17–50 percent of cases.[54] Confusion over diseases and pathogens, particularly in the case of nonvenereal (yaws) and venereal (syphilis) treponematoses, rendered screening an even murkier process. It led colonial officers and missionaries to overemphasize the role of sexuality in spreading so-called "venereal" diseases.[55] Effective biomedical control of yaws may have actually favored the spread of syphilis, by suppressing cross-immunity to sexually transmitted treponemas.[56]

Medical authorities sometimes proposed "indiscriminate treatment" (treating *everyone* with a standard cure) to counteract the diagnostic difficulties in sleeping sickness and yaws campaigns. High infection indexes, the need to treat all "contacts" and "cases" (potentially everyone in a high prevalence area), and the cost, inaccessibility, or unreliability of tests justified this approach.[57] Although it could expose healthy patients to invasive and toxic medical procedures, it also achieved some successes: the WHO in 1955 adopted indiscriminate mass treatment of yaws with efficient, relatively safe, long-acting intramuscular penicillin (PAM), a strategy that brought about the epidemic's rapid decline.[58]

But treatments could be imperfect. Even when drugs were relatively efficient, the organization of the campaigns offered few possibilities to follow up on secondary effects, therapeutic failures, and relapses. Treatment protocols typically consisted of a series of injections with arsenical drugs, administrated by mobile teams of nurses who regularly visited villages (for instance, once a week for ten weeks). Individualizing treatment schemes for yaws and sleeping sickness patients was difficult, and health services simply opted for a "standard cure" regardless of individual clinical status. Metropolitan specialists roundly criticized this practice, and heated debates erupted between "bush doctors" (who favored standard cures) and "armchair trypanologists" (who sought individualized treatment).[59]

Treatments often did not seek to cure, but rather to make the most visible disease symptoms disappear and, most important, to render patients noncontagious.[60] Medical authorities used such terms as "sterilization" or "*blanchiment*" to refer to this partial therapy, pragmatically adopted because it required fewer injections than a complete cure and would achieve the same "preventive effect" of reducing transmission to zero.[61] But it could also provoke increased drug resistance. Yaws treatment protocols offering a single injection, for instance, actually promoted relapses of more advanced, severe forms, which reached epidemic proportions in Kenya.[62] So long as the number of infectious cases declined, authorities did not consider this approach problematic.[63]

Health authorities rarely addressed the many weaknesses of the test-and-treat paradigm. Declining infection indexes suggested that eradication was within reach, and thus the rationale of "treatment as prevention" could accommodate therapeutic accidents, iatrogenic infections, inefficient drugs, incomplete cures and undetected infections.

Prevention as Treatment as Prevention: The Forgotten History of Pentamidine Prophylaxis

After 1945, the social prophylaxis paradigm was pushed to its limits—in both senses that it took an unprecedented scale and that it was more and more contested. Health authorities transformed and extended these test-and-treat programs in response to several developments. New "wonder drugs," including antibiotics, raised new hopes of eradication.[64] Health services and infrastructures received unprecedented funding, the fruits of new imperial development policies.[65] Transportation infrastructures and technologies also opened new possibilities for mobile medicine, ushering in the era of Land Rover public health.

Pentamidine's role in redefining sleeping sickness control after 1945 resembles many "prophylactic" programs of this period and illustrates how an unreflective adherence to the test-and-treat paradigm and to eradication blinded authorities to the drug's efficiency and safety. Discovered prior to World War II, pentamidine belonged to a new family of drugs, the diamidines. It was rapidly identified as an excellent treatment for early-stage sleeping sickness, and subsequently marketed by the British firm May&Baker as Pentamidine®, and by the French firm Spécia as Lomidine®. In the Belgian Congo, where chemoprophylaxis for sleeping sickness was well established, colonial doctors also found that pentamidine had *preventive* effects (sensu stricto).[66] Belgian authorities organized a trial testing the efficiency of preventive pentamidine in the Kwango District, a "heavily infected focus." Mobile teams recruited

GUILLAUME LACHENAL

more than nine hundred uninfected people, two-thirds of whom received one injection of pentamidine, and a third served as a control. Six months later, seven new sleeping sickness cases, all from the uninjected control group, were identified.[67] The study thus concluded "that . . . a single dose of [pentamidine] injected in the muscles protects the healthy individual for at least 6 months."[68]

From 1945, medical campaigns routinely used this method in the Congo, Nigeria, AEF, and Cameroon. A comparison of initial results some three years later concluded that administering pentamidine injections to an entire population of infected areas (*"lomidinisation"* or *"pentamidinisation totale"*) promised a rapid eradication of sleeping sickness. From 1945 to 1960, medical workers administered more than 10 million injections to healthy subjects, mostly in the French, Belgian, and Portuguese colonies of West and Central Africa.[69] Pentamidinization campaigns, combined with classic test-and-treat campaigns for sleeping sickness patients, coincided with a massive decline of the epidemic. From 1952, authorities repeatedly heralded the imminent eradication of sleeping sickness.[70]

Although medical authorities officially presented pentamidine as a chemo-prophylactic drug, several problems led experts to describe it with increasing ambiguity as a form of "collective prophylaxis," which above all protected the "group," "race," or "population" from new infection. Experts could not identify the biological mechanism that explained the drug's apparent effects.[71] Pentamidine appeared effective for more than one year, but this duration was inconsistent with the drug's pharmacokinetics. Reports of individual failures, in which subjects received treatment but were found to be infected a year later, also surfaced.[72] Rather than questioning the drug's efficacy, experts surmised that these infected subjects had managed to evade injection after their registration with the medical team; individual indiscipline thus explained individual failures. Others suggested that pentamidinization had not been applied with sufficient intensity or geographical extent. In response, French and Belgian doctors proposed scaling up these collective campaigns, by applying the same measures in unaffected "buffer zones."[73]

Pentamidine injections also caused significant side effects, inducing hypo-glycemia, hypotension (leading to nausea and collapse), pain, and edema. Because injections were given serially to several hundred people, the risks of error and contamination increased. Fatalities sometimes resulted. In 1953, for instance, Spécia, conducting an investigation in Cameroon to identify causes of fainting, concluded that it occurred where African subjects were known to be "little inclined to discipline."[74] Again, individual indiscipline—not the drug

A Genealogy of Treatment as Prevention

itself—was to blame; accidents even seemed to reinforce doctors' trust in the drug.[75] Post-injection gangrenes constituted a further concern. Mobile teams used the cheaper bulk powder of pentamidine, mixing it with running (but not sterile) water, instead of purchasing more expensive solutions prepared under sterile conditions. Yet rather than incriminating unsterile drug preparation, official interpretations instead blamed the victims for their gangrene, accusing them of rubbing earth or other preparations on their injection sites.[76]

In retrospect, the apparent preventive effects of pentamidine during the first trials raise some questions. Pentamidine's efficiency as chemoprophylaxis had been tested on the *individual* scale only once. Two "voluntary Congolese natives" received a single dose of pentamidine and were subjected daily to tsetse bites in 1941–42. The authors concluded that because they found trypanosomes in the subjects' blood only a few months later, this was proof of pentamidine's preventive powers. At the time, some experts observed that the trial design was weak, for it included no controls and only two cases.[77] But the debates ended before they even began: by the time the trial was published, the community-scaled trials in the Kwango district had demonstrated the success of preventive pentamidine.

Interpretations of these crucial experiments reveal that community constituted the only relevant scale on which to evaluate pentamidinization. This emphasis on collective health potentially contradicted the definition of chemoprophylaxis,[78] but at the time, this contradiction was not seen as problematic. The colonial medical profession unswervingly embraced the social prophylaxis approach.

The collective rationale of pentamidine prophylaxis had one racialized exception: authorities contended that pentamidinization of Europeans was inefficient and too risky and would potentially mask the disease's early development and complicate its treatment. Europeans thus benefited from an evaluation of their risks and rights at the individual scale, and medical authorities took considerable precautions (including written consent) when they gave Europeans the injections. Meanwhile, for "the health of their race" and the sake of eradication, Africans had to submit to compulsory pentamidinization. Those who protested or avoided the injections were criminalized as "individualistic."

Pentamidinization ceased in the 1960s for several reasons. Colonial medical services were dismantled, and sleeping sickness in most African countries nearly disappeared. The method proved highly unpopular among African populations. More generally, nationalist movements and the emergence of an African middle class ushered in a "liberal" critique of colonial public health and rejected its authoritarian and collectivist methods.

It now appears that pentamidinization did not prevent *individual* infection. Subsequent analysts reevaluated the campaigns' early successes of the late 1940s as the collective effect of indiscriminate treatment of *undiagnosed* parasite carriers. Mobile screening teams had missed up to 50 percent of trypanosome carriers, and subsequently treated them.[79] A single injection treatment could neither cure undiagnosed patients nor "protect" healthy patients for more than a few days, but it did interrupt transmission at the collective scale.[80] Pentamidinization therefore worked, but not as expected. As an involuntary indiscriminate treatment whose ethics went completely unexplored, it functioned as a classic treatment as prevention strategy. It was prevention as treatment as prevention.

❖

This brief genealogy of the current AIDS "treatment as prevention" efforts has two aims. The first is heuristic; it retraces the historical definitions and displacements of prevention and treatment in struggles against infectious diseases in African history. From quinine to pentamidine, a constant ambiguity prevailed between individual prophylaxis and collective prevention through "test-and-treat" strategies. Both experts at the time and present-day historians have never recognized this ambiguity. Yet it did not preclude that most of these programs were efficient, or at least that they fulfilled their self-defined aim: disease regression at the population scale. Race, both as the name of the "population" in the African colonial context, and as an operator of distinction between categories of humanity, gave its theoretical and ethical coherence to the "social prophylaxis" paradigm—what counted the most was to protect African collectives, or, in certain cases, European individuals. In this light, I find it useful to project back in the past the contemporary expression "treatment as prevention," as it captures the essentially shifting relationship between the two categories. Historically, the "as" in treatment as prevention could point to a series of gray zones and equivalences, ranging from "true" individual chemoprophylaxis (the quininization of Europeans) to indiscriminate mass treatments ("test and treat" for yaws . . . without testing), from "false chemoprophylaxis" (pentamidinization) to true "social prophylaxis" (the "méthode Jamot" against sleeping sickness).

The second aim of this work is critical. As several AIDS experts and activists have already noted, previous episodes of "test and treat" in this chapter are disquieting, particularly when the first large-scale TasP trials are now under way in Africa. Technically, over-treatment, under-diagnosis, undetectable carriers, drug resistance, migration, unforeseen accidents, and the fatigue of populations and governments have been continual sources of difficulty; TasP for HIV may potentially raise similar problems. More fundamentally, the lesson of the colonial history of public health is one of the danger of hubris, biomedical messianism, and prophetic announcements of eradication. Great ambitions and technological confidence "justified" arrangements with rationality and ethics, and generally ended in failure, if not catastrophe. Significantly, TasP enthusiasts' favorite historical reference, smallpox eradication through vaccination, appears to be an exception (and a problematic one)[81] in the landscape of test-and-treat schemes with diminished outcomes, at least when compared to their initial objectives. Retrospectively, it remains possible that the clearest colonial public health successes (such as the near elimination of yaws and sleeping sickness by 1960) resulted as much from "test-and-treat" schemes as from wider ecological and economic changes.[82] This is yet another lesson to keep in mind, particularly when TasP and other biomedical approaches to prevention may discredit or siphon off resources from wider social and political interventions.

Finally, I want to focus attention on the relationship between past and present that characterizes this "global health" moment in Africa. It is neither one of "continuity" (as in "clinical trials of TasP replicate colonial medicine") nor of "rupture" (as in "ethics committees and human rights now protect Africans from the excesses of the past"). Rather, it is about the politics of remembering (and forgetting). Test-and-treat schemes were founded on fragile theories, hubristic hopes, naïve faith in wonder drugs, and racial and colonial paternalism, all of which will sound familiar to many global health practitioners who are aware of public health history. Surprisingly, their knowledge of this history coexists with the hype for biomedical solutions to HIV prevention, as if remembering failures and promising miracles is not contradictory. Although TasP trials may well be successful, eliminating HIV through generalized TasP will not occur in 2050 in any "real" world. And while many recognize this reality, they nevertheless feel compelled to promise it. In contrast to mid-twentieth-century optimism, our global health present may be characterized by this strange way of telling stories of future redemption in which one only *pretends* to believe.[83]

Notes

1. R. M. Granich et al., "Universal Voluntary HIV Testing with Immediate Antiretroviral Therapy as a Strategy for Elimination of HIV Transmission: A Mathematical Model," *Lancet* 373, no. 9657 (2009): 48–57.

2. The announcement was made, for example, at the International AIDS Society Conference in Cape Town. Reuben Granich, "HAART as Prevention," plenary

GUILLAUME LACHENAL

session conference (20 July 2009), consulted 12 April 2011, http://www.ias2009.org/pag/PSession.aspx?s=2365#2.

3. For press coverage of these debates, see J. Cohen, "17th Conference on Retroviruses and Opportunistic Infections, 16–19 February, San Francisco, Ca. Treatment as Prevention," *Science* 327, no. 5970 (2010): 1196–97; Gilles Pialoux, "Casablanca 2010: Le traitement comme prévention au coeur des débats," Vih.org, consulted 25 February 2011, http://www.vih.org/20100329/casablanca-2010-traitement-comme-prevention-au-coeur-debats-13356.

4. See his contribution on TasP and the gay community on the website Minorités. Didier Lestrade, "Aux armes les folles," consulted 9 September 2010, http://www.minorites.org/index.php/2-la-revue/833-aux-armes-les-folles.html.

5. Here, "AIDS academy" refers to the large and multidisciplinary scientific field formed by AIDS specialists.

6. The *Lancet* invited several responses to Granich et al.'s publication: D. P. Wilson, "Universal Voluntary HIV Testing and Immediate Antiretroviral Therapy," *Lancet* 373, no. 9669 (2009): 1077–78; A. Ruark et al., "Universal Voluntary Hiv Testing and Immediate Antiretroviral Therapy," *Lancet* 373, no. 9669 (2009): 1078; R. Jurgens et al., "Universal Voluntary HIV Testing and Immediate Antiretroviral Therapy," *Lancet* 373, no. 9669 (2009): 1079; H. Jaffe, A. Smith, and T. Hope, "Universal Voluntary HIV Testing and Immediate Antiretroviral Therapy," *Lancet* 373, no. 9669 (2009): 1080; Y. H. Hsieh and H. de Arazoza, "Universal Voluntary HIV Testing and Immediate Antiretroviral Therapy," *Lancet* 373, no. 9669 (2009): 1079–80; G. P. Garnett and R. F. Baggaley, "Treating Our Way out of the HIV Pandemic: Could We, Would We, Should We?" *Lancet* 373, no. 9657 (2009): 9–11; H. Epstein, "Universal Voluntary HIV Testing and Immediate Antiretroviral Therapy," *Lancet* 373, no. 9669 (2009): 1078–79; M. S. Cohen, T. D. Mastro, and W. Cates, Jr., "Universal Voluntary HIV Testing and Immediate Antiretroviral Therapy," *Lancet* 373, no. 9669 (2009): 1077; Y. Assefa and M. Lera, "Universal Voluntary HIV Testing and Immediate Antiretroviral Therapy," *Lancet* 373, no. 9669 (2009): 1080.

7. See V. K. Nguyen et al., "Remedicalizing an Epidemic: From HIV Treatment as Prevention to HIV Treatment as Prevention," *AIDS* 25, no. 3 (2011): 291–93.

8. R. Granich, "HAART as Prevention," at Fifth IAS Conference on HIV Pathogenesis, Treatment and Prevention, 21 July 2009 (Cape Town, South Africa, 2009).

9. Harold Jaffe took part in the CDC task force that established the epidemiology of AIDS in 1982–83 and was a major figure in the book and movie, *And the Band Played On*. See Randy Shilts, *And the Band Played On: Politics, People, and the AIDS Epidemic* (New York: St. Martin's Press, 1987).

10. Jaffe, Smith, and Hope, "Universal Voluntary," 1080.

11. Highly active antiretroviral treatment.

12. Granich, "HAART as Prevention."

13. Roy Porter and Dorothy Porter, "The Enforcement of Health: The British Debate," in *AIDS: The Burdens of History,* ed. Elizabeth Fee and Daniel M. Fox (Berkeley: University of California Press, 1988), 97–116.

14. Garnett and Baggaley, "Treating Our Way," 11.

A Genealogy of Treatment as Prevention

15. *"Bref, qu'avons-nous retenu des exemples du passé vis-à-vis des politiques de santé publique à l'égard d'infections sexuellement transmissibles comme la syphilis?"* Georges Sideris, "Ethique et santé: L'idée d'éradiquer l'épidémie de VIH en mettant sous traitement antirétroviral toutes les personnes nouvellement dépistées et l'ensemble des séropositifs pose question," *Warning* (25 August 2010), consulted 12 November 2010, http://www.thewarning.info/spip.php?article311.

16. Jean-Pierre Dozon and Didier Fassin, "Raison épidémiologique et raisons d'etat: Les enjeux socio-politiques du sida en Afrique," *Sciences sociales et santé* 7, no. 1 (1989): 21–36; Randall M. Packard and Paul Epstein, "Epidemiologists, Social Scientists, and the Structure of Medical Research on AIDS in Africa," *Social Science and Medicine* 33, no. 7 (1991): 771–83; Didier Fassin, *When Bodies Remember: Experiences and Politics of AIDS in South Africa* (Berkeley: University of California Press, 2007).

17. Mitchell Dean, *Critical and Effective Histories Foucault's Methods and Historical Sociology* (London: Routledge, 1994), 35.

18. Ibid. For Foucault's main discussion of "genealogy," see Michel Foucault, "Nietzsche, la généalogie, l'histoire," in *Hommage à Jean Hyppolite,* ed. Collectif (Paris: PUF, 1971). See also Judith Revel, *Foucault, une pensée du discontinu,* Essais (Paris: Mille et une nuits, 2010).

19. From a European perspective, this claim may be true. See Porter and Porter, "Enforcement of Health," 97–98.

20. "Koch's method" stood in opposition to environmental interventions or vector control (e.g., "Ross's method").

21. Christoph Gradmann has recently revised this view, showing how Koch had earlier tested the concept of the carrier state and the "screening campaign" during his travels in colonial Africa and the Pacific. Christoph Gradmann, "Robert Koch and the Invention of the Carrier State: Tropical Medicine, Veterinary Infections and Epidemiology around 1900," *Studies in History and Philosophy of Biological and Biomedical Sciences* 41, no. 3 (2010): 232–40.

22. These key concepts were imported from veterinary medicine. James L. A. Webb, Jr., *Humanity's Burden: A Global History of Malaria* (Cambridge: Cambridge University Press, 2009), 133–36.

23. Robert Koch, "Address on Malaria to the Congress at Eastbourne," *Journal of State Medicine,* no. 10 (1901); Wolfgang U. Eckart, *Medizin und Kolonialimperialismus: Deutschland 1884–1945* (Paderborn: F. Schöningh, 1997), 401–9.

24. In German: "Chinisierung."

25. Webb, *Humanity's Burden,* 134–35; Wolfgang U. Eckart, "Malaria and Colonialism in the German Colonies New Guinea and the Cameroons: Research, Control, Thoughts of Eradication," *Parassitologia* 40, no. 1–2 (1998): 83–90; Ann Beck, "Medicine and Society in Tanganyika, 1890–1930: A Historical Inquiry," *Transactions of the American Philosophical Society* 67, no. 3 (1977): 1–59.

26. For an example of an ambiguous use of "prophylaxis," see Beck, "Medicine," 16.

27. Webb, *Humanity's Burden,* 127–28, 135.

28. Koch, "Address on Malaria to the Congress at Eastbourne."

29. See E. Collignon, "Sur le cout de la quinisation des réservoirs de virus paludéen en Algérie," *Bulletin de la Société de pathologie exotique* 29 (1936): 1090–93;

Edmond Sergent, "La quininisation en Algérie," *Bulletin de la Société de pathologie exotique* 1 (1908): 534–36.

30. Since then, the results and understandings of malaria chemoprophylaxis and mass treatment schemes have not helped to clarify the picture. A new approach to malaria control, "Intermittent Preventive Therapy" (note the resemblance with TasP), is based on the "blind" and repeated distribution of antimalarial treatments to pregnant women or infants (without prior testing) and has proven extraordinarily successful; its mechanism remains, to use its promoters' euphemism, "intriguing." D. Schellenberg et al., "Intermittent Preventive Antimalarial Treatment for Tanzanian Infants: Follow-up to Age 2 Years of a Randomised, Placebo-Controlled Trial," *Lancet* 365, no. 9469 (2005): 1482.

31. R. Koch, M. Beck, and F. Kleine, *Bericht über die Tätigkeit der zur Erforschung der Schlafkrankheit im Jahre 1906/07 nach Ostafrika entsandten Kommission* (Berlin: J. Springer, 1909).

32. Wolfgang U. Eckart, "The Colony as Laboratory: German Sleeping Sickness Campaigns in German East Africa and in Togo, 1900–1914," *History and Philosophy of the Life Sciences* 24, no. 1 (2002): 68–89.

33. Eckart, *Medizin;* Michael Worboys, "The Comparative History of Sleeping Sickness in East and Central Africa, 1900–1914," *History of Science* 32, no. 1=95 (1994): 89–102.

34. Jean-Pierre Dozon, "Quand les pastoriens traquaient la maladie du sommeil," *Sciences sociales et santé* 3, no. 3–4 (1985): 27–56; Maryinez Lyons, *The Colonial Disease: A Social History of Sleeping Sickness in Northern Zaire, 1900–1940* (Cambridge: Cambridge University Press, 1992); Jean-Paul Bado, *Les grandes endémies en Afrique, 1900–1960: Lèpre, Trypanosomiase humaine et onchocerchose* (Paris: Karthala, 1996); Heather Bell, *Frontiers of Medicine in the Anglo-Egyptian Sudan, 1899–1940* (Oxford: Oxford University Press, 1999); Rita Headrick, *Colonialism, Health and Illness in French Equatorial Africa, 1885–1935,* ed. Daniel Headrick (Atlanta: African Studies Association Press, 1994); Worboys, "Comparative History."

35. The British colonial health services' preference for vector-control and population resettlements partly resulted from the etiology of the East African sleeping sickness epidemic, *T. rhodesiense,* a different species of trypanosome, with an animal reservoir in wild game. Mass treatment of human beings was therefore insufficient. Kirk Arden Hoppe, *Lords of the Fly: Sleeping Sickness Control in British East Africa, 1900–1960* (Westport, CT: Praeger, 2003).

36. On the Mission Jamot, see Guillaume Lachenal and Bertrand Taithe, "Une généalogie missionnaire et coloniale de l'humanitaire: Le cas Aujoulat au Cameroun, 1935–1973," *Le mouvement social* 227, no. 1 (2009): 45–63; Marcel (Dr) Bebey-Eyidi, *Le vainqueur de la maladie du sommeil: Le docteur Eugène Jamot, 1879–1937* (Paris: L'auteur, 1951); Alain Froment, "Le docteur Jamot, sa vocation africaine, et l'épidémiologie," *Bulletin de liaison et de documentation de l'OCEAC* 85 (1988): 23–25; Blandine Gomart-Jacquet, "[Le] docteur Eugène Jamot et la maladie du sommeil, 1910–1937" (Thèse de doctorat nouveau régime, Université de Provence, 1995); Jean-Marie Milleliri, "Jamot, cet inconnu," *Bulletin de la Société de pathologie exotique* 94, no. 3 (2004): 214–18; Bertrand Taithe, "La trypanosomiase et l'expédition Jamot:

A Genealogy of Treatment as Prevention

Les pouvoirs ambigus de la prophylaxie militante," *Le concours médical* 130, no. 11 (2008): 558–59.

37. Quoted in Jean-Paul Bado, *Eugène Jamot, 1879–1937: Le médecin de la maladie du sommeil ou trypanosomiase* (Paris: Karthala, 2011), 71.

38. On health planning at the Brazzaville conference, see Danielle Domergue Cloarec, "Les problèmes de santé à la conférence de Brazzaville," in *Brazzaville, Janvier–Février 1944: Aux sources de la décolonisation*, ed. Institut Charles de Gaulle and Institut d'histoire du temps présent (France) (Paris: Plon, 1988), 157–69; more generally, Frederick Cooper, *Decolonization and African Society: The Labor Question in French and British Africa* (Cambridge: Cambridge University Press, 1996), 177–83.

39. See Guillaume Lachenal, "Biomédecine et décolonisation au Cameroun, 1944–1994: Technologies, figures et institutions médicales à l'épreuve" (Thèse de doctorat en epistémologie, histoire des sciences et des techniques, Université Paris 7 Denis-Diderot, 2006).

40. Anne Cornet, "Politiques sanitaires, état et missions religieuses au Rwanda (1920–1940): Une conception autoritaire de la médecine coloniale?" *Studium* 2, no. 2 (2009): 105–15; Mark Dawson, "The 1920s Anti-Yaws Campaigns and Colonial Medical Policy in Kenya," *International Journal of African Historical Studies* 20, no. 3 (1987): 417–35.

41. G. E. Samame, "Treponematosis Eradication, with Special Reference to Yaws Eradication in Haiti," *Bulletin of the World Health Organization* 15, no. 6 (1956): 897–910; C. J. Hackett, "Consolidation Phase of Yaws Control: Experiences in Africa," *Bulletin of the World Health Organization* 8, no. 1–3 (1953): 297–343.

42. The tuberculosis program focused on vaccination, syphilis on passive detection and therapy at dispensaries, and leprosy on segregation of cases and vector control.

43. Steven Palmer, "Migrant Clinics and Hookworm Science: Peripheral Origins of International Health, 1840–1920," *Bulletin of the History of Medicine* 83, no. 4 (2009): 676–709.

44. The programs frequently followed the discovery of these drugs.

45. L. Lapeyssonnie, *La médecine coloniale: Mythe et réalités* (Paris: Seghers, 1984).

46. Dozon, "Les pastoriens"; Bado, *Grandes endémies*.

47. See Alice L. Conklin, *A Mission to Civilize: The Republican Idea of Empire in France and West Africa, 1895–1930* (Stanford, Calif.: Stanford University Press, 1997), chap. 2.

48. Belgian doctors diagnosed exclusively based on clinical aspects (lymph node palpation); French physicians criticized this practice. On their debates, see P. G. Janssens, "Eugène Jamot et Emile Lejeune: Pages d'histoire," *Annales de la Société belge de médecine tropicale* 75, no. 1 (1995): 1–12; Headrick, *Colonialism,* 315–18.

49. Cornet, "Politiques sanitaires."

50. A work by French colonial doctors found that only one in six or seven "clinical suspects" were actually infected. Maurice Blanchard and G. Lefrou, "Résultats des plus récentes recherches faites à l'Institut Pasteur de Brazzaville sur le diagnostic et la prophylaxie de la maladie du sommeil," *Revista medical de Angola* 4 (1923), cited in Headrick, *Colonialism,* 317. On internment and repeated treatment of "suspects" without evidence of trypanosome infection, see G. Neujean and F. Evens, *Diagnostic et traitement*

de la maladie du sommeil à T. gambiense: Bilan de dix ans d'activité du centre de traitement de Léopoldville (Gembloux: Duculot, 1958).

51. H. Lester, "Further Progress in the Control of Sleeping Sickness in Nigeria," *Transactions of the Royal Society of Tropical Medicine and Hygiene* 38, no. 6 (1945): 425–44.

52. The most complete account of the Bafia accident is Gomart-Jacquet, "Eugène Jamot"; Cornet, "Politiques sanitaires," 109.

53. In Kenya, financial difficulties led to the use of more dangerous bismuth salts, instead of arsenicals. Dawson, "Anti-Yaws Campaigns," 427.

54. Marcel Vaucel, "Les acquisitions nouvelles dans l'étude des trypanosomiases," *Annales de médecine et de pharmacie coloniales*, no. 31 (1933): 40.

55. Megan Vaughan, "Syphilis in Colonial East and Central Africa: The Social Construction of an Epidemic," in *Epidemics and Ideas: Essays on the Historical Perception of Pestilence*, ed. Terence Ranger and Paul Slack (Cambridge: Cambridge University Press, 1992).

56. Dawson, "Anti-Yaws Campaigns," 433–34.

57. For example of shortages of diagnostic equipment, see Bado, *Grandes endémies*, 269.

58. On yaws eradication and indiscriminant mass treatment in Haiti, see David McBride, *Missions for Science: U.S. Technology and Medicine in America's African World* (New Brunswick, NJ: Rutgers University Press, 2002).

59. See G. Muraz, "A propos de la "cure-standard" appliquée: En Afrique Equatoriale Française, aux trypanosomés," *Bulletin de la Société de pathologie exotique et de ses filiales* 23 (1930): 917–22; G. Muraz, "Le traitement standard de la maladie du sommeil," *Bulletin de la Société de pathologie exotique et de ses filiales* 24, no. 7 (1931): 530–34; G. Muraz, "Quelques derniers mots au sujet de la "cure standard" de la maladie du sommeil," *Bulletin de la Société de pathologie exotique et de ses filiales* 25, no. 1 (1932): 39–43.

60. Dawson, "Anti-Yaws Campaigns," 420.

61. In Europe, the widely used term "*blanchiment*" had acquired the same meaning since the late nineteenth century for syphilis.

62. Dawson, "Anti-Yaws Campaigns," 433.

63. Ibid., 430.

64. Penicillin could be used to treat yaws, syphilis, and other venereal diseases; streptomycin for tuberculosis; sulfones for leprosy; and pentamidine for sleeping sickness.

65. Cooper, *Decolonization;* Frederick Cooper, *Africa since 1940: The Past of the Present* (Cambridge: Cambridge University Press, 2003).

66. From the late 1920s, Belgian mobile teams extensively used *preventive* injections of Bayer 205, although neither the British nor the French believed that "Bayerisation" was safe or efficient. See H. L. Duke, "On the Prophylactic Action of 'Bayer 205' against the Trypanosoma of Man," *Lancet* 227, no. 5870 (originally published as vol. 1, no. 5870) (1936): 463–69.

67. L. Van Hoof, C. Henrard, and E. Peel, "Pentamidine in the Prevention and Treatment of Trypanosomiasis," *Transactions of the Royal Society of Tropical Medicine and Hygiene* 37, no. 4 (1944): 271–80.

68. L. Van Hoof et al., "A Field Experiment on the Prophylactic Value of Pentamidine in Sleeping Sicknesss," *Transactions of the Royal Society of Tropical Medicine and Hygiene* 39, no. 4 (1946): 327–29.

69. On the pentamidine prophylaxis programs, see Archives of Institut de médecine tropicale du service de santé des armées (IMTSSA, Marseille, France), Boîte 249, J. Demarchi, "Rapport sur la chimioprophylaxie de la trypanosomiase à *T. gambiense*" (1958), 52–56; B. B. Waddy, "Chemoprophylaxis of Human Trypanosomiasis," in *The African Trypanosomiases,* ed. H. W. Mulligan and W. H. Potts (London: George Allen and Unwin, 1970), 711–25.

70. Muraz, "Des très larges mesures de chimioprophylaxie par injections intramusculaires de diamidines aromatiques (lomidine) mises en oeuvre depuis plusieurs années déjà et tendant à l'éradication de la maladie du sommeil dans les territoires de l'Afrique noire française (A.O.F., A.E.F., Cameroun et Togo Sous Mandat), Contaminés de cette endemie," *Bulletin de l'Académie nationale de médecine* 138, no. 33–34–35 (1954): 614–17.

71. For contemporary discussions, see D. Gall, "The Chemoprophylaxis of Sleeping Sickness with the Diamidines," *Annals of Tropical Medicine and Parasitology* 48, no. 3 (1954): 242–58.

72. A. J. Lotte, "Essai de codification de la prophylaxie chimique de la maladie du sommeil," *Médecine tropicale* 13 (1953): 889–948.

73. J. Burke, "Compte-rendu de la chimioprophylaxie dans la région du Kasai (Sous-secteur du Bas Kwilu, Foreami)," *Annales de la Société belge de médecine tropicale* 33, no. 1 (1953): 13–32.

74. Arch. IMTSSA, Boîte 253, "Rapport : Accidents de lomidinisation au Cameroun Français: Leur thérapeutique et leur prévention (Expérimentation du 4.891 RP) par R. Beaudiment—L. Cauvin—Ph. Leproux," 3.

75. Arch. IMTSSA, Boîte 253, "Rapport: Accidents de lomidinisation au Cameroun Français: Leur thérapeutique et leur prévention (Expérimentation du 4.891 RP) par R. Beaudiment—L. Cauvin—Ph. Leproux"; Waddy, "Chemoprophylaxis of Human Trypanosomiasis."

76. G. Muraz, "Oui, L'Afrique intertropicale peut et doit guérir de la maladie du sommeil en généralisant la lomidinisation de toutes ses régions contaminées," *L'essor médical dans l'union française* 3 (1954): 24.

77. Van Hoof, Henrard, and Peel, "Pentamidine."

78. Chemoprophylaxis is supposed to prevent disease on an individual level.

79. "Rapport final de la iième conférence technique de l'Occgeac (1967), Yaoundé (Cameroun)," in *Première conférence technique de l'OCEAC* (Arch. OCEAC 1967).

80. D. Kayembe and M. Wery, "Observations sur la sensibilité aux diamidines de souches de Trypanosoma gambiense récemment isolées en république du Zaire," *Annales de la Société belge de médecine tropicale* 52, no. 1 (1972): 1–8.

81. Sanjoy Bhattacharya, *Expunging Variola: The Control and Eradication of Smallpox in India, 1947–1977* (New Delhi: Orient Longman, 2006); Paul Greenough, "Intimidation, Coercion and Resistance in the Final Stages of the South Asian Smallpox Eradication Campaign, 1973–1975," *Social Science and Medicine* 41, no. 5 (1995): 633–45.

GUILLAUME LACHENAL

82. John Ford, *The Role of the Trypanosomiases in African Ecology: A Study of the Tsetse Fly Problem* (Oxford: Clarendon Press, 1971).

83. This regime of truth has many similarities with the scientific "economy of promise" that Kaushik Sunder Rajan analyzes in *Biocapital: The Constitution of Postgenomic Life* (Durham, NC: Duke University Press, 2006). The importance of ignorance in contemporary bioscientific research and interventions in Africa is addressed in P. W. Geissler, "Public Secrets in Public Health: Knowing Not to Know While Making Knowledge," *American Ethnologist* 40, no. 1 (2013): 13–34.

A Genealogy of Treatment as Prevention

4

THE TRUE FIASCO
The Treatment and Prevention of Severe Acute Malnutrition in Uganda, 1950–74

JENNIFER TAPPAN

Severe acute malnutrition is the most serious and fatal form of childhood malnutrition. Current global estimates indicate that the condition annually affects approximately ten million children and contributes to a significant proportion of annual deaths in children under the age of five.[1] The recent development and remarkable success of innovative forms of therapy and prevention, known as Ready-To-Use Therapeutic Foods (RUTF), have galvanized a renewed international interest in this significant threat to child health and well-being.

In the immediate post–World War II period, the problem of severe malnutrition had been at the forefront of global medicine. Efforts to combat childhood malnutrition were among the initial programs of the World Health Organization (WHO), the United Nations Children's Fund (UNICEF), and other international institutions. Key developments in the understanding and treatment of severe childhood malnutrition unfolded at the central Ugandan hospital on Mulago Hill, making the small East African country an international center of nutritional research and an important site in the evolution of global endeavors to prevent the condition. Many of these inaugural efforts centered on the distribution of skim-milk powder, which inadvertently served to encourage bottle feeding with deleterious consequences. This essay traces the events through which skim-milk powder distribution came to be seen as the best possible means of preventing severe malnutrition in young children for several decades following the Second World War. In contrast with the better-known controversies over the global marketing of infant formulas by multinational corporations, the following examination focuses on the work of biomedical experts in their efforts to save young lives. Moreover, physicians and scientists advancing dried skimmed milk as therapy and prevention in this period sought to encourage rather than discourage breastfeeding. This was not, however, the case in the Belgian Congo, where colonial authorities promoted skim-milk powder in order to explicitly replace breastfeeding, reduce birth-spacing, and thereby increase labor supplies.[2] Thus although the period under consideration bridges the late-colonial and immediate postcolonial period, the following analysis evaluates the scientific and medical rationale underlying the distribution of dried skimmed milk as an early chapter in the rise of global rather than colonial medicine. Revisiting the fiasco of skim-milk distribution reveals that earlier critiques of the postwar efforts to combat childhood malnutrition focused narrowly on questions of emphasis, missing an opportunity to interrogate the unintended consequences of specific initiatives and their underlying approach in order to ensure that future efforts are able to avoid the same mistakes.

Severe acute malnutrition encompasses a range of severely malnourished states that, in the period under consideration, were thought to be two distinct conditions—kwashiorkor and marasmus. According to this view, marasmus was essentially undernutrition or starvation with the extreme and highly visible wasting of both muscle and fat as the characteristic symptom. Kwashiorkor, however, was defined as a form of malnutrition and was attributed to a diet deficient in protein. In sharp contrast with the very thin appearance of children suffering from marasmus, the most important and consistent symptom of kwashiorkor was edema, or an accumulation of fluid in the tissues that gave severely malnourished children a swollen and fatty appearance. The telltale swelling was exacerbated by an extensive fatty build-up beneath the skin and in the liver. Many children with kwashiorkor developed a form of dermatosis in which the skin simply peeled away, and they often lost the pigment in their hair. One of the most distressing aspects of the condition was the extent to which children with kwashiorkor suffered. They were visibly miserable, apathetic, and anorexic. Their refusal to eat further contributed to their impaired ability to digest food, increasing the high mortality rates associated with the condition. The specific cause or set of causal factors that lead to kwashiorkor remains uncertain today, and the condition continues to have a high case fatality.[3] Kwashiorkor and marasmus are now seen as extreme manifestations at opposing ends of a spectrum of severe acute malnutrition.

Kwashiorkor Treatment and Prevention

Controversy over kwashiorkor began in the early 1930s when Cicely Williams proposed that the condition was a form of protein deficiency.[4] Established experts in the new field of nutritional science rejected the protein hypothesis. Figures such as Dr. Hugh Stannus remained convinced that they were dealing with a micronutrient deficiency.[5] Opposition to the protein hypothesis was partially a reflection of the heightened interest in micronutrients following the wave of vitamin and mineral discoveries in the initial decades of the twentieth century.[6] Over time, the heated disputes over the cause of protein deficiency ultimately centered on the therapeutic failure of dietary protein. In fact, the inability to treat severely malnourished children with protein rich food cast doubt upon the protein theory and the very high prevalence of "secondary" infections lent credence to a variety of alternative diagnoses.[7]

During the decades of controversy, mortality rates remained remarkably high. In the early 1930s, Dr. Hugh Trowell reported losing more than three-quarters of his kwashiorkor patients. The first WHO survey of kwashiorkor in Africa cited mortality rates in 1950 ranging from 40 to 90 percent.[8] The inability to alleviate the suffering and save the lives of severely malnourished children left physicians like Trowell desperate to determine the cause of this highly fatal condition. In a description of his work following his transfer to the central Ugandan hospital on Mulago Hill, Trowell explained, "Still we were losing 40% of our cases in hospital. And you expect a person to get better if you are giving all the known vitamins, and protein, and we were still having this enormous mortality."[9]

A breakthrough was finally made shortly after the end of the Second World War when the pathologist, Jack Davies joined Trowell at Mulago Hospital. Together Trowell and Davies conducted thorough autopsies of severely malnourished children immediately following death, which revealed that the pancreas had not been secreting digestive enzymes. This discovery provided the long-awaited evidence substantiating the protein theory, as enzyme synthesis depends on adequate supplies of dietary protein. Pancreatic atrophy explained why severely malnourished children were not easily treated through the provision of food alone. Without sufficient protein for the production of the digestive enzymes that are needed to break down and absorb essential nutrients, even protein-rich foods such as milk were of limited therapeutic value—severely malnourished children simply could no longer digest and absorb food.

This important development in the search for the etiology of kwashiorkor came at a significant moment in the rise of global medicine. In October of 1949, an Expert Committee on Nutrition formed jointly by the United Nations Food and Agricultural Organization (FAO) and the WHO held its first meeting in Geneva. Kwashiorkor, described as "one of the most widespread nutritional disorders in tropical and sub-tropical areas," was high on the agenda and Trowell was asked to prepare a memorandum on the condition for the committee's consideration.[10] The committee resolved to conduct an investigation of kwashiorkor in sub-Saharan Africa, beginning with a visit to Mulago Hospital in order to first consult Trowell and his colleagues in Uganda.

A subsequent WHO report, "Kwashiorkor in Africa," was based in large part on evidence from Mulago and became the seminal study in the growing international focus on protein malnutrition.[11] A second meeting of the Joint FAO/WHO Expert Committee on Nutrition centered largely on discussions of "Kwashiorkor in Africa," concluding with a resolution to conduct further surveys.[12] Delegations were then sent to Central America and Brazil, and the resulting reports confirmed the growing belief that kwashiorkor was a worldwide problem that required immediate action.[13]

With the etiology apparently established, the remaining challenge was to develop a protein-rich formula capable of reversing pancreatic atrophy or jump-starting digestive enzyme production. However, this task did not prove easy, for as Davies later explained, they simply "had no special high protein material to feed the children."[14] The man who did finally devise an effective therapy was Dr. Rex Dean, a veritable "giant in the field of nutritional science."[15] Under the auspices of the British Medical Research Council (MRC), Dean began working in Uganda in 1950 in order to apply his expertise toward the future prevention of kwashiorkor in Africa. Within a few years he was directing the MRC Infantile Malnutrition Research Unit on Mulago Hill, establishing Uganda's position as an international center of nutritional science. The aim of Dean's work was to build on the success he achieved developing mixtures of plant proteins "rivaling milk in nutritive value" for malnourished orphans and schoolchildren in postwar Germany.[16] Yet when he arrived in Uganda the immediate problem Dean faced was not the prevention of kwashiorkor but the appalling mortality rates among the severely malnourished children brought to Mulago Hospital.[17] Although he never lost sight of his goal to prevent malnutrition, Dean's major contribution to applied nutritional science was the development of a highly effective curative therapy. Moreover, given his mandate to develop a vegetable-based preventive mixture as he had done in Germany, Dean's "High Protein Therapy" ironically ended up being a milk-based formula that mixtures of vegetable proteins could never rival.

Dean turned to milk simply because the most inexpensive and accessible source of protein in Uganda at the time was dried skimmed milk. As a waste product in the manufacture of butter in Europe and the United States, ample supplies of dried skimmed milk were easily acquired in the postwar period.[18] Yet, even skim milk had its shortcomings. Many severely malnourished

Treatment and Prevention of Severe Acute Malnutrition in Uganda

children in Uganda were lactose-intolerant and developed diarrhea in response to the skim-milk-based formula. Although a very common symptom of lactose-intolerance, diarrhea is an extremely dangerous situation in already acutely malnourished children. Dean overcame this dilemma by reducing the amount of skim milk and supplementing the mixture with Casilin, a commercially produced preparation of calcium caseinate containing an 80 percent concentration of milk protein. Despite the cost, this high-protein therapeutic formula was a resounding success. Even before cottonseed oil was added to the formula in order to compensate for the diminished caloric content, Dean and his colleagues were able to celebrate the development of effective kwashiorkor therapy.[19]

The development of Dean's High Protein Therapy was only part of the story. As severely malnourished children had "grossly impaired" capacities to digest and absorb even essential nutrients, Dean insisted on the institution of what he called "dietary discipline." Coining the term "dietary discipline" emphasized that the provision of dietary therapy in severely malnourished patients was no different from the provision of drug therapy to treat infection.[20] In his regimented system of infant feeding, a precise amount of protein and calories, determined by the child's weight, was prescribed and administered at specific intervals. The daily provision of the high-protein therapy was prepared in a glass bottle and in order to avoid spoilage, Dean required that "the bottle must therefore be changed every 6 hours."[21] Under Dean's direction, all aspects of kwashiorkor treatment became standardized. Secondary infections were so prevalent that the routine therapeutic measures included daily injections of penicillin in the initial week of treatment whether or not an infection was evident. Children admitted with severe kwashiorkor were also automatically treated for malaria, anemia, dehydration, and potassium loss.[22] The "dietary discipline" transformed kwashiorkor treatment into a hospital-centered cure involving tubes, formulas, syringes, IVs, and injections.

Only two years after arriving in Uganda, Dean could report in *The Lancet* that the "concentrated milk-protein" formula had already succeeded in reducing the mortality rate to between 10 to 20 percent, a significant achievement given the 75 to 90 percent mortality reported in the 1930s and 1940s by Trowell and others.[23] Moreover, the phenomenal pace of recovery was equally striking. Even in very severe cases nearly all of the most prominent symptoms began to improve within seven to ten days. The anorexia that frequently made intragastric tube feeding necessary subsided so rapidly that tube-feeding was rarely continued beyond the second day of treatment.[24] The edema also promptly diminished, as did the skin lesions or dermatosis and the fatty buildup beneath the skin, and, by the end of a week, the child's demeanor also began to noticeably improve.[25] The formula's capacity to rapidly and visibly transform the health of severely malnourished children appears to have contributed to shifts in local acceptance of hospital treatment for kwashiorkor. In Uganda, earlier references to parents and guardians "absconding from hospital," "running away," or refusing treatment for their children gave way to signs of increasing demand for kwashiorkor therapy at Mulago. Unlike the 1940s and early 1950s, when "expeditions into the villages were necessary to convince mothers that their children . . . had an illness which could be treated in hospital,"[26] by the 1960s, "the dramatic intravenous and intragastric therapies, which were often lifesaving, were expected by mothers. In fact," according to one physician, "the fame of the hospital resulted in some mothers traveling hundreds of miles" in order to obtain kwashiorkor treatment for their children.[27]

Dean's work in Uganda provided further evidence in support of the protein hypothesis and contributed to the growing international concern that severe protein malnutrition was "the biggest menace to the future health of the nations in developing regions."[28] Experts then began to convene at a number of additional international conferences and meetings and when the Expert Committee on Nutrition met again in 1952, the proceedings were dedicated entirely to kwashiorkor.[29] In 1955, the WHO created a Protein Advisory Group and, in cooperation with the Committee on Protein Malnutrition of the US National Academy of Sciences/National Research Council, the Protein Advisory Group led the global effort to close the "protein gap."[30] The perception that the "deficiency of protein in the diet is the most serious and widespread problem in the world," became so pervasive that in 1968 the General Assembly of the United Nations even considered the creation of a United Nations Protein Board.[31]

Up until the mid-1950s, the international campaign to combat protein malnutrition focused primarily on the "emergency action" that the initial report on "Kwashiorkor in Africa" called for—namely a public campaign to spread awareness of the condition and the therapeutic efficacy of high-protein, skim-milk-based formulas. As part of this early emphasis on curative measures, it was recommended that "skim-milk powder should be made available to hospitals and maternity and child-welfare centres" and that UNICEF should coordinate with governments to secure supplies of skim milk for both curative and preventive purposes. The distribution of skim-milk powder as a means of preventing severe protein deficiency was always seen as a temporary measure.[32]

By 1955, the agenda shifted from short-term curative initiatives toward prevention. In international reports the vital need for educational programs designed to improve methods of infant feeding figured prominently, but the main thrust was the development of "milk substitutes," or protein-rich foods specifically formulated for infants and young children.[33]

The "protein-rich food programme" became a nascent industry centered on the research and development of commercially acceptable high-protein mixtures and ingredients. Both the WHO and FAO supplied ongoing finances and consultants to a number of international research centers involved in producing high-protein foods, including Guatemala's Institute of Nutrition for Central America and Panama (INCAP) and the MRC Unit in Uganda. Such funds were augmented by $860,000 in grants from the Rockefeller Foundation and UNICEF specifically earmarked for "research in protein-rich foods."[34] The apparent success of these endeavors over the course of the 1960s led the United Nations to call for a $75 million program in 1970.[35] Already by 1962, the Expert Committee on Nutrition could claim, "The stage has now been reached when it can be said with some confidence that one of the major, most promising and most rapid methods of improving nutrition in many countries lies in an effective and speedy programme for the production, distribution and consumption of protein-rich foods."[36] Confidence, in the early 1960s, appeared warranted. Commercial production of flours made from soybeans, groundnuts, cottonseeds, and refined fish had already achieved satisfactory results, and acceptability trials of these products and mixtures made from them were under way in more than twenty different countries around the globe.[37]

Not surprisingly, Dean was at the forefront of this work, and with assistance from the FAO and the WHO, the MRC Unit in Kampala coordinated with INCAP to lead the development and commercial production of mixtures suitable for supplementary infant feeding.[38] In the early 1950s Dean conducted promising trials with mixtures containing soy milk and sweet banana. In 1952, he wrote to Cicely Williams to announce "that we have just discharged from hospital the first child who has been successfully treated for fairly advanced Kwashiorkor by means of an all-plant diet. . . . We are pleased with this result because we think it proves that we are on the right lines: and that prevention cannot be impossibly difficult. There is plenty of soya here."[39]

In the end, nonmilk-based formulas met with very limited success. By the late 1950s, Dean abandoned the aim of devising an entirely milk-free mixture and began experimenting with formulas containing various quantities of milk powder. The primary ingredient of these mixtures was the groundnut or peanut. Unlike soy, groundnuts were grown in nearly every garden plot and had long been an integral component of the local diet. Mixtures of groundnuts, maize and wheat flour, cottonseed oil, sugar, and skim-milk powder proved to be just as effective as the high-protein therapy in the hospital treatment of kwashiorkor—suggesting to Dean and his colleagues that the mixture could also reduce the prevalence of protein malnutrition. By making the ingredients into a cooked biscuit that was later ground into a fine powder, it was thought that the meal could be stored in even "unsealed containers without apparent deterioration for many months."[40] As Dean noted, "A dry material has great advantages in an equatorial climate."[41] By 1959, plans were well under way for the commercial production of the groundnut biscuit by a local Ugandan company under the guidance of the biochemist at the MRC unit and an expert sent by the WHO.[42] By the later 1960s, a number of different high-protein mixtures had entered the market: from INCAP a product known as Incaparina, Fortifex in Brazil, Pronutro in South Africa, Arlac in Nigeria, Lac-Tone in India, and Surpro in East Africa. At the end of 1968, 162 tons of Superamine were ready for the market in Algeria.[43]

Yet, these high-protein mixtures failed as weaning foods capable of preventing kwashiorkor. A series of technical setbacks proved insurmountable. In Uganda, all work on the groundnut biscuit was immediately suspended when it was discovered in 1960 that a highly toxic and carcinogenic mold, aflatoxin, was frequently found on cereals and oilseeds, including groundnuts.[44] In other regions, high production costs made high-protein foods prohibitively expensive for the segments of the population most susceptible to protein malnutrition. Early success with Pronutro in South Africa, where approximately 600 tons were sold per month, was diminished when the rising cost of ingredients was passed on to consumers who could no longer afford the product.[45] A similar fate befell Incaparina. After nearly two decades of production in some countries, the director of INCAP insisted that without "subsidized distribution" or significant poverty reduction, "a commercially produced and marketed vegetable mixture could" not be expected to "'solve' the problem of protein-calorie malnutrition."[46] Prohibitive costs were compounded by the failure of acceptability trials or poorly planned initiatives such as the fortification of bread in South Africa with over 800 tons of fish flour only to discover that brown bread was not a significant component of the diet among poor, African children.[47]

Then in 1974, Dr. Donald S. McLaren published an article in the preeminent medical journal *The Lancet* titled "The Great Protein Fiasco."[48] McLaren criticized the emphasis placed on severe protein malnutrition by international agencies linked to the United Nations and effectively undermined the widespread view that there was an "impending protein crisis" of global proportions. His article triggered a decisive shift away from targeting protein malnutrition in order to improve nutritional health in young children. The pendulum swung so swiftly in the opposite direction that kwashiorkor research and programming ground to a virtual halt. Those who championed McLaren's critique represented a growing group of biomedical practitioners who, like McLaren, had been working in regions of the world where protein deficiency did not appear to be the most prevalent form of malnutrition. For McLaren and many others, it was marasmus or undernutrition that warranted greater attention but had been overshadowed by the international preoccupation with protein malnutrition.

Examining the causal role of infectious disease was also a growing focus, and at the MRC unit in Uganda the "nutrition-infection complex" became the center of ongoing research. Ironically, McLaren's intention had not been to question the science implicating protein deficiency as the cause of kwashiorkor, merely the general application of that evidence in the international arena. The interpretive error, as McLaren has repeatedly argued, was "the extrapolation by others of the atypical experience in Africa to the rest of the developing world."[49] As McLaren explained in a letter to Cicely Williams, it was not the evidence of protein malnutrition in Africa that was problematic, merely the translation of that evidence to a global scale.[50]

The True Fiasco

A closer look at the impact of the high-protein food program in Uganda suggests an alternative explanation of "The Great Protein Fiasco." When the discovery of aflatoxin left milk as the only source of protein that was known to be "safe" and effective in kwashiorkor treatment and prevention, Dean focused his energies on the distribution of dried skim milk and the commercial production of "reinforced milk packets." Dean's decision to abandon his efforts to develop a plant-based mixture after the failure of the groundnut biscuit was also influenced by his own deteriorating condition. Dean contracted transverse myelitis in 1956 while conducting a survey on "Kwashiorkor in Malaya" for the WHO, and by the early 1960s the illness began to take its toll.[51] The local commercial production of fortified and packaged dried skim milk was Dean's final effort to contribute to the prevention of kwashiorkor. Equivalent to one pint of full cream milk, "reinforced milk packets" contained a simple mixture of dried skimmed milk, cottonseed oil, and cane sugar. After carrying out "extensive trials on the efficiency of this preparation in the prevention and cure of kwashiorkor," Dean began to work with a local company, the "'Uganda Co-operative Creameries' about the possibility of their producing this 'reinforced milk' on a commercial basis."[52] Prior to Dean's death in 1964, the central Ugandan hospital reported that dried skimmed milk was "either issued plain in bags . . . or reinforced with additional calories . . . 'reinforced milk packets' as they are called."[53]

It was thus that in the 1950s and 1960s, parents and guardians who sought treatment for malnourished children in Uganda often returned to their homes with much healthier children and with a supply of dried skim milk. Health care professionals provided skim milk powder to forestall the possibility of relapse in children successfully treated for kwashiorkor and as part of their efforts to prevent severe malnutrition. With skim milk powder as the basis of both preventive and curative measures the distinction between prevention and cure broke down. Dried skimmed milk was either given or sold at hospitals and health centers in Uganda beginning in the early 1950s as an immediate, emergency measure until high-protein foods could be developed. Yet, the practice continued in Uganda through the late 1960s when, in the context of developing the first Nutrition Rehabilitation Program in Africa, physicians at Mulago decided to begin "weaning the mother from free milk powder."[54] In the interim, Dean and Derrick B. Jelliffe, the prominent professor of pediatrics at Uganda's Makerere University, recommended that in "mild" or "moderate cases," "Dried skimmed milk (D.S.M.) should be supplied to the mother either once or twice weekly, or fortnightly." When the "distance and timing of clinics" made the distribution of smaller quantities impractical, they advised the "monthly issue of powdered milk to mothers."[55] To prevent malnutrition in children not yet presenting symptoms, they suggested, "that a supply of special infant food, such as D.S.M., should be made available at child welfare centres for the majority of poorer parents."[56] As the Uganda Government Nutrition Advisor, Dean was in a position to advocate that the policy of distributing dried skimmed milk be implemented throughout the country. Moreover, missionary institutions historically at the forefront of medical provision in Uganda planned in 1958 to begin weekly distributions of a half-pound of milk powder per child and requested an initial shipment of 148 tons from the Church World Service.[57]

Biomedical practitioners were well aware that without access to clean water bottle feeding posed a significant hazard to the health of young children, for the

Treatment and Prevention of Severe Acute Malnutrition in Uganda

gastroenteritis that often followed the introduction of bottle feeding in impoverished regions of the world was widely known to be a leading contributor to marasmus or undernutrition. As a result, health education that emphasized the importance of breastfeeding was considered an essential component of preventing malnutrition in Uganda. The primary focus of health education geared toward the prevention of kwashiorkor was to convince mothers that breast milk was nutritionally insufficient and had to then be supplemented when a child reached the age of six months. A label created to accompany the reinforced milk packets instructed, in fine print: "Suckle your child until he is one and a half years old. In addition, from the age of six months onwards, give him some solid food such as eggs, beans, peas, groundnuts or green vegetables, also if possible some meat or fish."[58] However, the message conveyed in bold print on the label designed to accompany the milk packets read, "EMMERE Y'OMWANA EMMERE EKUZA OMWANA OBULUNGI" or "FOOD WHICH MAKES THE CHILD GROW WELL."[59]

Parents who received dried skim milk at Mulago were reportedly given explicit instructions to add it to a child's meal and not to reconstitute the powder as milk for the child to drink. The policy followed at the outpatient department was to "supply the child's mother with enough of these packets to last her until she next comes up, and, rather than ask her to dissolve the milk powder in water of doubtful safety, ask her to add it to the sauce that she would normally give her sick child, or to other items of his diet."[60] Yet, as this was precisely how physicians treated malnourished children in the pediatric wards, the message was essentially "Do as I say not as I do." Interviews with elderly women and men in a rural area approximately thirty miles north of Kampala confirm that the distribution of milk powder at hospitals and health centers was widespread, and two women interviewed even received milk packets from Mulago and remembered the accompanying label. When asked how they were instructed to feed the skim milk powder to their children, emphasis was always placed on the need to boil the water used to make the powder into milk for their children to drink, and not one informant could recall being instructed to add the powdered milk to a child's food.[61]

At the mobile child welfare clinics held on a regular basis in and around the Ugandan capital, Kampala, Dr. Hebe Welbourn sold dried skim milk to parents who participated in the "group demonstrations" on "mixing dried milk" that were offered "at most clinics."[62] In Welbourn's view, it was necessary to sell the skim milk powder for a nominal fee in order to ensure that the practice of feeding the milk to children became an established part of feeding

JENNIFER TAPPAN

practices. Welbourn even persuaded a psychologist studying child-rearing practices in Uganda, to "follow the same procedure as the clinic followed, buying the milk in large quantities wholesale and selling it at cost."[63] Due to her conviction that "highly educated" women were capable of bottle feeding successfully, Welbourn even explicitly encouraged bottle feeding among some parents. Evidence from the period suggests that many of the mothers who used bottles to supplement their child's diet did so upon the advice of the health clinic.[64] According to Catherine Nansamba, medical personnel at the local health center taught her that bottle feeding was advantageous if used correctly and only a problem for child health when mothers lacked knowledge of proper use. Moreover, Catherine, like all of the elderly informants consulted for this study remembered bottle feeding as a pervasive practice in Uganda during the period coinciding with skim milk distribution.[65]

As early as the mid-1950s, physicians in Uganda were troubled by the growing popularity of bottle feeding. The first to raise concern over generalized bottle feeding in Uganda was Dr. Hebe Welbourn. Through her mobile child welfare clinics, she was well placed to observe changing patterns in infant feeding, and the record cards kept for each child provided data for later analysis.[66] According to Welbourn, most mothers in Uganda exclusively breast-fed until the mid-1950s when she noted that "it has now become a common sight in Uganda to see an African baby being fed . . . with various mixtures of milk, cereal or tea from a bottle."[67] In comparing the records from 1955 with those taken in 1950, Welbourn found evidence of a distinct shift toward supplementary bottle feeding. Although most of the children were still breast-fed, the percentage of infants under one and six months of age who were also bottle-fed more than doubled in just six years. Furthermore, Welbourn's figures indicated that "supplementary feeding was nearly always followed by early weaning."[68] The infants who were given supplementary bottles were weaned, on average, six months earlier than those who were breast-fed alone.

This trend to supplement breastfeeding and to wean early was also emphasized by Dr. Latimer Musoke in his analysis of the pediatric admissions at Mulago in 1959. Like Welbourn, Musoke observed that among "the Baganda, although many do still breast-feed their babies, early supplementary feeding is increasing."[69] In a study of weaning practices in Buganda in the mid-1960s, Dr. Josephine Namboze also found that among mothers residing in Kampala or the surrounding area, nearly half weaned their infants before their first birthday and 34 percent gave their young children formula, milk, or cereal "instead of breast milk."[70] Moreover, Welbourn's clinic record cards, five years following

Treatment and Prevention of Severe Acute Malnutrition in Uganda

her first assessment, revealed that bottle feeding had risen a further 20 percent to the point that "in 1960, 42 percent of babies attending child welfare clinics were being given supplementary bottle feeds before the age of 6 months."[71]

Considering the hazards of bottle feeding in communities with insufficient supplies of safe drinking water, many characterized the growing popularity of bottle feeding in Uganda in alarmist terms. Bottle feeding did pose a number of very real dangers for infant health in Uganda.[72] The first was the fact that even supplementary bottle feeding "tended to replace breast feeds," and as a mother's supply of breast milk is directly determined by the demand of the suckling infant, less frequent nursing quickly translated into an often irreversible reduction of breast milk.[73] The result was that bottle-fed babies faced a significantly higher risk of consuming an insufficient diet, and "after a few months of supplementary bottle feeding," Welbourn found that, "most of the children showed signs of undernutrition."[74] In fact, the bottle-fed babies in Welbourn's sample were an average of one to two pounds lighter than those who were exclusively breast-fed, and two of the three children who developed kwashiorkor while attending Welbourn's clinics in 1955 were being fed with a bottle.[75]

Problems of undernutrition were exacerbated by the far greater frequency of infectious disease in bottle-fed infants. The prevalence of water-borne pathogens exposed bottle-fed infants to a host of infections that they might otherwise avoid, and the consequent reduction or absence of breast milk in the diet meant that these very same children were not acquiring the antibodies that passed from mother to child providing breast-fed babies with some protection from infection. Welbourn's evidence indicated that the children who were fed supplementary bottles were twice as likely to develop diarrhea, vomiting, and acute respiratory infections.[76] Such "disastrous consequences" of bottle feeding were also evident in the pediatric wards of Uganda's central hospital by the close of the 1950s, and physicians were well aware that the growing prevalence of gastroenteritis among Mulago's pediatric patients represented a shift from earlier disease patterns.[77] Musoke wrote for instance that, "It is significant that a disease which seven years ago was considered to be quite uncommon, now tops the list of admissions. Davies ... stated that [in 1950] diarrhoea and vomiting were relatively unimportant causes for admission of children in Mulago Hospital. . . . The present analysis shows that the diarrhoea and vomiting syndrome has become one of the major problems of the ward." Moreover, biomedical practitioners rightly attributed this epidemiological shift to the rise of supplementary bottle feeding; as Musoke pointed out, exclusively breast-fed children constituted less than 14 percent of the cases admitted for diarrhea and vomiting.[78]

However, the connection between the distribution of dried skim milk, skim-milk-based kwashiorkor therapy, and the growing use of nursing bottles in Uganda was not at first appreciated. Despite the widespread recognition that bottle feeding was on the rise, scientists and physicians uncritically accepted the view that bottle feeding was an inevitable result of urbanization, "Westernization," and "civilization." Thus Trowell, in the first edition of the classic text *Diseases of Children in the Subtropics and Tropics,* opened the chapter about infant feeding with a treatise on the "natural" progression from breast to bottle feeding: "The incidence and duration of breast feeding reflect the customs, social patterns, economic development and sophistication current in any community. Perhaps," he reasoned, "those who are nearest to nature are themselves most natural. . . . Under the impact of civilization and sophistication the movement at first is always away from breast feeding to bottle feeding."[79] Trapped within this teleological framework, biomedical personnel failed to register the role of their own therapeutic and preventive practices. In fact it was not until the late 1970s that Jelliffe and his wife regretfully acknowledged: "It was a nutritional tragedy that the well-intentioned, widespread feeding programmes in developing countries in the 1940s and 1950s should have been primarily concerned with the distribution of dry skimmed-milk powder. . . . As far as mothers of young children are concerned, this can only have appeared as endorsement of bottle feeding, with a resulting displacement effect on breast-feeding."[80] The true fiasco of the international preoccupation with protein was not misplaced focus on the wrong condition. In Uganda, the tragedy was that well-intentioned biomedical efforts to prevent kwashiorkor inadvertently increased the prevalence of marasmus.

McLaren concluded his indictment of international efforts to combat the "worldwide protein crisis" by insisting that the true costs be measured in terms of the children "lost in the unchecked scourge of malnutrition."[81] To this we must add many of the children who died as a result of bottle feeding in this period. Unlike the scandalous global marketing of infant formulas, medical providers distributed dried skim milk as part of well-meaning efforts to treat and prevent severe malnutrition in young children. Skim milk distribution was initially meant to be only an immediate emergency measure until high-protein weaning foods could be developed. The failure of the high-protein food program meant that widespread distribution of milk powder continued to be the basis of prevention much longer than originally planned. What is more, skim milk powder, reconstituted as a liquid formula for malnourished children to drink, was the basis of the first highly curative and effective therapeutic regimen capable of reversing the many symptoms associated with the severe malnutrition and significantly reducing mortality rates. It was thus that an unintended reliance on dried skim milk in the prevention and cure of kwashiorkor served to endorse bottle feeding in Uganda and increase the prevalence of marasmus.

McLaren's article in *The Lancet* ended an era of international emphasis on severe protein malnutrition, but it did not end the practice of distributing dried skim milk, and Dean's milk-based forms of treatment remained the basis of curative therapies until the advent of RUTF. Defining the problem as misplaced emphasis on the wrong condition diverted further critical appraisals of the high-protein food program and left later efforts to treat and prevent childhood malnutrition with little knowledge of past initiatives and the reasons for their failure. The recent development of ready-to-use-therapeutic foods can, therefore, be seen as having succeeded where previous efforts failed. Now that kwashiorkor and marasmus are viewed as extreme manifestations of a single condition and the efficacy of RUTF appears established, solving the problem of severe acute malnutrition in young children seems to require simply returning childhood malnutrition to the international limelight.

Recognizing that McLaren's critique in "The Great Protein Fiasco" missed the unintended consequences of the high-protein food program in Uganda is therefore crucial as a new generation of physicians and scientists, emboldened by the curative and preventive promise of RUTF, works to combat severe malnutrition around the globe. Few would question the fact that RUTF was a long overdue improvement on Dean's milk-based forms of treatment. The nutrient-rich packages of peanut butter provide a significant savings over hospital-based therapy and rehabilitation, and local production of RUTF offers an even cheaper and thus more sustainable alternative. As a prepackaged paste that does not require reconstitution in water of questionable safety, ready-to-use-therapeutic foods can also be safely administered outside of hospitals and clinics, significantly lessening the drain on already overextended health services.[82] The enthusiasm appears at first glance to be warranted as RUTF expand the potential reach of both curative and preventive initiatives—fulfilling the dream that Dean and others had for the high-protein food program in the immediate postwar period.

Yet the parallels between RUTF and the high-protein food program should give us pause. Both originated in the remarkable success of curative strategies developed in desperate efforts to save lives. Using the cure to achieve prevention, as the foregoing analysis illustrates, relies on the commercial production of nutritional therapy within a framework of "drug" provision. It is a model in which companies supply and profit from therapeutic foods purchased with often limited and fluctuating supplies of foreign aid, making nutritional health and child survival even more dependent on maintaining international awareness in order to secure scarce resources, as Médecins sans frontières' campaign "Starved for Attention" makes explicit.[83] Despite the emphasis placed on the reduced cost of RUTF-based treatment, large-scale prevention programs in the most impoverished regions of the world come at fairly hefty costs, and local production schemes do not eliminate questions of expense among populations subsisting on less than a dollar per day and within contexts of diminishing resources for medical provision.[84] Moreover, the reliance on technological solutions and the "magic-bullet" approach reinforce the misconception that malnutrition is a "disease" within medical communities and the populations they serve, leaving current efforts equally susceptible to unintended consequences, failure and "donor fatigue." Innovative approaches to prevention later developed at the Nutrition Rehabilitation Program in Uganda empowered mothers and guardians with knowledge of how to prevent malnutrition independent of hospitals, hand-outs, and expensive commercial therapies.[85] Revisiting "The Great Protein Fiasco" suggests that establishing sustained initiatives to promote nutritional health in young children entails acknowledging the limitations of targeted, technological fixes and working instead toward a more comprehensive, integrated, and constantly evolving set of strategies.

The efforts to prevent severe protein malnutrition in the 1950s and 1960s through the high-protein food program and the widespread distribution of dried skim milk have direct relevance for the contemporary endeavors to combat severe acute malnutrition in young children around the globe because the fundamental approach remains unchanged. The development of RUTF appears to pick up precisely where physicians and scientists left off in the wake of "The Great Protein Fiasco"—focused on the curative and preventive potential of particular formulas of nutritionally dense therapeutic foods. Malnutrition is again recast as a "disease" requiring the further development

Treatment and Prevention of Severe Acute Malnutrition in Uganda

and commercial production of effective "drugs" suitable for both cure and prevention. Although some thought is given to questions of expense and who ultimately benefits from framing the problem of malnutrition in this way, questions of long-term impact are rarely raised. Although the RUTF program runs little risk of inadvertently serving to endorse bottle feeding, the consequences of widespread and continuous use of RUTF and similar therapeutic products to prevent malnutrition in young children should be subjected to serious and ongoing scrutiny. In addition to evaluating the impact of therapeutic mixtures in the bodies of already or potentially malnourished children, routine investigations of the broader consequences are necessary and must include critical appraisals of how populations interpret and incorporate public health interventions. The history of skim milk distribution in Uganda illustrates that the danger is not simply failure and waning international investment, but unforeseen adverse health impacts that could lead to further loss of young lives.

Notes

1. André Briend et al., "Putting the Management of Severe Malnutrition Back on the International Health Agenda," *Food and Nutrition Bulletin* 27, no. 3 (2006): S3.

2. Nancy Rose Hunt, "'Le Bébé en Brusse': European Women, African Birth Spacing and Colonial Intervention in Breast Feeding in the Belgian Congo," *International Journal of African Historical Studies* 21, no. 3 (1988): 401–32.

3. Michael Krawinkel, "Kwashiorkor Is Still Not Fully Understood," *Bulletin of the World Health Organization* 81, no. 12 (2003): 910; Snezana Nena Osorio, "Reconsidering Kwashiorkor," *Topical Clinical Nutrition* 26, no. 1 (2011): 10–13. Recent research on aflatoxins and antioxidants remains inconclusive. As in the late 1960s, kwashiorkor continues to be seen as a form of protein-energy malnutrition aggravated by infection. See, for instance, Olaf Müller and Michael Krawinkel, "Malnutrition and Health in Developing Countries," *Canadian Medical Association Journal* 173, no. 3 (2005): 279–86.

4. C. D. Williams, "A Nutritional Disease of Childhood Associated with a Maize Diet," *Archives of Disease in Childhood* 8, no. 48 (1933): 423–33; and C. D. Williams, "Kwashiorkor: A Nutritional Disease of Children Associated with a Maize Diet," *Lancet* 2 (16 November 1935): 1151–52.

5. H. S. Stannus, "A Nutritional Disease of Childhood Associated with a Maize Diet—and Pellagra," *Archives of Disease in Childhood* 9, no. 50 (1934): 115–18.

6. Celia Petty, "Primary Research and Public Health: The Prioritization of Nutrition Research in Inter-war Britain," in *Historical Perspectives on the Role of the MRC*, ed. J. Austoker and L. Bryder (New York: Oxford University Press, 1989), 83–108; E. V. McCollum, *The Newer Knowledge of Nutrition* (New York: Macmillan, 1918).

7. Interview with Hugh Trowell by Elizabeth Bray, MSS.Afr.s.1872 (144B), Rhodes House Library, Oxford University (hereafter RHL); "Dr. Hebe Flower Welbourn: Reminiscences of My Career in Uganda," Personal Memoir, MSS.Afr.s.1872 (152), RHL.

8. Hugh Trowell, "Food, Protein and Kwashiorkor (Presidential Address)," *Uganda Journal* 21 (1957): 84; J. F. Brock and M. Autret, "Kwashiorkor in Africa," *Bulletin of World Health Organization*, Monograph Series 8 (1952): 24.

9. Interview with Hugh Trowell by Elizabeth Bray, MSS.Afr.s.1872 (144B), RHL: 33–34.

10. "Joint FAO/WHO Expert Committee on Nutrition: Report on the First Session," World Health Organization Technical Report Series No. 16 (Geneva, 1950), 15; Interview with Hugh Trowell by Elizabeth Bray, RHL MSS.Afr.s.1872 (144B), 56–57.

11. Brock and Autret, "Kwashiorkor in Africa."

12. "Joint FAO/WHO Expert Committee on Nutrition: Report on the Second Session," World Health Organization Technical Report Series No. 44 (Geneva, 1951), 29.

13. M. Autret and M. Behar, "Sindrome Policarencial Infantil (Kwashiorkor) and Its Prevention in Central America," *FAO Nutritional Studies*, no. 13 (1954); J. C. Waterlow and A. Vergara, "Protein Malnutrition in Brazil," *FAO Nutritional Studies*, no. 14 (1956).

14. "Davies, Dr. J.N.P.," Personal Memoir, MSS.Afr.s.1872(40), RHL, 76.

15. Interview with Dr. Roger Whitehead, Kampala, Uganda, 9 December 2003.

16. R. F. A. Dean, "Plant Proteins in Child Feeding," Medical Research Council Special Report Series, No. 279 (London, 1953), see "Preface"; Members of the Department of Experimental Medicine, Cambridge, and Associated Workers. "Studies of Undernutrition, Wuppertal 1946–9," Medical Research Council Special Report Series, No. 275 (London, 1951).

17. R. G. Whitehead, "Kwashiorkor in Uganda," in *The Contribution of Nutrition to Human and Animal Health,* ed. E. M. Widdowson and J. C. Mathers (Cambridge: Cambridge University Press, 1992), 307.

18. Whitehead, "Kwashiorkor in Uganda," 307; interview with Dr. Roger Whitehead, Kampala, Uganda, 9 December 2003.

19. R. F. A. Dean, "The Treatment of Kwashiorkor with Milk and Vegetable Proteins," *British Medical Journal* 2, no. 478 (11 October 1952): 792; R. F. A. Dean and B. Weinbren, "Fat Absorption in Chronic Severe Malnutrition in Children," *Lancet* 268, no. 6936 (1956): 252; R. F. A. Dean and M. Skinner, "A Note on the Treatment of Kwashiorkor," *Journal of Tropical Pediatrics* 2, no. 4 (March 1957): 215–16.

20. Whitehead, "Kwashiorkor in Uganda," 307; "MRC Child Nutrition Unit: A Progress Report from October 1968–December 1970 Presented to the Tropical Medical Research Board of the Medical Research Council of the United Kingdom and the National Research Council of Uganda." Public Record Office (hereafter PRO), The National Archives, formerly Kew; FD 12/282: 25.

21. R. F. A. Dean and D. B. Jelliffe, "Diagnosis and Treatment of Protein-Calorie Malnutrition," *Courrier* 10, no. 7 (1960): 433.

22. Ibid. "The Hospital Treatment of Severe Kwashiorkor," January 1967, Personal Papers of Dr. Mike Church.

23. Dean, "Treatment of Kwashiorkor," 792.

24. For more on the importance of a child's appetite and acceptance of the formula see Barbara Cooper, "Chronic Malnutrition and the Trope of the Bad Mother,"

in *A Not-So Natural Disaster: Niger 2005,* ed. Xavier Crombé and Jean-Hervé Jézéquel (New York: Columbia University Press, 2009), 147–68.

25. Dean, "Treatment of Kwashiorkor," 792–93.

26. H. C. Trowell, J. N. P. Davies, and R. F. A. Dean, *Kwashiorkor* (1954; London: Academic Press, 1982), 63.

27. M. A. Church, "Evaluation as an Integral Aspect of Nutrition Education" (September 1982), 4, Personal Papers of Dr. Mike Church.

28. "Lives in Peril: Protein and the Child," FAO/WHO/UNICEF Protein Advisory Group, World Food Problems No. 12 (Rome, 1970), 25.

29. "Joint FAO/WHO Expert Committee on Nutrition: Report on the Second Session," (1951): 22–27; "Joint FAO/WHO Expert Committee on Nutrition: Report on the Third Session," World Health Organization Technical Report Series No. 72 (Geneva, 1953). In addition to the regular meetings of the Joint FAO/WHO Expert Committee on Nutrition see J. C. Waterlow, ed., *Protein Malnutrition,* proceedings of a conference in Jamaica, sponsored jointly by the FAO, WHO and the Josiah Macy Jr. Foundation (New York: Cambridge University Press, 1953); "Nutrition Seminar for English-speaking Countries and Territories in Africa South of the Sahara," organized jointly by the Uganda Government, WHO, and FAO at Kampala, Uganda, 25–29 November 1957; "Report of the FAO/WHO Seminar on Problems of Food and Nutrition in Africa South of the Sahara," Lwira, Bukavu (Congo), 18–29 May 1959, FAO Nutrition Meeting Report Series No. 25 (Rome, 1961); "Progress in Meeting Protein Needs of Infants and Preschool Children," proceedings of an international conference held in Washington, DC, 21–24 August 1960.

30. "Lives in Peril," 51.

31. Quote cited from K. J. Carpenter, *Protein and Energy: A Study of Changing Ideas in Nutrition* (New York: Cambridge University Press, 1994): 160; "Lives in Peril," 52.

32. Brock and Autret, "Kwashiorkor in Africa," 69–70; "Joint FAO/WHO Expert Committee on Nutrition: Report on the Second Session," 22–27; "Joint FAO/WHO Expert Committee on Nutrition: Report on the Third Session," 11–15.

33. The distinction is important as protein-rich foods need not resemble milk in regions where milk was not a "traditional" weaning food. "Joint FAO/WHO Expert Committee on Nutrition: Report on the Third Session," 14–15.

34. "Joint FAO/WHO Expert Committee on Nutrition: Fifth Report," World Health Organization Technical Report Series No. 149 (Geneva, 1958), 19–25; "Joint FAO/WHO Expert Committee on Nutrition: Sixth Report," World Health Organization Technical Report Series No. 245 (Geneva, 1962), 55–61.

35. Carpenter, *Protein and Energy,* 178.

36. "Joint FAO/WHO Expert Committee on Nutrition: Sixth Report," 56.

37. Ibid., 40.

38. R. F. A. Dean, "Use of Processed Plant Proteins as Human Food," in *Processed Plant Protein Foodstuffs,* ed. Aaron M. Altschul (New York: Academic Press, 1958), 205–47; "Joint FAO/WHO Expert Committee on Nutrition: Fifth Report," World Health Organization Technical Report Series No. 97 (Geneva, 1955), 8–9.

39. Dean to Williams, 19 June 1952, Wellcome Library PP/CDW L.1. Although further trials proved equally promising, enthusiasm surrounding soy dissipated when

Dean and his colleagues discovered that soy beans were grown locally only as cash crops for export. Dean, "Treatment of Kwashiorkor," 795; Interviews with Ephraim Musoke, Luteete, Uganda, April, 2004 and 3 June 2004.

40. K. Mary Clegg, "The Availability of Lysine in Groundnut Biscuits Used in the Treatment of Kwashiorkor," *British Journal of Nutrition* 14, no. 3 (1960): 325–29; K. M. Clegg and R. F. A. Dean, "Balance Studies on Peanut Biscuit in the Treatment of Kwashiorkor," *American Journal of Clinical Nutrition* 8, no. 6 (1960): 885–95.

41. Dean, "Treatment of Kwashiorkor with Moderate Amounts of Protein," 675.

42. Interview with Dr. Roger Whitehead, Kampala, Uganda, 9 December 2003.

43. "Lives in Peril," 33–39.

44. Interview with Dr. Roger Whitehead, Kampala, Uganda, 9 December 2003.

45. Carpenter, *Protein and Energy*, 178–79.

46. Nevin S. Scrimshaw, "A Look at the Incaparina Experience in Guatemala: The Background and History of Incaparina," *Food and Nutrition Bulletin* 2, no. 2 (1980): 1; also quoted in Carpenter, *Protein and Energy*, 175.

47. Carpenter, *Protein and Energy*, 164.

48. Donald S. McLaren, "The Great Protein Fiasco," *Lancet* 304, no. 7872 (July 1974): 93–96.

49. Donald S. McLaren, "The Great Protein Fiasco Revisited," *Nutrition* 16, no. 6 (2000): 464. For the original articulation of this argument see McLaren, "Great Protein Fiasco," 95.

50. "Correspondence re Kwashiorkor—with DS McLaren, 1972–1975," 1980, PP/CDW, Box 32: H.2/1, Wellcome Library.

51. R. F. A. Dean, "Kwashiorkor in Malaya: The Clinical Evidence (Parts I and II)" *Journal of Tropical Pediatrics* 7, no. 1 (1961): 3–15; "Child Research Unit—Future of the Unit, I," PRO FD 12/274; "Future of Dr. R. G. Whitehead," 24 July 1963, PRO FD 12/274.

52. Whitehead to Lush, 30 November 1964, PRO FD 12/274.

53. "Protein Calorie Malnutrition," in *Medical Care in Developing Countries: A Primer on the Medicine of Poverty and a Symposium from Makerere,* ed. Maurice King (Nairobi: Oxford University Press, 1966), 14:14.

54. D. C. Robinson, "The Nutrition Rehabilitation Unit at Mulago Hospital, Kampala: Further Development and Evaluation, 1967–69," in "Recent Approaches to Malnutrition in Uganda" Monograph No. 13, *Journal of Tropical Pediatrics and Environmental Child Health* 17, no. 1 (1971): 37.

55. D. B. Jelliffe and R. F. A. Dean, "Protein-Calorie Malnutrition in Early Childhood (Practical Notes)," *Journal of Tropical Pediatrics* 5 (December 1959): 98; Dean and Jelliffe, "Diagnosis and Treatment of Protein-Calorie Malnutrition," 429–39.

56. Jelliffe and Dean, "Protein-Calorie Malnutrition in Early Childhood," 103.

57. Minutes of meeting held at the Bishop's House, Namirembe, 9 August 1957, "To Consider the Acceptance and Distribution of Gifts from Church World Service," and Minutes of Welfare Committee, 20 August 1957, Uganda Christian University (UCU) Archives, RG 1/BP/187/3.

58. "Protein Calorie Malnutrition," in *Medical Care in Developing Countries,* ed. King, 14:14.

59. Ibid.

60. Ibid.

61. Interview with Joyce Lukwago Nakidalu, Kisaaku, Uganda, 21 July 2012; Interview with Daisy Nakyejwe, Luteete Uganda, 20 July 2012.

62. Hebe F. Welbourn, "Child Welfare in Mengo District, Uganda," *Journal of Tropical Pediatrics* 2, no. 1 (June 1956): 29.

63. Mary D. Salter Ainsworth, *Infancy in Uganda: Infant Care and the Growth of Love* (Baltimore: Johns Hopkins University Press, 1967), 23.

64. Hebe F. Welbourn, "Bottle Feeding: A Problem of Modern Civilization," *Journal of Tropical Pediatrics* 3, no. 4 (March 1958): 157–66; Ainsworth, *Infancy in Uganda,* 285.

65. Interview with Catherine Nansamba, Luteete, Uganda, 20 July 2012.

66. Welbourn, "Child Welfare in Mengo District, Uganda." Clinics were held in Kampala and in "peri-urban" villages within twenty miles of the capital on a weekly, biweekly or monthly schedule with 7,719 children attending in 1954 alone.

67. Welbourn, "Bottle Feeding," 157.

68. Ibid., 158.

69. Latimer K. Musoke, "An Analysis of Admissions to the Paediatric Division, Mulago Hospital in 1959," *Archives of Disease in Childhood* 36, no. 187 (1961): 310.

70. Josephine M. Namboze, "Weaning Practices in Buganda," *Tropical and Geographical Medicine* 19, no. 2 (1967): 154–56.

71. Hebe F. Welbourn, "Weaning among the Baganda," *Journal of Tropical Pediatrics and African Child Health* 9, no. 1 (June 1963): 17.

72. Musoke, "Analysis of Admissions," 314; "Appendix: Subjects That Might Be Included in a Programme of Nutritional Research in Adults in Kampala," from Dean to Himsworth, 18 January 1963, PRO FD 12/274; D. B. Jelliffe, "The Need for Health Education," in "Health Education and the Mother and Child in East Africa," report of a seminar organized by the Departments of Paediatrics and Child Health, and of Preventive Medicine, with the co-operation of UNICEF, at Makerere Medical School, Kampala Uganda, 12–16 November 1961, 1.

73. Ainsworth, *Infancy in Uganda,* 69.

74. Welbourn, "Weaning among the Baganda," 17; Welbourn, "Bottle Feeding," 164. In children weighing on average between seven and twenty pounds, a one- to two-pound difference was significant.

75. Welbourn, "Bottle Feeding," 162, 165.

76. Ibid., 161–62.

77. Ibid., 165.

78. Musoke, "Analysis of Admissions," 309–10.

79. H. C. Trowell and D. B. Jelliffe, eds., *Diseases of Children in the Subtropics and Tropics* (London: Edward Arnold, 1958): 118–19.

80. Derrick B. Jelliffe and E. F. Patrice Jelliffe, *Human Milk in the Modern World: Psychosocial, Nutritional and Economic Significance* (1978; Oxford: Oxford University Press, 1979), 234.

81. McLaren, "Great Protein Fiasco," 95.

82. Isabelle Defourny et al., "Management of Moderate Acute Malnutrition with RUTF in Niger," *Field Exchange* 31 (2007): 3, http://fex.ennonline.net/31/rutfinniger

JENNIFER TAPPAN

.aspx; Claudine Prudhon et al., eds., "WHO, UNICEF, and SCN Informal Consultation on Community-Based Management of Severe Malnutrition in Children," *Food and Nutrition Bulletin* 27, no. 3 (2006), Supplement-SCN Nutrition Policy Paper no 21; "Severe Malnutrition: Report of a Consultation to Review Current Literature, 6–7 September 2004," Nutrition for Health and Development: World Health Organization (2005).

83. Médecins Sans Frontières (MSF) and VII Photo, "Starved for Attention," accessed 19 September 2011, http://starvedforattention.org/.

84. Locally produced RUTF cost an estimated $3.00/kilogram and treatment for severe acute malnutrition would therefore cost roughly $30 to $45. "Community-Based Management of Severe Acute Malnutrition," a joint statement of the World Health Organization, the World Food Programme, the United Nations System Standing Committee on Nutrition, and the United Nations Children Fund (May 2007). When purchased from Plumpy'nut, the French company holding the international patent, treatment costs an estimated $60. Andrew Rice, "The Peanut Solution," *New York Times Magazine*, 2 September 2010. These figures pertain to treatment and not long-term or ongoing prevention. http://www.nytimes.com/2010/09/05/magazine/05Plumpy-t.html

85. See Jennifer Tappan, "'A Healthy Child Comes from a Healthy Mother': Mwanamugimu and Nutritional Science in Uganda, 1935–1973," PhD diss., Columbia University, 2010.

PART II

❖

The Past in the Present

5

PEOPLE, GREAT APES, DISEASE, AND GLOBAL HEALTH IN THE NORTHERN FORESTS OF EQUATORIAL AFRICA

TAMARA GILES-VERNICK AND STEPHANIE RUPP

Cross-species transmissions—that is, when pathogens infecting one species "jump" to infect another species[1]—pose considerable challenges to global health.[2] As the consequence of complex, dynamic, ongoing interactions between pathogens, people, other mammals, and forest ecologies, cross-species disease transmissions are not unusual in human history; indeed, many human pathogens have animal origins.[3] Moreover, some zoonoses and human diseases of animal origin have developed into devastating global pandemics through the centuries. Consider, for instance, the bubonic plague pandemics, facilitated by global mobility and trades, that ravaged populations from China to Europe from the thirteenth and fourteenth centuries, and wreaked havoc in the late nineteenth century.[4]

But over the last several decades, cross-species transmissions have acquired a singular importance as a major source of "emerging infectious diseases."[5] Studies tell us, for instance, that emerging infectious diseases have increased since 1940, and that more than 60.3 percent of these events are zoonoses.[6] Such alarming reports have only bolstered what Andrew Lakoff and Stephen Collier have described as "a growing perception ... that new biological threats challenge existing ways of understanding and managing collective health and security."[7]

Public health planners perceive the cross-species transmissions that generate new human illnesses as a threat to biosecurity, a preoccupation with securing health that commentators identify as one of global health's central features.[8] Experiences of SARS and other coronaviruses and avian and H1N1 influenza demonstrate all too compellingly that disease transmission between animals and human beings, facilitated by the intensified circulation of people, capital, animals, pathogens, and technologies, are a recurrent aspect of life on earth, often in highly uneven and unpredictable ways. But this alarm may have more to do with contemporary politics of biosecurity preparedness and the exigencies of preparing for the worst possible scenario than it does with genuinely new health threats.[9] Anticipating through surveillance or managing a future threat is patently impossible, inherently incomplete, and extraordinarily costly.[10] But some biomedical researchers and their funders still find that the promise of identifying uncertain future threats justifies funding for research on host shifts.[11]

Central Africa has acquired a notable role in contemporary biomedical analyses, as a site of pathogen sharing, infectious disease emergence, and potential threat to global health security.[12] In central Africa, people, great apes, pathogens, and their broader ecologies have all been significant actors in a dynamic, complex evolutionary history that has produced some of the most devastating pathogens to human beings and nonhuman primates alike. Many diseases afflict both people and great apes, including retroviruses (HIV and SIV), but also hemorrhagic fevers (Ebola and Marburg viruses), falciparum malaria, yellow fever, shigella and salmonella, tuberculosis, filariasis, polio, and anthrax.[13]

Some biomedical researchers, conservation and public health planners, and funding institutions have contended that the threat of cross-species transmissions between people and apes has escalated with intensified "contact" from the early twentieth century—primarily in the form of "anthropogenic change" (more intensive hunting and other forest exploitation practices, population increase, and urbanization), which renders human beings all-powerful (and self-destructive) and great apes defenseless. A historical, anthropological analysis modifies this claim: it shows that "contact" has changed in different ways over time.

This essay examines the implications for global health of integrating longer-term perspectives and local narratives with biomedical understandings about human-ape disease transmission in equatorial Africa's northern forest. It presents evidence that the northern forests where great apes live and where some notable host shifts have occurred have had a lengthy history of human mobility, settlement, trade, and forest exploitation. This history reveals the complexity, variability, and nonlinearity of human–great ape and human-environmental relations. These dynamic processes are at odds with the unilinear assumptions embedded in biomedical and global health analyses of host shifts and epidemic outbreaks in equatorial Africa. These historical patterns underscore the limitations of global health initiatives in predicting and controlling cross-species transmissions. Moreover, northern forest narratives show that "contact" with great apes has been fluid and multifaceted. In contrast to biomedical and global health narratives, not all contact is pathogenic.

This essay is organized in two sections. The first critically evaluates the temporalities used by biomedical (virological, epidemiological, and primatological) researchers and conservation planners, who focus on the uniqueness of recent anthropogenic change in order to project an increased risk of future

TAMARA GILES-VERNICK AND STEPHANIE RUPP

cross-species transmissions and escalating global circulation of pathogens and epidemic disease.[14] The second section analyzes the narratives of people–great ape relations by Africans of the northern forest.

Cross-Species Transmissions, People, and Great Apes

Virologists, primatologists, evolutionary biologists, and epidemiologists have investigated the transmission of pathogenic agents between humans and great apes in the equatorial African forest.[15] A 2010 study identifies Central Africa as a "hotspot" of pathogen sharing and infectious disease emergence, a region where people, chimpanzees, and gorillas engage in frequent, close contact.[16] Some pathogens have shifted from nonhuman primate reservoirs into human populations and vice versa; other infectious diseases have emerged from other animal reservoirs but then infected human and/or nonhuman primates. The role of human-ape contact in provoking cross-species disease transmission is widely debated. According to some evolutionary biologists, virologists, and epidemiologists, contact between people and apes is one factor among many that facilitates disease emergence. Pedersen and Davies, for instance, enumerate three "drivers," all of which *could,* but do not necessarily, implicate human beings: "(1) an increase in host population density and contact rates, (2) environmental changes that effect host quality and demography, and (3) changes in host mobility and behavior."[17]

For pathogens with nonhuman primate origins, some biomedical researchers have placed considerable weight on recent anthropogenic change and emphasize the destructive and deadly consequences of human interventions that facilitate closer contact between people and apes in the equatorial forest, even when they lack compelling virological, epidemiological, or historical evidence of increased encroachment of people on primate habitats. One group of ecological and primatological researchers asserted that "within the last several decades, humans have been responsible for massive, irrevocable changes to primate habitats. . . . As anthropogenic habitat change forces humans and primates into closer and more frequent contact, the risks of interspecific disease transmission increase."[18] Similarly, biomedical researchers studying the origins of HIV have used molecular clocks to suggest that the simian ancestor (SIVcpz) of the pandemic strain of HIV first infected human beings in the early twentieth century.[19] They explain HIV's emergence by identifying "historical" developments occurring at the same time: colonial rule, increased hunting of all game, but especially chimpanzees and gorillas, intensified urbanization, and human migration.[20]

A similar temporality is found in some virological and primatological explanations of Ebola hemorrhagic fever. Wolfe and colleagues cite the escalation of twentieth century hunting and butchering of wild animals (including chimpanzees and other nonhuman primates) as a contributing factor to Ebola transmission and outbreaks in the first decade of the 2000s, observing that

> during the 20th century, firearms increased the efficiency and frequency
> of hunting. Both subsistence and commercial hunting with wire snares
> and firearms are widespread activities through the forests of central
> Africa. . . . In addition, road networks and increasing opportunities for
> transporting hunted game have led to an increase in sales and the rate
> of hunting.[21]

Nonetheless, virologists conducting a phylogenetic analysis of the Ebola viruses circulating among people and great apes in previous outbreaks have presented models of "multiple independent emergence" of the virus lineages.[22] The authors suggest that complex patterns of mobility and contact within the animal reservoir (fruit bats), but also movement and contact of "susceptible species" (great apes, people, or other susceptible animals) triggered these outbreaks.[23] In this view, nonanthropogenic change may have contributed to or triggered Ebola's emergence.

The degree to which human action contributes to the spread of Ebola hemorrhagic fever outbreaks once they have erupted in human populations is unclear. Multiple modes of transmission sustain these outbreaks. Human contact with meat or bodily fluids of great apes (and other forest animals) in contexts of hunting, trapping, and butchering is an important risk factor, but scientific research also brings human beings in proximity to apes and can facilitate virus transmission. In addition, human contact with sick patients in health care settings and with the deceased during funerary rites is especially risky.[24]

Some researchers have projected uncertainties about contemporary host shifts, emergence, and transmission and projected them into future threats. They argue that understanding the dynamics of any cross-species transmission is of critical *future* importance, since it permits insight into the emergence of new viruses and provides the impetus for epidemiological surveillance to detect them.[25] Biomedical researchers have used these arguments to rally popular support for their research. Primatologists have worried in the pages of the journal *Nature* that these host shifts threaten the future of chimpanzee and gorilla populations in Africa.

Fundamentally, such arguments about unidirectional disease transmission between apes and humans rest on erroneous historical and cultural assumptions.

TAMARA GILES-VERNICK AND STEPHANIE RUPP

By focusing on twentieth-century changes to the equatorial African rain forest, such analyses presume that colonial rule violently wrested the entire forest and its population from a precolonial equilibrium, and that hunting of great apes has escalated steadily ever since.

Long-Term Historical Change in the Equatorial African Forests

Human–great ape contact has a very long history in equatorial Africa. Human habitation of the equatorial African rain forests extends as far back as 40,000 to 35,000 B.P., and development and growth of forest villages and agriculture in present-day southern Cameroon date to the mid-to-late second millennium B.C.E.[26] The forest-farming complex, which included forest disturbance through fire and clearing, provided a habitat conducive to breeding of *Anopheles gambiae*, the mosquito "complex" most heavily involved in falciparum malaria transmission in Africa.[27] Some groups of forest-dwelling peoples practiced sedentary lives, whereas others were more mobile, but Kairn Klieman finds linguistic evidence of much larger human settlements that came with the cultivation of yams, bananas/plantains, and flourishing regional trade developing in the equatorial African rain forest between 1500 and 500 B.C.E.[28] This evidence, though distant from contemporary debates, highlights that mobility, hunting, trade, settlement, and forest disturbance have a very long history in the equatorial forests.

Viewing African history over the *longue durée* also offers insight into an earlier host shift between human beings and nonhuman primates. The nonhuman primate origins of *Plasmodium falciparum* (malaria) have come under scrutiny in the past several years, with researchers debating whether falciparum malaria crossed from western lowland gorillas, chimpanzees, or bonobos to people or through contact with other non-ape primates.[29] Despite controversy over methods and interpretations of results, these studies attest to very long term, intensive contact between human and nonhuman primates, with the significant host shift of falciparum malaria from nonhuman primates to people. The date of this shift remains the subject of ongoing research and debate, with hypotheses as of 2013 ranging from 50,000 years ago, when human beings left Africa; to between the second and first millennia B.C.E., with the expansion of plantain/banana cultivation and of larger human settlements in the rainforests; to between 112,000 and 1,036,000 years ago (median 365,000 years ago).[30]

Even in more recent centuries, human mobility, settlement, trade, and contact with great apes were all features of this dynamic forest region. In the nineteenth century, pressures on northern equatorial forest inhabitants came from the north, south, and east, precipitating a period of intensive warfare, flight, and slave raiding, as well as hunting and trade in food crops and forest bark products for bodily adornment.[31]

During the nineteenth century, some social groups within the Sangha basin forests and further south hunted chimpanzees and gorillas.[32] In the nineteenth century, big game hunting and trapping were sufficiently effective to supply a dynamic regional and international trade in ivory and meat, and in some parts of central Africa to deplete elephant populations.[33]

This brief historical sketch suggests that late twentieth-century political ecological changes are part of a much longer history. The "scientific" assumption that human beings had little or no contact with great apes in the equatorial forests prior to the twentieth century is naive and uninformed.

People and Apes: Narratives from the Northern Equatorial African Forests

African narratives reflect on the interactions between people and apes over at least the past century and a half in the northern forest societies of equatorial Africa.[34] In contrast to biomedical assumptions presuming that "contact" comes only in the form of destructive "anthropogenic change" with inherently devastating consequences, northern forest narratives suggest a greater range of and fluidity in human interactions with apes and some monkeys. These narratives reveal great apes and some monkeys as simultaneously part of and distinct from human worlds; the narratives elicit a sense of familiarity with great apes and monkeys, recount recollections of a distant shared past, and reveal exchanged knowledge of forest spaces and resources, but they also evoke fierce competition for forest resources, and sometimes the risk of illness and death.[35] The equatorial African narratives suggest that people-ape contact is intimate and of long standing.

In this analysis, "northern forest societies" refer to a region of northern Gabon and the Sangha River basin that has long been peopled by a mosaic of interacting language groups (including Bantu A.80 and C.10 groups as well as the Bangando-Ngombe subgroup of the Gbaya branch of Ubangian languages). In the nineteenth century, these groups shared patterns of political and social organization: they were small-scale, geographically scattered, highly mobile collectivities (frequently patriclans), often organized around an open shelter (council house) where male kin would gather, allocate labor and food from a constellation of wives' kitchens, and adjudicate disputes. They developed close relations with neighboring communities, leading to sustained economic, linguistic, agricultural, and cultural exchanges that interwove this complex cultural

TAMARA GILES-VERNICK AND STEPHANIE RUPP

mosaic. Prior to the mid-nineteenth century, middle and upper Sangha basin peoples engaged in small-scale trade, concluded blood brotherhoods and marriages, exchanged different varieties of maize, cassava, and yams, and shared other forms of cultural expressions.[36] After midcentury, increased competition for slave labor and forest resources precipitated small-scale flight among upper and middle Sangha basin peoples. Oral and explorers' accounts attest to warfare, shifting alliances, and mutual enslavement among Mpiemu and Bakwele, Gbaya, Bangando, and Kako speakers within the Sangha forests—relations that both divided and brought communities together in complex, dynamic consociation.

GREAT APES AND HUMAN ORIGIN STORIES

The northern forest narratives portray past dynamics of collaboration, competition, exchange, and expropriation between people and great apes, and the varied consequences of ape-human contact. Bulu and Beti peoples living in southeastern Cameroon in the early twentieth century invoked a distant, undated past in which people and gorillas were connected by kin ties and mutual rights and obligation and occupied the same domestic spaces. Families included both people and apes, and relatives were expected to behave according to rules of respect, sharing, and mutual support. One gorilla's rapacity for meat and women, however, ruptured this peaceful cohabitation between people and gorillas. The gorilla demanded more than his share of family resources, staking a claim to the prized head of a killed elephant and sleeping with one of his human uncle's wives, when he had rights only to the meat or the woman. His voracious appetite sparked hostilities between people and gorillas and resulted in human banishment of gorillas to the forest.[37]

Baka forest peoples, also living in the southeastern Cameroon and northern Gabon, similarly populated their origin stories with gorillas and chimpanzees. They contended that among the original Baka ancestors was Chimpanzee (*seko*), whose "crazy" behavior offended all: "He acted out of control. He lashed out in every direction, broke everything, climbed everywhere, cried out for no reason, jumped everywhere, without being aware of the dangers."[38] When he abducted the baby girl of the Baka deity Komba, the deity punished him, relegating him to the level of animals. Although this origin story again reflects on the common origins and social lives that people and great apes once shared, it also comments on the rapacity and lack of restraint of chimpanzees and gorillas in order to explain their exile from human society. Even after Chimpanzee's exile, Baka human ancestors continued to interact with the neighboring village of "fur-bearing primates," which included Chimpanzee (*seko*), Gorilla

People, Great Apes, and Disease in Equatorial Africa

(*ebobo*), and Monkey (*kema*). This story, too, reveals a fluidity between human and animal worlds. In contrast to the previous narrative, a deity—not people—wielded the authority to cast Chimpanzee from human society because of his rapacity and lack of restraint. But that exile was incomplete, because the human-ape interactions continued.

Great apes also appear as powerful actors in human history. Bangando peoples of southeastern Cameroon have recounted their nineteenth-century migrations, when their ancestors were subject to violence precipitated by the Sokoto Caliphate's centralization and ensuing competition for slaves and trade in forest resources in the grasslands north of the forest zone. The Caliphate's activities exerted pressures on savanna and northern forest societies, which in turn engaged in mutual slave raiding and competition for forest resources. Oral historical testimonies recount that Bangando clans fled through the forest-grassland mosaic of the Sangha River region, moving deeper into the forest of the Congo River basin. Members of the *bo dawa* clan (clan of primates) recount that their ancestors were rescued by chimpanzees, which heard the people's calls of distress. From their vantage point high in the forest canopy, the chimpanzees were able to guide Bangando ancestors away from the invaders, leading them to safety deep in the forest. *Bo dawa* clans members still abstain from eating the meat of all monkeys and great apes, citing continuing respect for the ancestral chimpanzees that rescued their vulnerable forebears.[39]

Some northern forest societies have expressed respect for great apes' knowledge of forest plants and trees. In both southwestern Central African Republic, Mpiemu healers contended in the 1990s that they would observe the behavior of gorillas and chimpanzees to learn about the locations and properties of foods and medicinal plants in the forest.[40]

Societies in the northern forest have sought to appropriate great ape power, but this time to bolster male authority. During the 1960s, Fang people in northern Gabon symbolically integrated gorillas' power into men's council houses, the sites of male reproduction, by placing gorilla skulls on the central support poles. This central support served as a spatial and symbolic anchor for ceremonies; people entering or leaving the council house would lay a hand on the pole, hoping to appropriate some of the gorilla's power.[41] The integration of gorilla body parts into social and symbolic spaces echoes human domination of gorillas described in biomedical narratives. Violence undergirded this appropriation of power: the skull was an object of power, but the gorilla itself was dead. This practice is not isolated to northern Gabon: the anthropologist Axel Kohler, working in nearby southern Congo in the early 2000s, observed

TAMARA GILES-VERNICK AND STEPHANIE RUPP

that gorilla skulls in council houses served as a display of political authority and to highlight a hunter's prowess.[42]

Interactions between great apes and human beings also came with the threat of dangerous, even disastrous consequences, including violence and death. One account from northern Gabon explored the potential for interspecies collaboration, even as it quarried human (and perhaps simian) fears of interspecies contact. In this story, a mother could not undertake work in her garden day after day because her sobbing, inconsolable baby required constant and undivided attention. An empathetic gorilla, however, emerged from the forest and offered to care for the baby so that the mother could finish her work. But the gorilla warned the woman, "Never tell anyone [of my help] . . . or else bad things will happen to you and your child. Death does not come from the forest, but from the village."[43] The gorilla comforted the woman's baby throughout the day, allowing the woman to work in her field. That night, unable to resist telling her husband of the extraordinary events, she confided in him. The man surreptitiously followed his wife to the field the following day, to find the gorilla calming the baby in her arms, just as his wife had described. Gripped by the fear that the gorilla would harm the baby, the husband fired his rifle at the gorilla, accidentally killing his own child. By highlighting the gorilla's capacity for empathy and the woman's capacity for trust, the tale suggests that people and apes shared qualities that made interspecies intimacy and cooperation possible. However, the tale's tragic conclusion emphasizes that despite these shared capacities, ultimately people and apes simply could not engage in such close interactions, which would result only in violence, destruction, and tragedy.

Fears about the mingling of humans and great apes may also reflect and be buttressed by long-term material struggles between people and apes over forest spaces and resources. In the middle Sangha river basin forest, stories of gorillas becoming ensnared in hunting nets and then attacking and injuring hunters have circulated for many decades, among Swedish missionaries in the 1930s and '40s and among hunters and trappers in the 1990s. In southeastern Cameroon in the late 1990s, Bangando peoples explained a particular instance of interspecies competition. During the short, dry season, the ripening bush mangoes (*Irvingia excelsa*) attract apes and smaller monkeys but also bring Bangando and Baka families into the forest to harvest them. To prevent direct contact between people and apes, parents exhorted their children to sing songs, dance, and play games rambunctiously while they lived in forest camps, frightening the apes away. People expressed considerable urgency in keeping gorillas and chimpanzees at a safe distance from the stands of mango trees, not only because these apes posed competition for food but also because in the context of contemporary ape (and other bushmeat) hunting, parents feared gorillas' aggressive attacks on their families.[44] Like some of the preceding narratives, this one portrays human beings and great apes alike as powerful actors in a competition for food and forest spaces, and it reflects an abiding anxiety over the potentially violent consequences of this competition.

GREAT APES AND INFECTIOUS SPACES

A sense of anxiety and danger manifested itself in certain narratives that linked space and resource competition between people and great apes with human illness. Some of the evidence from naturalist and missionary archives in the 1930s and '40s, and from ethnographic accounts in the late 1990s and 2000s, indicate that contact with great apes can sometimes bring nefarious health consequences, ranging from persistent coughs and dysentery to sleeping sickness. At other times, such interspecies contact may affect human health but for reasons that have less to do with destructive human "contact" with apes and more to do with active competition among people, or between people and great apes. We explore here the logic behind these etiologies by examining sleeping sickness in the 1930s and '40s and Ebola virus in the first decade of the 2000s.

From the early twentieth century through the 1940s, parts of the northern equatorial African forest experienced persistent epidemics of sleeping sickness.[45] In 1929, Henry Raven, a curator for the American Museum of Natural History and a zoology lecturer at Columbia University, traveled to the forests of Lomié, Dja, and Abong Mbang in southeastern Cameroon to collect gorilla and chimpanzee specimens for the museum. In one chapter of *In Quest of Gorillas* titled "Gorillas, Men and Sleeping Sickness," Raven maintained that gorillas and Africans competed for the same ecological spaces, but that the introduction of firearms and Western medicine to control sleeping sickness gave human beings an advantage over gorillas:

> As the native population increased, new villages would be formed and more clearings made. Then epidemics would occur, killing off great numbers of natives, and their gardens would be neglected to run into secondary growth. The gorillas, with a constitution so nearly like that of man that they can find more food in human plantations than in the virgin forest, would move into these deserted clearings. There with an abundance of food they throve and congregated, to such an extent

TAMARA GILES-VERNICK AND STEPHANIE RUPP

eventually that if only a few natives remained they were actually driven out because of their inability to protect their crops against gorillas. But with the advent of the white men's government, with the distribution of firearms among the natives, preventive medicine and the treatment for epidemic and infective diseases, man has the upper hand at present in this age-long struggle.[46]

Raven thus celebrated the triumph of colonial medicine and technology over disease, and of human dominion over animals. But this triumph was seemingly undercut by another dynamic, described by African assistants to the expedition and to villagers visiting Raven's camp: the ravages of sleeping sickness and shifting frontiers of gorilla and human habitation.[47] Raven's central African assistants alerted him to these patterns of sleeping sickness and gorilla and human colonization of forest sites. Indeed they warned him not to investigate a part of the forest with high gorilla population densities because

> people that went there died of sleeping sickness. I had been told that there were no inhabitants. . . . When we reached there I found a deserted hut by the roadside, but all about was the densest type of jungle and the remains of a great many native houses that had tumbled down. (Emphasis added)[48]

What then happened must have convinced Raven's assistants that their fears were well founded. The day after arriving in the forest inhabited by gorillas, Raven fell sick with a host of illnesses, including sleeping sickness.[49] It appears, however, that the assistants' etiology of sleeping sickness differed from Raven's. Raven contended that people and great apes competed for specific forest spaces, but then sleeping sickness epidemics ravaged human populations, so that they could no longer cope with an advancing frontier of gorilla settlement. But his assistants suggested something different: that people traveling to particular sites with high gorilla densities could fall ill from sleeping sickness. Whether the site was "sick"—or whether the presence of gorillas made it so—is unclear.

This linkage between human-ape competition for habitable spaces and illness was echoed on the other bank of the Sangha river, in southwestern Ubangi-Shari (now Central African Republic). According to the Catholic priest Monseigneur Sintas, gorillas far outnumbered people in the upper Sangha basin forest, and these great apes "love[d] to amuse themselves by terrorizing women and children."[50] Commenting on the ravages of sleeping sickness and the consequent human depopulation of the forests, Sintas observed, "For hundreds of kilometers, one encounters no other inhabitants except for gorillas and chimpanzees, who establish their habitats among the old villages and old plantations of those who were once called the Mbimous."[51] Sintas's writings suggest that his assistants and Catholic followers influenced considerably his perceptions, although we can only speculate whether they suggested that sleeping sickness cleared these spaces of human habitation, leaving them open for recolonization by gorillas.

Hence, whereas Raven optimistically highlighted the role of weapons and medicines in giving humans an ultimate upper hand in the competition for forest resources, Sintas, writing a decade later, emphasized the receding frontier of human habitation, and a concomitant wave of gorilla colonization as the result of sleeping sickness epidemics. Although their assistants' and followers' influence remains murky, it appears that in both cases, gorillas were clearly the more powerful agents of change, possibly by "infecting" spaces or by reaping the rewards of human mortality from repeated epidemics.

Sleeping sickness epidemics in the Sangha basin waned in the 1950s, but have reemerged in recent decades.[52] No biomedical studies to our knowledge link gorillas and sleeping sickness, but ethnohistorical research may nonetheless prove useful. It would be possible, for instance, to investigate these sites heavily populated by gorillas. Is there something about the tsetse vector and local ecologies, for instance, that facilitates trypanosomiasis transmission? Such a study might permit researchers to study further the complex and changing relations between forest ecologies, tsetse vectors, and changing gorilla and human use of these zones.[53] Such questions, however, involve a radical decontextualization of this "local knowledge," extracting a single claim from a variegated body of knowledge about gorillas and other great apes. If we isolate this single claim (gorillas compete with people to inhabit particular "sick" landscapes) from a broader range of conceptions of great apes, we risk losing sight of other equally important concerns: people's shared but ruptured histories with great apes, as well as people's anxieties about competition for forest resources with apes.

A second example addresses Ebola hemorrhagic fever outbreaks, which many epidemiological and virological studies have traced to contact with infected great apes.[54] The sole published ethnographic studies of equatorial Africans affected by these outbreaks in the 2000s are by medical anthropologists Barry Hewlett and Bonnie Hewlett. We draw heavily from their work below to show how great apes figure into local etiologies of outbreak, but in ways that differ substantially from evaluations by virologists and epidemiologists.[55]

The place that equatorial Africans attributed to great apes in Ebola virus outbreaks varied across the region and over time. In southeastern Cameroon where Stephanie Rupp conducted field research, hunters were aware of the

TAMARA GILES-VERNICK AND STEPHANIE RUPP

1999 outbreak in Gabon through a shortwave radio broadcast of an international news report, but expressed doubt that contact with bodily fluids of infected chimpanzees and gorillas could make them sick. Nevertheless, when the Hewletts were conducting "outbreak ethnography" in the Republic of Congo in 2003 and northern Gabon in 1997[56] (where the outbreak's origins began with hunters exposed to the infected flesh of gorillas or antelopes), informants did recognize that great apes were also afflicted by Ebola virus.[57] Moreover, in the Gabonese outbreak, they had detailed knowledge of the index case—a hunter who had found a dead gorilla in the forest and had brought it back to his village to share it with others.

But the Hewletts' informants in Gabon and Congo explained the illness in diverse ways, although we focus here primarily on great apes.[58] In Gabon, *ezanga* ("bad human-like sprits that cause illness in people who accumulate [things] and do not share") figured prominently in explanations. As the Hewletts explained, "Persons who are jealous of the material wealth or sociopolitical power of others can secretly send *ezanga* to eat their internal organs, making them sick or die."[59] Significantly, *ezanga* "can also transform people into chimps, gorillas, or elephants—agents that can cause sickness in others."[60] Hence, we see again a much older fluidity between human and ape realms, wherein human contact with a dead ape can cause devastating illness, but the agent of that illness is neither a chimp nor a gorilla, but rather another (envious) person. In Congo the researchers found that explanations shifted over a relatively short period of time. Some informants began to argue against sorcery or other supernatural explanations, arguing that the outbreak was caused by an *ekono,* an illness caused by contact with polluted people or substances, or more gravely, by an *opepe,* an epidemic in which the infective substances is transmitted by air or wind.[61] As Barry Hewlett and Melissa Leach later observed, these explanations for Ebola combine local cultural models for the infection and disease—contact with pollution and transmission by malevolent wind—with biomedical models of hemorrhagic fevers as spread by contact with contaminated body fluids of great apes.[62]

Specific claims about gorilla or great ape involvement in transmitting a particular illness are part of a broader, complex, and varied body of knowledge (and practice) about great apes in the northern equatorial forest. It may be possible to extract specific claims, for instance, about gorillas and diseased spaces, to be investigated by specialists exploring changing disease ecology. But this effort would also isolate a single claim from a complex and sometimes contradictory body of knowledge of these nonhuman primates. It would elide the deep ambivalence that northern forest peoples appear to express—their

People, Great Apes, and Disease in Equatorial Africa

anxieties over the risky and potentially treacherous consequences of contact, but also the shared histories and the promise of social and material benefits. This decontextualization would thus suppress the range of rich social, cultural, and historical understandings of great apes.

Nevertheless, the Hewletts do identify numerous important contributions that "outbreak anthropology" can make to efforts at outbreak control.[63] Although people normally eat dead animals found in the forest, they did not object to avoiding dead gorillas and chimpanzees during outbreaks. Complete bans on game meat consumption, however, posed huge difficulties because of a dearth of affordable protein; in the Republic of Congo, it also fanned mistrust of game park officials. Among their many recommendations, the Hewletts argued for continuing a ban on chimpanzee and gorilla consumption, but not outlawing all game meat consumption during outbreaks. We would add here that public health workers could mobilize this long-standing ambivalence about great apes; they could communicate the risks of contact with infected apes by drawing on the past and present stories that people tell about gorillas and chimpanzees. And over the longer term, these understandings could help initiate local and national reflection about great ape hunting in equatorial African forests and its control, particularly now that gorilla and chimpanzee populations have been decimated by Ebola virus.[64] To be sure, ministry officials, local authorities, antipoaching patrols, and conservationists all attest to the difficulty of controlling great ape hunting, particularly when hunters come from outside of these forest regions and are so heavily armed. Allocating resources not just for antipoaching efforts but also for developing alternative economic opportunities could lighten hunting pressure on great apes. But most important, the multifaceted narratives about contact with great apes could draw attention away from stigmatizing criticisms of equatorial African hunting practices, and instead focus attention on the poverty and political marginalization that populations in the northern forest face.[65] At the very least, international investment in local health infrastructures and personnel could make a major difference in the precarious health of northern forest populations.

This chapter offers some ethnographic and historical perspectives on human-ape contact as the source of host shifts, infectious disease epidemics, and mortality. We show that biomedical researchers have asserted that in the recent past anthropogenic change has provoked host shifts that have

TAMARA GILES-VERNICK AND STEPHANIE RUPP

devastated human and great ape populations alike; from these assertions, they project an uncertain future of further host shifts, epidemics, and dwindling great ape populations in the equatorial African rain forests. This imagined future has critical global health implications, for it justifies additional funding for future research, and it is used to exert political pressure on central African states to suppress great ape hunting.

The foreshortened time frame is deeply misleading. It fails to consider twentieth-century human mobility and great ape hunting in the context of longer historical continuities. A longer-term historical perspective casts doubt on these suppositions of an early twentieth-century watershed in people-ape relations. It can also signal other important changes contributing to cross-species transmission: climatic and environmental changes, shifting land uses, local institutions, poverty, and changing health care resources and personnel.[66] Investigating these changes is important because it may well lead to more nuanced, locally contextualized understandings of patterns of host shifts and infectious disease outbreaks. At the same time, global health efforts to predict and control host shifts will invariably fall short; these shifts are too complex, too varied, and too unpredictable to manage.

Some northern equatorial forest societies have understood their interactions with great apes as characterized by long-term material and sociocultural exchanges and expropriations. Northern forest peoples have emphasized that they share much with apes: histories of origin and kinship, cohabitation, and forest knowledge, but they also have long engaged in competition fraught with anxiety and danger. Their narratives express a deep ambivalence about gorillas and chimpanzees, because these animals are active agents in human lives, capable of making their actions felt in human worlds. Etiologies of infectious diseases, including sleeping sickness and Ebola virus, seem to draw from these foundations.

Such insights can be integrated into global health interventions. People living in the forests in proximity to great apes and near sites of outbreaks frequently know much about local ecologies and epidemiologies. Such local claims should also be understood in the terms through which they are expressed, as part of a broad, varied body of knowledge about great apes. We have suggested above some productive ways that this knowledge may be used to communicate the risks of zoonotic disease transmission, to raise debates about hunting practices within the northern forest, or to deflect attentions from these practices to genuinely pressing concerns about woefully inadequate health care infrastructures in this region.

Notes

1. "Zoonotic diseases," which infect a particular animal population but then leap directly to infect human populations, are but one type of cross-species transmission. Rabies, Ebola virus, and influenza are examples of zoonoses. Not all host shifts are considered zoonoses; instead, they require some form of adaptation in order to be transmitted between people. Personal communication, François Simon, September 2012; P. A. Marx, C. Apetrei, and E. Drucker, "AIDS as a Zoonosis? Confusion over the Origin of the Virus and the Origin of the Epidemics," *Journal of Medical Primatology* 33, no. 5–6 (2004): 220–26.

2. Many definitions of global health explicitly or implicitly rely on Yach and Bettcher's characterization of the globalization of public health in terms of a "process of increasing political, economic, and social interdependence and global integration that occurs as capital, traded goods, people, concepts, images, ideas and values diffuse across national boundaries." D. Yach and D. Bettcher, "The Globalization of Public Health," *American Journal of Public Health* 88, no. 5 (1998): 735–38; quoted in T. Brown, M. Cueto, and E. Fee, "The World Health Organization and the Transition from 'International' to 'Global' Public Health," *American Journal of Public Health* 96, no. 1(2006): 62–72; L. Gostin and E. Mok, "Grand Challenges in Global Health Governance," *British Medical Bulletin* 90 (2009), 7–8; C. Janes and K. Corbett, "Anthropology and Global Health," *Annual Review of Anthropology* 38 (2009), 167–83. Some historians have roundly criticized the ahistoricity of this definition, contending that these processes of interdependence and integration have existed for centuries (see F. Cooper, "What Is the Concept of Globalization Good For? An African Historian's Perspective," *African Affairs* 100, no. 399 [2001]: 55–71). Adams, Novotny, and Leslie have noted some genuinely new features that characterize global health: "the changing environment of funding for health development, particularly the growth in non-governmental structures alongside traditional multilateral and bilateral organizations; . . . an increase in pharmaceutical and clinical research in global health; the emergence of new concerns for 'biosecurity.'" V. Adams, T. Novotny, and H. Leslie, "Global Health Diplomacy," *Medical Anthropology* 27, no. 4 (2008): 315–23.

3. J. O. Lloyd-Smith et al., "Epidemic Dynamics at the Human-Animal Interface," *Science* 326, no. 1362 (2009): 1362–67; N. D. Wolfe et al., "Bushmeat Hunting, Deforestation, and Prediction of Zoonotic Disease Emergence," *Emerging Infectious Diseases* 11, no. 12 (2005): 1822–27; S. S. Morse, "Factors in the Emergence of Infectious Diseases," *Emerging Infectious Diseases* 1, no. 1 (1995): 7–15.

4. M. Echenberg, *Plague Ports: The Global Urban Impact of Bubonic Plague, 1894–1901* (New York: New York University Press, 2008).

5. Morse, "Emergence," 7.

6. K. E. Jones et al., "Global Trends in Emerging Infectious Diseases," *Nature* 451, no. 7181 (2008): 990–93.

7. S. Collier and A. Lakoff, "The Problem of Securing Health," in *Biosecurity Interventions: Global Health and Security in Question,* ed. A. Lakoff and S. Collier (New York: Columbia University Press, 2008), 8.

8. WHO/FAO/OIE, 2004; Adams, Novotny, and Leslie, "Global Health."

9. A. Lakoff, "Preparing for the Next Emergency," *Public Culture* 19, no. 2 (2007): 246–71.

10. For an influential analysis of "biosecuring" ("attempts to manage the movement of . . . diseases" and the "unfinished business of making safe"), see S. Hinchliffe and N. Bingham, "Securing Life: The Emerging Practices of Biosecurity," *Environment and Planning A* 40, no. 7 (2008): 1535–42.

11. T. MacPhail, "A Predictable Unpredictability: The 2009 H1N1 Pandemic and the Concept of 'Strategic Uncertainty' within the Concept of Global Health," *Behemoth* 3, no. 3 (2010): 57–77.

12. A. G. Pedersen and T. J. Davies, "Cross-Species Pathogen Transmission and Disease Emergence in Primates," *EcoHealth* 6, no. 4 (2010): 496–508; P. Wald, *Contagious: Cultures, Carriers, and the Outbreak Narrative* (Durham, NC: Duke University Press, 2008).

13. S. Calattini et al., "Simian Foamy Virus Transmission from Apes to Humans, Rural Cameroon," *Emerging Infectious Diseases* 13, no. 9 (2007): 1314–20; C. A. Chapman, T. R. Gillespie, and T. L. Goldberg, "Primates and the Ecology of Their Infectious Diseases: How Will Anthropogenic Change Affect Host-Parasite Interactions?" *Evolutionary Anthropology* 14 (2005): 134–35; R. Prugnolle et al., "African Monkeys Are Infected by *Plasmodium falciparum* Non-Human Primate Specific Strains," *Proceedings of the National Academy of Sciences* 108, no. 29 (2011): 11948–53; W. Liu et al., "Origins of the Human Malaria Parasite *Plasmodium falciparum* in Gorillas," *Nature* 467, no. 7314 (2010), downloaded 31 March 2011, www.nature.com/nature/journal /v467/n7314/full/nature09442.html; more broadly, see Lloyd-Smith et al., "Epidemic Dynamics."

14. N. D. Wolfe et al., "Exposure to Nonhuman Primates in Rural Cameroon," *Emerging Infectious Diseases* 10, no. 12 (2004), 2094–99; Wolfe et al., "Bushmeat Hunting"; P. D. Walsh et al., "Catastrophic Ape Decline in Western Equatorial Africa," *Nature* 422, no. 6932 (2003): 611–14; Jones et al., "Global Trends."

15. Pedersen and Davies, "Cross-Species Pathogen"; Lloyd-Smith et al., "Epidemic Dynamics"; Calattini et al., "Simian Foamy Virus."

16. Pedersen and Davis, "Cross-Species Pathogen."

17. Ibid., 497; see also Morse, "Emergence."

18. Chapman, Gillespie, and Goldberg, "Primates," 134.

19. D. M. Tebit and E. J. Arts, "Tracking a Century of Global Expansion and Evolution of HIV to Drive Understanding and to Combat Disease: Review Article," *Lancet Infectious Diseases* 11, no. 1 (2011): 45–56; J. D. de Sousa et al., "High GUD Incidence in the Early 20th Century Created a Particularly Permissive Time Window for the Origin and Initial Spread of Epidemic HIV Strains," *PLoS One* 5, no. 4 (2010): e9936; M. Worobey et al., "Direct Evidence of Extensive Diversity of HIV-1 in Kinshasa by 1960," *Nature* 455, no. 7213 (2008): 661–65.

20. T. Giles-Vernick is working with Guillaume Lachenal, William Schneider, and Didier Gondola to write a fuller, more historically grounded context in which to situate the emergence of HIV/AIDS. J. Takehisa et al., "Origin and Biology of Simian Immunodeficiency Virus in Wild-Living Western Gorillas," *Journal of Virology* 83, no. 4 (2009): 1635–48; Worobey et al., "Direct Evidence"; Wolfe et al., "Bushmeat Hunting"; Wolfe et al., "Exposure"; A. Chitnis, D. Rawls, and J. Moore, "Origin of HIV Type 1 in Colonial French Equatorial Africa?" *AIDS Research and Human Retroviruses* 16, no.

1 (2000): 5–8; B. H. Hahn et al., "AIDS as a Zoonosis: Scientific and Public Health Implications," *Science* 287, no. 5453 (2000): 607–14.

21. Wolfe et al., "Exposure"; see also Walsh et al., "Catastrophic Ape Decline."

22. T. J. Wittmann et al., "Isolates of Zaire Ebolavirus from Wild Apes Reveal Genetic Lineage and Recombinants," *Proceedings of the National Academy of Sciences* 104, no. 43 (2007): 17125.

23. Wittmann, "Isolates," 17126; P. D. Walsh et al., "Potential for Ebola Transmission between Gorilla and Chimpanzee Social Groups," *American Naturalist* 169, no. 5 (2007): 684–89.

24. M. Leach and B. Hewlett, "Haemorrhagic Fevers: Narratives, Politics and Pathways," in *Epidemics: Science, Governance and Social Justice*, ed. S. Dry and M. Leach (London: Earthscan, 2010), 43–69; B. L. Hewlett and B. S. Hewlett, *Ebola, Culture, and Politics: The Anthropology of an Emerging Disease* (Belmont, CA: Thomson Wadsworth, 2008); E. M. Leroy et al., "Multiple Ebola Transmission Events and Rapid Decline of Central African Wildlife. *Science* 202, no. 5656 (2004): 387–90; B. S. Hewlett and R. P. Amola, "Cultural Contexts of Ebola in Northern Uganda," *Emerging Infectious Diseases* 9, no. 10 (2003): 1242–48.

25. See N. D. Wolfe, C. P. Dunavan, and J. Diamond, "Origins of Major Human Infectious Diseases," *Nature* 447, no. 7142 (2007): 279–83. This argument, undergirded by what MacPhail has called a "strategic uncertainty" offers compelling reasons for institutions to support this research, although one virologist admitted to me that he thought that his own research on simian viruses had "no public health implications." But many researchers argue that the poorly understood nature of cross-species transmission and the future threats that they pose amply justify funding. A consortium of researchers from the United States and the UK has made a similar argument, receiving some £1.8 million to study the emergence of HIV in Uganda during the 1970s, on the grounds that the study will illuminate "how retroviruses are maintained in primate populations" and how human practices and beliefs may facilitate retrovirus host shifts between red colobus monkeys and people. MacPhail, "Predictable Unpredictability"; "£300,000 for New Study into the Origin of AIDS," University of Bristol, 13 September 2011, http://bristol.ac.uk/news/2011/7892.html.

26. See A. Holl, "Cameroun," in *Aux origines de l'Afrique Centrale*, ed. R. Lanfrachi and B. Clist (Libreville: Centre culturel français, 1981), 149–54, 193–96, cited in Kairn Klieman, *"The Pygmies Were Our Compass": Bantu and Batwa in the History of West Central Africa, Early Times to c. 1900 C.E.* (Portsmouth: Heinemann, 2003), 40.

27. See James L. A. Webb, Jr., *Humanity's Burden: A Global History of Malaria* (Cambridge: Cambridge University Press, 2009) for an extended discussion of how forest agriculture facilitated the transmission of falciparum malaria.

28. Klieman, *Pygmies*; see also Webb, *Humanity's Burden*.

29. Liu et al., "Origins"; Prugnolle at al., "African Monkeys." See also Loretta A. Cormier, *The Ten-Thousand Year Fever: Rethinking Human and Wild-Primate Malaria* (Walnut Creek, CA: Left Coast Press, 2011), 63–70.

30. K. Tanabe et al., "*Plasmodium falciparum* Accompanied the Human Expansion out of Africa," *Current Biology* 20, no. 14 (2010): 1283–89; Webb, *Humanity's Burden;* Cormier, *Ten-Thousand Year Fever,* 55–70; J. M. Baron, J. M. Higgins, and W. H. Dzik,

"A Revised Timeline for the Origin of *Plasmodium falciparum* as a Human Pathogen," *Journal of Molecular Evolution* 73, no. 5–6 (2011): 297–304.

31. Congo river trading activities that developed in the seventeenth and eighteenth centuries encompassed part of the Sangha basin during much of the nineteenth century, with a highly active exchanges in guns, local slaves, ivory, foods, and other commodities. Riverine societies along the Sangha, Alima, and Likouala Rivers were major providers of manioc and palm oil, which fueled these long- and short-distance trades. The Sangha basin supplied enormous quantities of ivory for the Congo trade during this period. Some riverine societies along the lower and middle Sangha banks took advantage of trade networks to accumulate firearms and to provoke the flight of neighboring forest peoples whom they sought to enslave. S. Rupp, *Forests of Belonging: Identities, Ethnicities, and Stereotypes in the Congo River Basin* (Seattle: University of Washington Press, 2011); T. Giles-Vernick, *Cutting the Vines of the Past: Environmental Histories of the Central African Rain Forest* (Charlottesville: University of Virginia Press, 2002); E. Copet-Rougier, "Political-Economic History of the Upper Sangha," in *Resource Use in the Trinational Sangha River region of Equatorial Africa: Histories, Knowledge Forms, and Institutions*, ed. H. Eves, R. Hardin, and S. Rupp, Bulletin Series, Yale School of Forestry and Environmental Studies, no. 102 (1998), 41–84; R. Harms, *Games against Nature: and Eco-cultural History of the Nunu of Equatorial Africa* (Cambridge: Cambridge University Press, 1987); R. Harms, *River of Wealth, River of Sorrow: The Central Zaire Basin in the Era of the Slave and Ivory Trade, 1500–1891* (New Haven: Yale University Press, 1981).

32. T. Giles-Vernick and S. Rupp, "Visions of Apes, Reflections on Change: Telling Tales of Great Apes in Equatorial Africa," *African Studies Review* 49, no. 1 (2006): 51–73.

33. J. MacKenzie, "Chivalry, Social Darwinism, and Ritualized Killing: The Hunting Ethos in Central Africa up to 1914," in *Conservation in Africa: People, Policies, and Practice*, ed. D. Anderson and R. Grove (Cambridge, Cambridge University Press, 1987).

34. Giles-Vernick and Rupp, "Visions of Apes."

35. In addition to chimpanzees and gorillas, pangolins, crocodiles, leopards, and elephants have also occupied an important place in the practices and imaginations of equatorial Africans. M. Douglas, "Animals in Lele Religious Thought," *Africa* 27, no. 1 (1957): 46–58; N. R. Hunt, *A Colonial Lexicon of Birth Ritual, Medicalization, and Mortality in the Congo* (Durham, NC: Duke University Press, 1999); J. Fabian, *Remembering the Present: Painting and Popular History in Zaire* (Berkeley: University of California Press, 1996); C. Gray, *Colonial Rule and Crisis in Equatorial Africa: Southern Gabon ca. 1850–1940* (Rochester, NY: University of Rochester Press, 2002); D. Joiris, "Baka Pygmy Hunting Rituals in Southern Cameroon: How to Walk Side by Side with the Elephant," *Civilizations* 41, no. 2 (1993): 51–82.

36. See G. Balandier, *Sociologie actuelle de l'Afrique noire* (1955; Paris: PUF, 1992); M. Mveng-Ayi, "Rapport du synthèse: Echanges précoloniaux et diffusion des plantes au Sud-Cameroun," in *Contribution de la recherche ethnologique à l'histoire des civilisations de Cameroun*, ed. C. Tardits (Paris: CNRS, 1981), 587–91; S. Bahuchet, *Les pygmées Aka et la forêt centrafricaine* (Paris: Peeters, 1985); E. Copet-Rougier, "Les Kakas," in *Contribution de la recherche ethnologique à l'histoire des civilisations de Cameroun*, ed. C. Tardits (Paris: CNRS, 1981), 511–16; Klieman, *Pygmies*. Generally, see J. Vansina, *Paths in the*

Rainforest: Toward a History of Political Tradition in Equatorial Africa (Madison: University of Wisconsin Press, 1990).

37. P. Laburthe-Tolra, *Les seigneurs de la forêt: Essai sur le passé historique, organisation sociale, et les normes éthiques des anciens Bëti du Cameroun* (Paris: Publications de la Sorbonne, 1981).

38. R. Brisson, *Mythologie des pygmées Baka* (Paris: SELAF, Editions Peeters, 1999), 144.

39. Rupp, *Forests of Belonging*.

40. Giles-Vernick, *Cutting the Vines;* elsewhere, see O. Ebiatsa-Hopiel, *Les Teke: Peuples et nation* (Montpellier, 1990).

41. J. Fernandez, *Bwiti: An Ethnography of the Religious Imagination in Africa* (Princeton: Princeton University Press, 1982).

42. A. Kohler, "Of Apes and Men: Baka and Bantu Attitudes toward Wildlife and the Making of Eco-Goodies and Baddies," *Conservation and Society* 3, no. 2 (2005): 407–35. See also D. Peterson, "Great Apes as Food," *Gastronomica: The Journal of Food and Culture* 3, no. 2 (2003): 64–70.

43. J. B. Abessolo-Nguema et al., *Contes du Gabon* (Paris: Éditions Fernand Nathan Afrique, 1985), 52.

44. These anxieties over contact and competition with apes intensified as conservation interventions in some parts of equatorial Africa protected apes from hunters. It may be that this protection has enabled great apes to roam more freely without fear of being hunted, but their mobility may have simultaneously increased their contact with people living in the forest. Rupp, *Forests of Belonging;* R. Ruggiero, "Phantom of the Forests," *Wildlife Conservation* 103, no. 5 (2000): 50–55.

45. G. Lachenal, "Le médecin qui voulut être roi: Médecine coloniale et utopie au Cameroun," *Annales: Histoire, sciences sociales* 1 (2010): 121–56; Giles-Vernick, *Cutting the Vines;* R. Headrick, *Colonialism, Health and Illness in French Equatorial Africa, 1885–1935* (Atlanta: African Studies Association, 1994); J.-P. Dozon, "Quand les Pastoriens traquaient la maladie du sommeil," *Sciences sociales et santé* 3, no. 3–4 (1985): 27–56.

46. W. K. Gregory and H. C. Raven, *In Quest of Gorillas* (New Bedford, MA: Darwin Press, 1937), 229.

47. H. C. Raven, "Meshie, the Child of a Chimpanzee," *Natural History Magazine* (1932), www.naturalhistorymag.com/picks-from-the-past/16178/meshie-the-child-of-a -chimpanzee?page2.

48. Gregory and Raven, *In Quest of Gorillas,* 223.

49. It is likely that Raven had been incubating some of these pathogens prior to his arrival at this site.

50. Quoted in Giles-Vernick, *Cutting the Vines,* 178.

51. Sintas referred here to a linguistic and ethnic group, currently identified as Mpiemu, who lived in large concentrations in the upper Sangha basin and who had been particularly affected by twentieth-century sleeping sickness epidemics. A. Sintas, "Extrait du rapport de visite pastorale de Mgr Sintas en pays Mbimou du 8 au 16 octobre 1944," personal archives of Père G. de Banville, Congrégation Spiritaine, Chevilly-la-rue (France); Giles-Vernick, *Cutting the Vines.*

TAMARA GILES-VERNICK AND STEPHANIE RUPP

52. F. Chappuis et al., "Human African Trypanosomiaisis in Areas without Surveillance," *Emerging Infectious Diseases* 16, no. 2 (2010): 354–55.

53. Leach and Hewlett, "Haemorrhagic Fevers."

54. P. Formenty et al., "L'épidémie de fièvre hémorragique à virus Ebola en République du Congo, 2003," *Médecine tropicale* 63, no. 3 (2003): 291–95; A. J. Georges et al., "Ebola Hemorrhagic Fever Outbreaks in Gabon, 1994–1997: Epidemiologic and Health Control Issues," *Journal of Infectious Diseases* 179, Supp. 1 (Ebola: The Virus and the Disease) (1999): S65–S75. See also S. Lahm et al., "Morbidity and Mortality of Wild Animals in Relation to Outbreaks of Ebola Haemorrhagic Fever in Gabon, 1994–2003," *Transactions of the Royal Society of Tropical Medicine and Hygiene* 101, no. 1 (2007): 64–78.

55. In 2012, two distinct Ebola outbreaks took place in Uganda and the Democratic Republic of Congo.

56. The Hewletts also conducted research in Uganda in 2000–2001.

57. Hewlett and Hewlett, *Ebola, Culture, and Politics;* B. S. Hewlett et al., "Medical Anthropology and Ebola in Congo: Cultural Models and Humanistic Care," *Bulletin de la Société de pathologie exotique* 98, no. 3 (2005): 230–36.

58. Still other important explanations centered on certain individuals' manipulation of supernatural powers, either by outright sorcery or through membership in the Rose Croix, a mystical Christian organization, with the aim of accumulating wealth and political authority. Struggles over political, economic, and environmental control also figured into these explanations, as informants reflected on their circumstances of political powerlessness, economic impoverishment and stymied opportunities. Hewlett and Hewlett, *Ebola, Culture, and Politics;* B. L. Hewlett and B. S. Hewlett, "Providing Care and Facing Death: Nursing during Ebola Outbreaks in Central Africa," *Journal of Transcultural Nursing* 16, no. 4 (2005): 289–97; Hewlett et al., "Medical Anthropology."

59. Hewlett and Hewlett, *Ebola, Culture, and Politics,* 6.

60. Ibid., 7.

61. Hewlett and Hewlett, "Providing Care," 292; see also Hewlett and Hewlett, *Ebola, Culture, and Politics.*

62. Leach and Hewlett, "Haemorrhagic Fevers."

63. See particularly Hewlett and Hewlett, *Ebola, Culture, and Politics.*

64. Walsh et al., "Catastrophic Ape Decline."

65. Leach and Hewlett, "Haemorrhagic Fevers"; Hewlett and Hewlett, *Ebola, Culture, and Politics.*

66. Leach and Hewlett, "Haemorrhagic Fevers."

People, Great Apes, and Disease in Equatorial Africa

6 DEFENSELESS BODIES AND VIOLENT AFFLICTIONS IN A GLOBAL WORLD

Blood, Iatrogenesis, and Hepatitis C Transmission in Egypt

ANNE MARIE MOULIN

Hepatitis C means "miles to go before we sleep."

—M. J. Alter et al., "The Natural History of Community-Acquired Hepatitis C in the United States"

In the wake of the political and intellectual ebullience of 1968, Ivan Illich offered a provocative assessment of medical progress: he insisted that more than medicine, hygiene could account for much of the world's population explosion during the twentieth century, including in the so-called developing world.[1] More than any other intervention, the provision of potable water and elimination of waste were responsible for a momentous decline in infectious disease. Illich rebuked doctors for their arrogance for claiming to have effected these changes, and he used the term *iatrogenesis* to refer to the ill-fated consequences of some medical therapies. In the last years, iatrogenesis has caused several crises in industrialized countries, including the early 1980s contaminated blood affair,[2] which profoundly unsettled blood banks and forced a reconsideration of blood transfusion indications in ways that had once been unthinkable by decision makers.[3] Injections are one such therapeutic practice that can provoke disasters, nullifying the positive effects of medicalization,[4] an oft-celebrated gift of modernity.

Iatrogenesis is a global epidemic, yet it has stricken Egypt more severely than other countries through the new plague of hepatitis C. Its citizens face the catastrophe with stoicism, and the epidemic has not yet triggered an outright political response adapted to the long-term coexistence with the epidemic.

The global history of iatrogenesis in Africa, however, is still in its infancy. The history of medical treatments and their unintended consequences remain insufficiently documented. Although some researchers have assumed that most iatrogenesis occurred in hypermedicalized contexts, several examples suggest otherwise. Early in the HIV epidemic, some social scientists rightly observed that it was not only sexual contact, but also blood transfusions (frequently given to anemic pregnant women) that facilitated HIV's spread throughout Africa.[5] The anthropologist Richard Rottenburg has recently argued that twenty-first-century Africa has become the focal point for new forms of social and scientific experimentation; it is, in Helen Tilley's words, a "laboratory" for myriad social, political, economic, juridical, and scientific experiments.[6]

With its historical experience of the hepatitis C propagation, Egypt represents the laboratory sheltering the most flamboyant episodes of contemporary iatrogenesis. Long occupying a strategic place on the African continent and in the Mediterranean, Egypt embraced scientific modernity in the nineteenth century and sought above all to regain its central place as *Oumm el-Dounya,* the mother of the world, a name evoking its glorious and ancient past. Egypt wanted to join the mainstream of a cosmopolitan medicine that it had long ago helped to found.

This chapter explores one major event in the history of iatrogenesis, by focusing on schistosomiasis treatment and the hepatitis C epidemic in Egypt. Evaluating this history, I discuss how and why this event and its consequences might be potentially subversive both scientifically and politically in Egypt, as has been the case in many countries of Africa, by questioning the foundations of health policy and opening up a new awareness of disease and of how social movements are linked to it. Indeed, this history may figure importantly in the future of Egypt's present Revolution.

The History of Hepatitis C in Egypt

Hepatitis C has been dubbed the "eleventh Egyptian plague."[7] With a population of 82 million,[8] Egypt has the largest proportion of hepatitis C cases known in the world.[9] The last Egyptian Demographic and Health Survey in 2008[10] estimated seroprevalence (anti-HCV antibodies) to be 14.7 percent of the population between fifteen and fifty-nine years old. In some villages, prevalence among adults exceeds 30 percent, especially among men and individuals older than forty. Not a single Egyptian family has remained untouched by cases of "*firous Ci*" infection or by *maradh al kabed,* the liver disease that is often a sequella of hepatitis C infection. HCV is not simply a problem among poor, agrarian populations; rural-urban linkages are intense, and the disease also afflicts wealthier classes, and notably health care professionals, surgeons, doctors, and nurses.

Blood, Iatrogenesis, and Hepatitis C Transmission in Egypt

First identified in the laboratory in 1989,[11] hepatitis C is an acute viral infection, frequently unnoticed at its onset. Some infected people are spontaneously cured, but the disease can be unpredictable in its evolution. HCV will become chronic in 55–85 percent of those infected;[12] some 20 percent of these carriers will develop cirrhosis, and between 1 and 4 percent will die of liver carcinoma.[13] This frequency of liver carcinoma (*saratan*) has triggered a massive upsurge in liver transplants.[14]

HCV's place in Egypt's modern history cannot be understood in isolation, for it has been deeply intertwined with another, more ancient affliction that also targets the liver: schistosomiasis.[15] The accepted explanation for Egypt's massive epidemic, first unofficially acknowledged in 1994, is the mass campaign of schistosomiasis treatment (late 1950s–70s) that used infected needles. Mass schistosomiasis treatment is assumed to have created within one generation a cohort infected with HCV; then unsafe injection practices in hospitals, health centers, pharmacies, and homes contributed to its dissemination throughout Egypt's population.[16] Long before ordinary citizens were aware of this disaster, the Egyptian medical press wrote of it, but it was not until 2000, with the publication of a widely cited paper in the *Lancet*,[17] that the Egyptian government admitted the hepatitis C epidemic and the chronology of events.

The HCV epidemic thus appears to be a dramatic, but also classic, case of iatrogenesis, revealing modern medicine's Janus face as simultaneously effective and dangerous. The story has all the elements of contemporary iatrogenesis: the "emergence" (both an ecological and epistemic development) of previously unknown infectious agents revealed by new diagnostic tools,[18] catalyzed by medical advances that both "produce" and illuminate new infectious agents. Yet this epidemic also demonstrates features that are specific to Egypt's historical, epidemiological, and sociocultural context.

Schistosomiasis: A Legacy from the Past or a Modern Plague?

Schistosomiasis dates back to Pharaonic times in Egypt. Indeed, parasitologists easily identify in the visceral remains of ancient Egyptian mummies the eggs with the spikes familiar to them, typical of the flatworm *Schistosoma haematobium,* a species within the class of Trematodes. The parasite's eggs, excreted through human urine and feces, enter freshwater and then hatch, penetrating particular species of river snails, the parasite's vectors. Upon completing part of their life cycle within the snails, the parasites then give birth to larvae—swimming "cercaria" (embryos) which in turn penetrate the human host's skin. Adult schistosoma worms subsequently mate in the blood vessels of the bladder;

ANNE MARIE MOULIN

female worms lay eggs, which are then released into the environment. Within the human body, most eggs remain encysted, causing inflammation and at times leading to liver or bladder cancer.

Schistosoma haematobium's life cycle requires that it passes through freshwater, and for this reason, it has long been linked to irrigation. For many centuries, male *fellahs* (farmers) have been in constant contact with water from the Nile River or irrigation canals, while women have washed clothes, bedding, and plates in these waters, or carried the water home for consumption and cleaning.

Beginning in the nineteenth century, with the accession to power of Pasha Mohammed Ali (1811–1849), and subsequently Khedive Ismaïl (1863–1879), irrigation developed on a massive scale. Mohammed Ali, the so-called founder of modern Egypt, wanted to industrialize the country and to transform it into one of the world's leading nations.[19] Cotton would offer that path to industrialization, and its cultivation demanded much water. The historian John Farley has thus called schistosomiasis an "industrial disease"[20]—not a rural affliction, or the result of the fellah's immersion in "nature."[21]

Because of their constant contact with infested water, fellahs harbored heavy *Schistosoma* parasite loads. These exceptional loads may have permitted the Austrian physician Theodor Bilharz, working in 1851 in the Medical School of Cairo, to see without a microscope the worms in the vessels of the *vena porta* in autopsied bodies.[22] When British colonizers took over Cairo's medical school following their occupation of Egypt in 1882, they immediately focused on this disease causing "Egyptian haematuria," for which prevalence exceeded 80 percent in the population.[23] The Scottish doctor Robert Leiper, working in Egypt from 1914 to 1918, identified a snail (*Bulinus* species) as the parasite's vector in freshwater. His discovery effectively transformed the British target in schistosomiasis control and the plans for improving sanitation, for he contended that the disease "should now be treated as one of those diseases for which the individual is mainly, if not entirely, personally responsible."[24] British authorities' intense interest in the disease vanished when they realized that an effective prophylactic measure was to forbid soldiers to bathe and to enter barefooted into irrigation canals.[25]

Hence following the First World War, the control strategy focused on treating waters with various molluscicides, which allowed the British to avoid direct interference with colonized populations, in keeping with their principles of Indirect Rule. During the Second World War, a malaria epidemic prompted the American military to establish in 1943 the research station NAMRU-3 (US Naval Medical Research Unit).[26] NAMRU-3 linked modern laboratory facilities with a Cairo hospital and the Sindbis village serving as an experimental station. It became the center of a network for virological research and included Egypt's most renowned infectious disease specialists.[27]

Human treatment for bilharzia dates back to 1918,[28] when antimony tartrate, long known as an emetic agent, was introduced into Egypt. At the time, it was considered a landmark drug, and over the next three years, some 500,000 peasants were reportedly treated with a series of intravenous injections in Cairo and Delta hospital annexes.[29] Following the Anglo-Egyptian treaty of 1936, which officially brought the end of the Egypt occupation,[30] Egyptians gradually assumed leadership over these schistosomiasis treatment campaigns. As the drug's toxicity and treatment duration rendered unattractive the notion of "irrigating the veins (of millions of people) with tartar emetic,"[31] public health experts preferred then to eradicate schistosome-carrying snails.

But following the 1952 "Free Officers" coup that evicted the king and brought Gamal Abdel Nasser to power, public health authorities within the new regime, espousing a socialist line and influenced by the Soviet model, reconsidered mass schistosomiasis treatment in the population at large. Although the mechanism of its therapeutic action was unclear, emetin tartrate became the treatment of choice. In 1959, Nasser's state developed mass campaigns using the emetin tartrate produced by the local Egyptian pharmaceutical industry. The treatment was first administered on a daily basis, but from 1960, the recommended regimen was sixteen intravenous injections over a period of three weeks, followed by one injection per week to lessen the burden on the patients. The campaigns took place chiefly in schools, hospitals, health centers, and other places of collective gatherings. After Western countries had adopted oral treatment for schistosomiasis, Egypt interrupted its injection treatment campaign only in 1982, some twenty years after it had commenced. Then the Egyptian Ministry of Health distributed the new wonder drug, praziquantel, as the Bayer pharmaceutical formulation, *Biltricid,* or as the South Korean product, *Distocid,* and it became the standard treatment in hospitals.

In 1989, assessing over fifty years of treatment (1932–89), Qalyub researchers in collaboration with the American Centers for Disease Control in Atlanta (CDC), indicated that *S. haemotobium* prevalence had declined substantially in Egypt, but that prevalence of *S. mansoni,* another schistosome parasite that causes liver cirrhosis and portal hypertension, had significantly increased.[32] With the replacement of *S. haematobium* with *S. mansoni,* bilharziosis now targeted a new organ in the body, the liver. Experts have repeatedly observed *S. mansoni's* expansion and replacement of *S. haematobium* in Africa, particularly with the strategy of building large dams.[33] Dam construction frequently brings about the disappearance of *Bulinus truncatus,* the snail host of *S. haematobium,* which is replaced by another snail, *Biomphalaria alexandrina, S. mansoni's* host, and a more difficult one to kill with chemical molluscicides. Most likely after the construction of the Great Aswan Dam in 1970, the chemical content of riverine silts altered, modifying the distributions of both snail species. It is unclear how and when people became aware of the increasing number of jaundice, the most flamboyant symptom of liver damage.

Jaundice and Iatrogenesis

Doctors have long suspected a link between jaundice (icterus) and medical procedures, which include the injection of human fluids. In 1885, for example, A. Lürman conducted an epidemiological study on 1,289 Bremen (Germany) shipyard workers, who had been inoculated against smallpox with human vaccine lymph stored in glycerine: one-sixth of the men experienced jaundice over the following eight months, and all had been vaccinated with the same vaccine batch.[34] Such were the *Hazards of Immunisation,* according to G. S. Wilson's review of the untoward effects of vaccination.[35] In the interwar period and during the Second World War, researchers found jaundice in patients treated with hyperimmune sera and in those receiving yellow fever vaccinations with human serum.[36] During the war several million people suffered from hepatitis with no definite cause, probably augmented by the expansion of blood transfusions and intravenous injections for the treatment of rheumatism as well as venereal diseases.[37] Human experimentation during the war on "volunteers," conscientious objectors, handicapped children, prisoners, and hospital patients confirmed the hypothesis.[38]

In the 1980s, as new virology techniques enabled the identification of new, previously unknown hepatitis viruses, Egyptian clinicians frequently began to identify patients with acute fevers and jaundices, signaling that these patients suffered simultaneously from the hepatitis B virus (already known) and the liver parasite *S. mansoni.* They thus wondered whether a link existed between the virus and parasite.[39] The interaction between these pathogens could work in two ways: heavy infestation by *Schistosoma* could impair local immunity and favor liver inflammation, or the hepatitis virus could trigger an immune reaction that facilitated Schistosoma-linked cirrhotic evolution.[40] An obsessive concern with schistosomiasis in Egypt sustained the conviction that hepatitis was more frequent and severe because human livers had for so long been impaired by the parasite seated in the organ,[41] although some specialists remained uncertain about the consequences of the parasite-virus interaction.[42]

Around 1980, the link between jaundice caused by the hepatitis B virus and the parenteral treatment of schistosomiasis began to echo earlier observations concerning possible consequences of blood transfusions. Where transfusion was once perceived as a life-saving intervention, medical specialists now eyed this sword of Damocles with considerable suspicion. But it was not only blood transfusion or injection of human serum that was hazardous; any previously used needle could transmit invisible viruses. This story has played out repeatedly throughout the world. Ernest Drucker derisively called the twentieth century the "injection century,"[43] and the WHO has officially recognized the "millions of deaths occurring through such infections."[44] Many cases of hepatitis in other African campaigns may be linked to vaccine campaigns or mass treaments,[45] but in 2003 Egypt represented "the world's largest iatrogenic transmission of blood borne pathogens known to this date."[46]

An Epidemic Discovered from the Outside

Pursuing his posttransfusion studies, in 1974 Alfred Prince had provided the first indirect evidence of NANB (non A-non B) hepatitis viruses. The name he proposed for the virus, "hepatitis C," was not officially adopted until 1989. With the availability of reagents in 1990 came extensive epidemiological studies among blood donors throughout the world.

Thanks to these new techniques, an early indication of Egypt's problem emerged in 1991 from Riyadh, Saudi Arabia, where a surprisingly high percentage of paid blood donors (most of whom were poor Egyptian migrants) tested positive for hepatitis C virus, particularly when compared with donors from elsewhere in the region.[47] In 1990–91, a study of multitransfused Egyptian children (versus nontransfused) showed that half presented antibodies against hepatitis C virus.[48] The following year, Dr. Yasin Abdel Ghaffar presented some of these findings at a Riyadh congress[49] to an incredulous audience. When Saudi authorities asked to test departing Egyptian migrants for HCV, the Egyptian government responded with rage. Abdel Ghaffar was openly contradicted, threatened, and insulted for the apparent blemish he had inflicted on Egypt's reputation.[50] In 1992–93, however, M. A. Darwish, one of the luminaries of Egyptian virology,[51] conducted a study among Egyptian blood donors in the country and found that HCV prevalence exceeded 13 percent. He concluded loudly that testing all donors was urgent and suggested that a history of schistosomiasis should be one criterion for excluding blood donors.[52]

An understanding of HCV risk groups was thus taking shape as discussions about the link between hepatitis C and schistosomiasis treatment with unsterile needles appeared in the *Journal of the Egyptian Public Health Association,* the *Egyptian Journal of Parasitology,* and the *Journal of the Egyptian Medical Association.* The authors still hesitated to acknowledge fully the causal link, but also refused to conclude that "injections were entirely free of risk."[53] It was difficult for Egyptian professionals to confront the notion that well-intended schistosomiasis campaigns had such deadly consequences. Instead, these articles indicated that the practices of barbers-circumcisers and traditional midwives (*dayas*) were an (undocumented) source of contamination. Nevertheless, in 1996, the late Mostafa Kamel Mohamed acknowledged in the professional Egyptian press the magnitude of the hepatitis problem, regardless of the mechanism of contamination, and in 1997, a study demonstrated the frequency of positive serologies for hepatitis B and C at Alexandria and attributed this frequency to parenteral transmission.[54]

In 2000, a landmark paper appeared in the *Lancet,* defining Egypt's hepatitis C epidemic as a *local epidemic.*[55] The result of a collaboration between scientists from the University of Maryland and Ain Shams University in Cairo, the article's authors had carefully included two WHO members (for an international dimension), two officers of Egypt's Ministry of Health, who had received access to the ministry's treatment files and had "authorized the report."[56] This seminal article solemnly stated: "This is the world's *largest iatrogenic transmission of blood borne pathogens known* to date, which probably led to a massive increase in the reservoir for HCV and HBV in the general population"[57] (emphasis added). The paper quoted 1964 World Health Organization evaluation of Egypt's mass schistosomiasis treatment.[58] Full attention was given to the account of the procedures by the WHO expert, Brian Maegraith, the well-known and respected dean of the Liverpool School of Tropical Medicine:

> The skilful doctor began injecting (intravenously) (tartrate emetin) at 9.30 a.m. and completed 504 injections of men, women and children by 10.10 a.m. Allowing for a 10-minute rest, the time taken to give these injections was 40 minutes. The average time for each injection was thus just under five seconds.[59]

Interestingly, the expert put the emphasis on the performance in front of his eyes and gave the following comment: "This remarkable performance is being repeated *at various tempos all over Egypt*" (emphasis mine). Further, the report detailed the procedure, which is the crucial point to assess the chances of proper sterilization. "The individual injection is given with a small all-glass syringe. . . . The doctor finds a vein, inserts the needle . . . , and injects the syringe contents quickly (in one or two seconds). . . . The used syringe is placed in an 'out' tray, from which it is taken by the nurse, washed through and boiled for a minute or two. As soon as the syringe is cold, it is filled with a volume of the drug solution. . . . It is then placed on the 'in' tray, which contains other syringes already filled. There are usually 20 to 30 syringes in rotation, and needles are sharpened after each day's performance."[60]

Although experts debate the figures, some 4 million people are said to have been treated between 1930 and 1961, and an additional 7 million received treatment between 1961 and 1963.[61] Between 1964 and 1982, 2 million infections by year took place.[62]

Schistosomiasis treatment played a foundational role in this epidemic. Because much of the campaign was conducted in schools, what epidemiologists call a cohort effect has clearly developed. Children were infected between 1950 and 1980, and the peak of morbidity and mortality occurred in the year 2000 among age groups from 30 to 60 years old; epidemiologists expect the cohort effect to continue until 2020.[63] In the years that followed, genetic analyses more clearly delineated this cohort effect. The homogeneity of virus genotypes (mainly the so-called type four) suggested a common origin of the epidemic, founded on an event or a series of events that were specific to Egypt.[64]

Were procedures during Egypt's schistosomiasis campaign especially sloppy, or did they simply conform to good clinical practices of the time? For WHO experts in 1964, the conduct of the mass treatment was poorly standardized and controlled. The experts acknowledged that there were "human mistakes" and were embarrassed by the variability of medical procedures, which were supposed to be uniform and standardized.[65] Doctors wary of the drug's toxicity offered different dosages to different patients; some patients passed out after treatment, while in many cases, the intravenous treatments frequently incapacitated a patient for a few hours.[66] Patients received instruction not to leave the hospital before defecating, because "maintaining . . . [the vermicide] in your bowels would be deadly poisonous."[67]

Whereas epidemiological studies performed contemporaneously in the United States detected that injection drug use was a risk factor in 50 percent of cases, the epidemiological study conducted in Egypt in 1996 among expatriate workers detected them in only 10 percent of the cases.[68] This discrepancy may result for various reasons: individual case information were not collected with the same level of detail as in the United States; Egyptian

ANNE MARIE MOULIN

patients were thought to be less accustomed to providing detailed narratives of their illnesses, be less cooperative with such administrative investigation, and less willing to divulge intimate, highly sensitive details of their lives. Limited communication between investigator and patient could also render the interpretation of results problematic, due to a long past of defiance toward state (or assimilated) intervention.

"Public Health" in Egypt or an Oxymoron for Violence

Public health in Egypt has had a long record of violence. When I discussed the hepatitis epidemic with aging people in Cairo in 2009–10, most had heard of the contamination by needles. They recalled that during their childhood, they had been "vaccinated" against the worms (*dud*). When I protested that there had never been a vaccine against *Schistosoma,* they sternly replied that they were dead certain of it, because the vaccine was forcibly administered to all people, healthy or unhealthy, and only vaccines fitted such criteria.[69]

Egypt's history of public health has long been characterized by numerous episodes of state violence and top-down programs applied without explanation, and for many Egyptians, submission and bribery have appeared to be the best responses to avoid trouble. Nineteenth-century examples are rife with such violent, oppressive measures: Mohammed Ali's compulsory vaccination against smallpox,[70] forced labor during the construction of the Suez Canal, and the oppression of peasants and merchants in contrast to Westerners' exorbitant privileges, during Ismail's administration (1863–79),[71] leading to Urabi's revolt in 1881.[72] The fear, resentment, and misunderstanding that people once expressed of these harsh and seemingly absurd interventions are echoed in more recent popular recollections of public health, illustrated by the mass treatment campaigns against schistosomiasis. The radical thinker Sayyid Qutb, later arrested and hanged by Nasser for participating in a plot with the Muslim Brotherhood, wrote in his autobiography *A Child from the Village* (1946) about his intense fear of the school doctor's visits. For Qutb and his classmates, the event could mean nothing but humiliation and physical violence, and Qutb chose to miss school and hide himself in the village.[73]

Similarly, when anthropologists Susan Watts and Samiha El Katscha researched rural schistosomiasis in 2000, they noted girls' absences from school when physicians visited, in an attempt to avoid unpleasant physical contact or breaches of privacy.[74] Their absence retrospectively explains the gender asymmetry in the population contaminated by HCV.[75] It also means that schistosomiasis prevalence measures, and even parasitological test results, were unreliable.

Blood, Iatrogenesis, and Hepatitis C Transmission in Egypt

Had not al-Qutb told stories about schoolboys, faced with demands to provide a feces specimen, who supplied instead animal manure from the street?

During mass treatment campaigns, doctors themselves explained that tartrate was a "poison," so that patients had to rest and to eat a meal in order to eliminate this poison from the body as quickly as possible.[76] Although the denomination of "poison" evokes the Greek etymology of pharmacy (poison as remedy), it illustrates here the ambivalent nature of medical cure, as well as the ambivalent feelings among the population toward public health programs.

The Local Memory of the Global Emergence of Viruses

Although there has been a tradition of violence exerted by the state, medical violence as such has been less addressed than the more political forms. Concerning the drama of schistosomiasis treatment and its role in the hepatitis C epidemic, no book or journal has yet provided a full narrative. No organized state hearing has ever been held. No evaluation of state responsibility for the schistosomiasis campaigns, blood transfusions (supervised by the state), or unsafe medical practices has ever been offered. Memory of the past has been suppressed. Beginning in 2000, Parliament broached the question of state responsibility several times; the Muslim Brotherhood (a forbidden party until January 2011, but which nonetheless constituted a major political force) seized the opportunity to blame the Mubarak government. But the debate over the "facts"[77] was aborted. In order to receive compensation, victims needed to supply proof that they had received the schistosomiasis treatment injections. Although patients normally received a numbered card to bring to each visit, most never kept their documents, nor were treatment registers properly maintained. Moreover, most victims were too poor or too busy to pursue their claims through the judicial system. In addition, some patients did not want their illnesses publicized. Although hepatitis does not carry the same stigma as HIV/AIDS,[78] its diagnosis nonetheless can have negative consequences; it can prevent marriages by raising suspicions about a young woman's virtue, and it can jeopardize a patient's professional and personal relations.

The state's reluctance to face its responsibility has been facilitated by scientific uncertainties concerning the disease's natural course. Charting this natural history is a difficult task, primarily because in order to determine the gravity of the disease and predict its course in individual patients, it is necessary to know the illness's date of onset,[79] which is seldom available. Most (70 percent) acute infections are asymptomatic and therefore cannot be detected at onset. Anti-HCV antibodies can be detected in blood only some two months after

ANNE MARIE MOULIN

infection. In some cases, patients admitted to a hospital for other reasons years later find that they are infected with HCV. Still others discover that they have HCV ten to twenty years after infection, when they develop complications of end-stage liver disease. There are many factors associated with chronicity, "predictors," including older age, male sex, asymptomatic acute infection, and immune deficiency.[80]

But no one can determine with certainty how the disease will progress in an individual. Nor are there definitive conclusions about the relationship between the mode of contamination and the disease's evolution. Yet, the discussion about past events remains more necessary than ever for a much-needed renovation of Egypt's health care system and the establishment of trust between the health profession and patients.

Medical Remembering as a Revolutionary Process

The historical past is a treasure that cannot be overestimated in Egypt. Pharaonic monuments remain one of the principal resources of the country, and tourism constitutes a major source of income for both state and particular populations. Monuments attesting to Egypt's ancient civilization are carefully preserved, despite ambivalence about this distant past. Radical Islamic thinkers sometimes refer to the Pharaonic period as a time of polytheism, or as *Jahiliya*, a pre-Islamic era of what they term "Ignorance," and they debase statues of gods and Pharaohs.

The history of a more recent past remains sidelined to the official version, which is filled with such positive episodes as Egypt's victorious war of 1973. Although Anwar el Sadat, in one version of his memoirs, continually celebrates his "People" for their immemorial virtues of patience and endurance, there is little attention paid to the material living conditions and well-being of Egypt's population.[81] Sadat postulates that his People possess an immutable identity, an essence that transcends the centuries from the Pharaonic to the present. His selective rendering of the past elides the considerable changes that the People have endured, and Egypt's medical history is altogether ignored.

Egypt's official history maintains a strong hagiographic tradition, relegating any critique to complicity with external enemies. However, criticisms can be found in journals with a tradition of cartoons that humorously refer to controversial events,[82] while ferocious *noqta* (jokes) permit the public to vent popular derision, anger, and frustration (*kabt*). But these expressions are only ephemeral reactions, not detailed analyses of social and political situations.[83] Theater can also offer critique, but its audience is limited.[84] As for medicine, films frequently express a popular mistrust of doctors, as well as overblown hopes and desires for magical drugs. More generally, health professionals have long invited popular ambivalence or even defiance. Nurses have not enjoyed the same professional valorization as their Western counterparts: there are no popular heroines akin to Florence Nightingale, the "Lady of the Lamp" during the Crimean War, or the Angels immortalized on postcards during the world wars. Doctors retain prestige as healers and upper-class idols, but are simultaneously resented as arrogant and avaricious.[85] Surgeons are suspected of lopping off useless organs without clear instructions, so that patients now try to confirm the precise nature and object of their surgeries before entering the operating room.[86] In the face of the present epidemic and the scarcity of available drugs, various therapies inspired by the Medicine of the Prophet, medieval Arabic tradition, or folk recipes have been revived in popular journals and the media. Egyptian diasporic populations in affluent countries such as Canada have sent home remedies (such as the "yellow pill") claiming to cure HCV.[87] Egyptians have also revived the ancient prophylactics of the *tasat al-sihhat* (the "bowl of health"), or the *tasat al-khadda* ("bowl of fright") to defend themselves against jaundice. The magical bowl, covered with passages from Koran and magical squares, contains holy water, which must be swallowed directly following psychological shock.[88] Markets currently sell many such bowls. Once relegated to folklore in Nasser's times,[89] the *tasat* now has reemerged to palliate a distraught population searching for new (and old) ways of healing itself.

A few months after the events of January 2011, Egypt's transitional government conferred upon medical historian Khaled Fahmy the mission of collecting all items and testimonies related to the "Revolution." It may be no coincidence that Fahmy and his students have emphasized the destructive effects of the state enterprises on human bodies.[90]

In some respects, Egypt occupies a place apart from the rest of the African continent. Since the early nineteenth century, its leaders actively promoted initiatives to stop epidemics, imposed quarantines and vaccination, and celebrated a renaissance of ancient Arab medicine revitalized by modernization. In the second part of the twentieth century, hepatitis C invaded the daily lives of people in part because of Egypt's embrace of the modern technologies of public health, whereas for the rest of the African continent, colonial history and its cultural legacy may have made it easier to point to colonial medicine as a source of contamination. The drama of iatrogenesis confronts Egypt with the perverse consequences of an unreflective, sweeping medical modernization.

In many African countries, facing HIV and hepatitis epidemics, patients' associations now occupy a newfound and growing place in public debates over treatment, social justice, and transparency in public health policies. Centralized, state-organized efforts to build infrastructures and institutions in Africa have been replaced by crisis-oriented humanitarian interventions that explicitly bypass African states. This new type of intervention focuses on the direct relief of endangered people, who are increasingly perceived as medical bodies and biologically defined populations. According to official sources, Egypt's blood supply has been screened for hepatitis C since 1995, but the epidemic continues.[91] Subsequent years have witnessed the launching of prospective studies that registered hepatitis C cases in two Cairo Ministry of Health "Fever" hospitals.[92] Unsafe injections are still likely to occur in hospitals and clinics, as well as in urban and rural settings, where informal medical attendants, maids, doormen, and barbers, offer injections. Unsafe surgery may have been responsible for new cases among children.[93]

But in contrast to many African countries such as Senegal or Ivory Coast,[94] Egypt has not witnessed the rise of patients' strategies of empowerment, despite their high number. In Egypt, no civil society groups have emerged compared to the numerous associations of "People living with AIDS" in sub-Saharan Africa. It does not resemble many African states, which suffer from weak governments, and which experience the growing influence of foreign nongovernmental organizations that bypass these weak states and interfere with human rights.

The idea of citizen surveillance on the health system is of recent vintage.[95] The Mubarak government's inadequate response to the epidemic could be perceived as paradigmatic of its inability to deal with crisis and with emerging health threats. In contrast, in 2009, in its management of the avian and H1N1 influenza pandemics, the Mubarak state seized the opportunity to join international exhortations for pandemic preparedness, but did so at the expense of its citizens, first by destroying domestic poultry, and later during the H1N1 pandemic, by slaughtering pigs raised by Copts.[96] The global surveillance network initiated appeared to many as a renewed instrument of domination by multinational companies and experts. Today in Egypt, the growing awareness of nosocomial infections may have helped undermine the foundations of Mubarak's power. Popular resentment of the state and its medical institutions created by the hepatitis C epidemic may be one of many elements that led to the revolution of January 2011. Demonstrations castigated government corruption and ineffectiveness, including those of the hospitals and Social Security, and they manifested the popular desire of transparency and citizen control, including of the medical sphere.

The archives of Egypt's medical past are not primarily stored in libraries. Instead, Egyptian "silent bodies"[97] are living archives of a mass campaign targeting the eradication of a millenary evil, schistosomiasis, a generation ago. That material evidence—the remains of those ruined bodies attacked by hepatitis—requires a historically based anthropological approach. The archaeology of contemporary bodies is a potentially revolutionary enterprise, one that might help shake the very foundations of Egyptian power and society, and open up new forms of curing and care. Medical archaeology would thus not only assist Egyptians in taking full stock of their past, but it might also forge a new future, helping the fruits of the revolution to mature and to bring more transparency and trust.[98] Will a form of sanitary governance emerge in the coming years, and will it resemble African experiments? If the political events of 2011 bring about genuine social revolution, people living with hepatitis will have their piece to say as well.

Notes

The epigraph is from M. J. Alter et al., "The Natural History of Community-Acquired Hepatitis C in the United States," *New England Journal of Medicine* 327 (1992): 1899.

1. Ivan Illich, *Medical Nemesis: The Expropriation of Health* (New York: Pantheon, 1976).

2. Anne Marie Casteret, *L'affaire du sang* (Paris: La Découverte, 1992); Marie-Angèle Hermitte, *Le sang et le droit: Essai sur la transfusion sanguine* (Paris: Le Seuil, 1995).

3. Harvey M. Sapolsky, "AIDS, Blood Banking, and the Bonds of Community," *Daedalus* 118, no. 3 (1989): 287–309.

4. Jean-Pierre Goubert, ed., *La médicalisation de la société française, 1770–1830* (Waterloo: Historical Reflections Press, 1982).

5. J.-P. Dozon and D. Fassin, "Raison épidémiologique et raisons d'état: Les enjeux socio-politiques du sida en Afrique," *Sciences sociales et santé* 7, no. 1 (1989): 21–36; J.-P. Dozon, "Sciences sociales et sida en Afrique," *Bulletin de l'ANRS* 17 (1996): 56–58; William H. Schneider and Ernest Drucker, "Blood Transfusions in the Early Years of AIDS in Sub-Saharan Africa," *American Journal of Public Health* 96, no. 6 (2006): 984–94.

6. R. Rottenburg, "Social and Public Experiments and New Figurations of Science and Politics in Postcolonial Africa," *Postcolonial Studies* 12, no. 4 (2009): 423–40; Helen Tilley, *Africa as a Living Laboratory: Empire, Development, and the Problem of Scientific Knowledge, 1870–1950* (Chicago: University of Chicago Press, 2011).

7. E. Favereau, "La onzième plaie d'Egypte," *Libération,* 13 July 2007.

8. P. Fargues, "Croissance et mutations démographiques au XXᵉ siècle," in *L'Egypte au présent—Inventaire d'une société avant révolution,* ed. V. Battesti and F. Ireton (Arles: Actes-Sud, 2011), 41–74.

9. A. G. Farghali and R. M. Barakat, "Prevalence, Impact, and Risk Factors of Hepatitis C Infection," *Journal of the Egyptian Public Health Association* 68, no. 1–2 (1993): 63–79; M. K. Mohamed et al., "A. HCV-Related Morbidity in a Rural Community of Egypt," *Journal of Medical Virology* 78, no. 9 (2006): 1185–89.

10. F. El-Zanati and A. Way, *Egyptian Demographic and Health Survey, 2008.* Cairo, Egypt: Ministry of Health and Macro International, 2009.

11. Q. Choo et al., "Isolation of a DNA Clone Derived from a Blood-Borne nonA-nonB Viral Hepatitis Genome," *Science* 244 (1989): 359–62.

12. J. H. Hofnagle, "Course and Outcome of Hepatitis C," *Hepatology* 36, no. 5, supp. (2002): S21–29.

13. H. J. Alter and J. B. Seeff, "Recovery, Persistence, and Sequelae in Hepatitis C Virus Infection: A Perspective on Long-Term Outcome," *Seminars in Liver Disease* 20, no. 1 (2000): 17–35.

14. Although transplantation with cadaver organs was legalized in Egypt in 2010, it is not functioning to the present (too costly and too controversial for religious reasons). Surgeons still currently perform liver transplants using exclusively living donors. Cairo's organ traffic is a lucrative business, with a ready supply from populations of increasingly impoverished urban dwellers and one million Sudanese and Ethiopian refugees. D. Budiani, "Transplantation," *Body and Society* 13, no. 3 (2007): 125–49; D. Budiani-Saberi, "Organ Trafficking and Transplant Tourism," *American Journal of Transplantation* 8, no. 5 (2008): 925–29; A. M. Moulin, "Changeante modernité: L'état égyptien et la modernisation de la santé publique (19e–20e siècles)," in *Perilous Modernity: History of Medicine in the Middle East, from the nineteenth Century Onwards,* ed. A. M. Moulin and Y. I. Ulman (Istanbul: Isis, 2010), 159–79.

15. J. L. Payen, *De la jaunisse à l'hépatite C: 5000 ans d'histoire* (Paris: EDK, 2002).

16. M. Habib, M. K. Mohamed, et al. "Hepatitis C Virus Infection in a Community in the Nile Delta: Risk Factors for Seropositivity," *Hepatology* 33, no. 1 (2001): 248–53; Ahmed Medhat et al., "Hepatitis C in a Community in Upper Egypt: Risk Factors for Infection, *American Journal of Tropical Medicine and Hygiene* 66, no. 5 (2002): 633–38.

17. C. Frank et al., "The Role of Parenteral Antischistosomal Therapy in the Spread of Hepatitis C Virus in Egypt," *Lancet* 355 (2000): 887–91.

18. S. S. Morse and A. Schluederberg, "Emerging Viruses: The Evolution of Viruses and Viral Diseases," *Journal of Infectious Diseases* 162, no. 1 (1990): 1–7.

19. K. Fahmy, *All the Pasha's Men: Mehmed Ali and the Making of Modern Egypt* (Cambridge: Cambridge University Press, 1997); Gilbert Sinoue, *Le dernier Pharaon: Méhémet-Ali, 1770–1849* (Paris: Pygmalion, 1997); Rauf Abbas, *Islâh am Tahdîth? Misr fî 'asr Muhammad 'Ali* (Réforme ou modernisation? L'Egypte à l'époque de Muhammad Ali) (Cairo: Supreme Council for Culture, 2000); S. Moussa, "Mohammed Ali: Barbare ou civilisé?" in *Le voyage en Egypte: Anthologie de voyageurs européens, de Bonaparte à l'occupation anglaise* (Paris: Laffont, 2004), 778–810.

20. J. Farley, *Bilharzia: A History of Imperial Tropical Medicine* (Cambridge: Cambridge University Press, 1991), 47.

21. On the discussion of the link between tropical disease and both luxuriant and hostile nature, see H. Naraindas, "Poisons, Putrescence, and the Weather: A Genealogy

Blood, Iatrogenesis, and Hepatitis C Transmission in Egypt

of the Advent of Tropical Medicine," in *Médecines et santé*, ed. A. M. Moulin (Paris: Editions de l'Orstom, 1995), 31–56.

22. T. Bilharz, "Ein Beitrag zur Helminthographia humana, aus brieflichen Mitteilungen des Dr Bilharz in Cairo," *Zeitschrift für wissenschaftliche Zoologie* (1853): 59–62; English translation in *Tropical Medicine and Parasitology: Classic Investigations*, ed. B. H. Kean, Kenneth E. Mott, and Adair J. Russell (Ithaca, NY: Cornell University Press, 1978), 2:475.

23. F. S. Sandwith, *The Medical Diseases of Egypt* (London: Henry Kimpton, 1905).

24. R. Leiper, "Report on the Results of the *Bilharzia* Mission in Egypt, 1915, Part V," *Journal of the Royal Army Medical Corps* 30 (1918): 248.

25. Farley, *Bilharzia*, 71.

26. M. Fintz, "De l'éradication à la surveillance épidémiologique: Les moustiques, l'Egypte et la santé publique internationale," *Maghreb-Machrek* 182 (Winter 2004–5): 111–24.

27. Even today, NAMRU-3 remains Egypt's main laboratory for identifying viruses, particularly for hepatitis.

28. Wagida Anwar, *Assessment of Efficacy of Praziquantel against Schistosoma Infection*, medical thesis, Ayn Chams University, Cairo, 1981, 40.

29. F. O. Lasbrey and R. B. Coleman, "Notes on One Thousand Cases of Bilharziasis Treated by Antimony Tartrate," *British Medical Journal* (26 February 1921): 299–301; M. Khalil, *Ankylostomiasis and Bilharziasis in Egypt: Reports and Notes of the Public Health Laboratories* (Cairo: Cairo Government Press, 1924).

30. Farley, *Bilharzia*, 98.

31. R. T. Leiper, *Report to the Undersecretary of Public Health on the Problems of Bilharzia Control in Egypt*, 1928, quoted in Farley, *Bilharzia*, 101.

32. J. A. Scott, "The Incidence and Distribution of Human Schistosomiasis in Egypt," *American Journal of Hygiene* 25, no. 3 (1937): 566–614; B. L. Cline et al., "Nile Delta Schistosomiasis Survey: 48 Years after Scott," *American Journal of Tropical Medicine and Hygiene* 4, no. 1 (1989): 56–62.

33. A. M. Moulin, "Les stratégies de lutte contre les bilharzioses en l'an 2000," in *La lutte contre les schistosomes en Afrique de l'Ouest*, ed. J.-F. Chippaux (Paris: IRD éditions, 2000), 9–17.

34. A Lürman, "Eine Icterusepidemie," *Berliner klinische Wochenschrift* 22, no. 2 (1885): 20–23.

35. G. S. Wilson, *The Hazards of Immunisation* (London: Athlone Press, 1967). See A. M. Moulin, *Le dernier langage de la médecine: Histoire de l'immunologie de Pasteur au sida* (Paris: PUF, 1991): 378–82.

36. G. M. Findlay and F. O. MacCallum, "Note on Acute Hepatitis and Yellow Fever Immunization," *Transactions of the Royal Society of Tropical Medicine and Hygiene* 31, no. 3 (1937): 297–308.

37. L. F. Barker et al., "Acute Infectious Hepatitis in the Mediterranean Theatre, Including Acute Hepatitis without Jaundice," *JAMA* 128 (1945): 997–1003; J. H. S. Gear, "Historical Perspectives of Viral Hepatitis," *Canadian Medical Association Journal* 106, no. 423 (1972): 1156–61; P. B. Beeson et al., "Hepatitis Following Injection of Mumps Convalescent Plasma: The Use of Plasma in Mumps Epidemics," *Lancet* 243,

no. 6304 (1944): 814–15; T. E. Anderson, "Jaundice in Syphilitics," *British Journal of Venereal Diseases* 19 (1943): 58–67.

38. H. Voegt, "Zur Etiologie der Hepatitis Epidemia," *Münchener medizinische Wochenschrift* 89 (1942): 76. J. D. S. Cameron et al., "Infective Hepatitis," *Quarterly Journal of Medicine* 12 (1943): 139–55 ; J. W. Oliphant, "Jaundice following Administration of Human Serum," *Bulletin of the New York Academy of Medicine* 20, no. 8 (1944): 429–45; J. R. Neefe et al., "Homologous Serum Hepatitis and Infectious Epidemic Hepatitis— Experimental Study of Immunity and Cross-Immunity in Volunteers, A Preliminary Report," *American Journal of the Medical Sciences* 210, no. 5 (1945): 561–75.

39. E. H. El-Raziky et al., "Prevalence of HBs Ag and Schistosomiasis: General Aspects," *Egyptian Journal of Bilharzia* 6 (1979): 1–20; A. El-Zayadi et al., "Prevalence of Hepatitis B Surface Antigen among Urinary Schistosomal Patients Receiving Frequent Parenteral Antischistosomal Therapy," *Journal of the Egyptian Society of Parasitology* 14 (1984): 61–64.

40. Immunologists hypothesize that the parasitic burden may cause an imbalance in the Th1Th2 response of the immune system and trigger inflammatory reactions. Parasitologists suggest that parasitic infection can downregulate the immune system and thus facilitate the multiplication of the virus.

41. Yasin A. Ghaffar, "The Impact of Endemic Schistosomiasis on Acute Viral Hepatitis," *American Journal of Tropical Medicine and Hygiene* 45, no. 6 (1991): 743–50. M. A. Kamel et al., "The Epidemiology of *Schistosoma mansoni,* Hepatitis B and Hepatitis C in Egypt," *Annals of Tropical Medicine and Parasitology* 88, no. 5 (1994): 501–9; A. El-Zayadi et al., "Does Schistosomiasis Play a Role in the High Seroprevalence of HCV Antibody among Egyptians?" *Tropical Gastroenterology* 18, no. 3 (1997): 98–100.

42. Amal Gad et al., "Relationship between Hepatitis C Virus Infection and Schistosomal Liver Disease: Not Simply an Additive Effect," *Journal of Gastroenterology* 36, no. 11 (2001): 753–58.

43. E. Drucker, P. G. Alcabes, and P. A. Marx, "The Injection Century: Massive Unsterile Injections and the Emergence of Human Pathogens," *Lancet* 358, no. 9297 (2001): 1989–92.

44. I. Simonsen et al., "Unsafe Injections in the Developing World and Transmission of Blood-Borne Pathogens: A Review," *Bulletin of the World Health Organization* 77 (1999), 789–800.

45. R. M. Packard, *Visions of Postwar Health and Development and their Impact on Public Health Interventions in the Developing World* (Berkeley: University of California Press, 1997), 93–118.

46. Drucker, Alcabes, and Marx, "Injection Century," 1990.

47. A. A. Saeed et al., "Hepatitis C Virus Infection in Egyptian Volunteer Blood Donors in Riyadh," *Lancet* 338 (1991): 459–60; S. E. Fathalla, "Hepatitis C Virus Infection among Egyptians in Dammam," *Annals of Saudi Medicine* 12, no. 4 (1992), 418–19.

48. A. S. Khalifa et al., "Prevalence of Hepatitis C Antibody in Transfused and Nontransfused Egyptian Children," *American Journal of Tropical Medicine and Hygiene* 49 (1993): 316–21. Tewhida Yassin Abdel Ghaffar, "Prevalence of non-A non-B Hepatitis in Egyptian Children Receiving Repeated Transfusions of Blood or Blood Fractions," MD thesis in pediatrics, Aïn Shams University, 1983.

49. A. El-Zayadi et al., "Prevalence of Hepatitis C Virus among Non-A, Non-B Related Liver Disease in Egypt," *Journal of Hepatology* 14, no. 2–3 (1992): 416–17.

50. His daughter suggests that his death in 1999 was a consequence of the grief and sorrow he suffered at the hands of critics. Dr. Tewhida Yassin Abdel Ghaffar, personal interviews, Cairo, April and July 2011.

51. N. M. Darwish et al., "Hepatitis C Virus Infection in Blood Donors in Egypt," *Journal of the Egyptian Public Health Association* 67 (1992): 223–36.

52. M. A. Darwish et al., "Risk Factors Associated with a High Seroprevalence of Hepatitis C Virus Infection in Egyptian Blood Donors," *American Journal of Tropical Medicine and Hygiene* 49, no. 4 (1993): 440–47.

53. Darwish et al., "Risk Factors."

54. M. K. Mohamed et al., "Viral Hepatitis C Infection among Egyptians: The Magnitude of the Problem: Epidemiological and Laboratory Approach," *Journal of the Egyptian Public Health Association* 71, no. 1–2 (1996): 79–111; M. Angelico et al., "Chronic Liver Disease in the Alexandria Governorate, Egypt: Contribution of Hepatitis and Schistosomiasis Virus Infections," *Journal of Hepatology* 26, no. 2 (1997): 236–43.

55. Frank et al., "Role of Parenteral Therapy," 887–91.

56. Ibid., 891.

57. Ibid.

58. B. G. Maegraith, "Treatment of Bilharziasis in Egypt, UAR, November 1962, Report to WHO" (Geneva: WHO, 1964), MNP/PA/269. 63. Rev.1; A. Abdallah, "Resume of Some Pilot Projects Carried Out in Egypt in the Past Twenty Years" (Geneva: WHO, 1972), SCHISTO/WP/(72.41).

59. Maegraith, "Treatment of Bilharzia," 3.

60. Ibid., 4.

61. Ibid., 7, 21.

62. Frank et al., "Role of Parenteral Therapy."

63. N. Arafa et al., "Changing Pattern of Hepatitis C Virus Spread in Rural Areas of Egypt," *Journal of Hepatology* 43, no. 3 (2005): 418–24.

64. D. L. Thomas et al., "Genetic Variation in IL28B and Specific Clearance of Hepatitis C Viruses," *Nature* 461 (2009), 798–801.

65. Maegraith, "Treatment of Bilharzia," 18.

66. Abdallah, "Resume of Some Pilot Projects," SCHISTO WP/72.41.

67. Maegraith, "Treatment of Bilharzia," 28.

68. M. K. Mohamed et al., "Study of Risk Factors for Viral Hepatitis C Infection among Egyptians Applying for Work Abroad," *Egyptian Journal of the Public Health Association* 71, no. 1–2 (1996): 113–47.

69. Vaccines at an experimental stage are still currently being tested. Maegraith notes that "some villages were treated, whether infected or not." Maegraith, "Treatment of Bilharzia," 45.

70. See S. Chiffoleau, "Un siècle de vaccination antivariolique en Égypte (1827–1927): Politiques de santé publique et pédagogie de la modernisation," in *Islam et révolutions médicales: Le labyrinthe du corps,* ed. A. M. Moulin (Paris: Karthala, 2013), 59–94; N. Gallagher, *Egypt's Other Wars: Epidemics and the Politics of Public Health* (Syracuse, NY: Syracuse University Press, 1990); L. Kuhnke, *Lives at Risk: Public Health in*

ANNE MARIE MOULIN

Nineteenth-Century Egypt (Berkeley: University of California Press, 1990). See also C. Cuny, *Propositions d'hygiène, de médecine et de chirurgie relatives à l'Égypte,* Thèse de médecine, Paris University, 1853, p. 12.

71. Popular resistance to this new oppression formed the roots of 'Urabi's revolutionary movement in 1881 J. Cole, *Colonialism and Revolution in the Middle East: Social and Cultural Origins of Egypt's 'Urabi Movement* (Cairo: American University in Cairo Press, 1999). Cf. T. Mitchell, *Colonizing Egypt* (Cambridge: Cambridge University Press, 1988).

72. T. Mostyn, *Egypt's Belle Epoque: Cairo and the Hedonists* (London: Tauris, 2006).

73. S. Qutb, *A Child from the Village* (Tifl min al-Qarya, 1946; Syracuse, NY: Syracuse University Press, 2000).

74. Susan Watts and Samiha El-Katscha, *Gender, Behaviour and Health: Schistosomiasis Transmission and Control in Rural Egypt* (Cairo: American University in Cairo, 2002).

75. Frank et al., "Role of Parenteral Therapy."

76. Maegraith, "Treatment of Bilharzia," 28.

77. Alleged facts are complex products, resulting from the assembling and packaging of items from various sources. Medical truths are currently negotiated between such social groups as scientists, authorities, and societies. A. M. Moulin, "The Transformations of Medical Truths in History in Light of Ludwik Fleck's Epistemology," in *Vérité, Widerstand, Development: At Work with / Arbeiten mit / Travailler avec Ludwik Fleck,* ed. R. Egloff and J. Fehr (Zürich: Collegium Helveticum Heft 12, 2011), 17–28.

78. H. A. S. Khatttab, *Report on a Study of Women Living with HIV in Egypt* (Cairo: Egyptian Society for Population Studies and Reproductive Health, 2007).

79. Leonard B. Seeff, "Why Is There Such Difficulty in Defining the Natural History of Hepatitis C?" *Transfusion* 40 (2000): 1161–64.

80. J. H. Hoofnagle, "Course and Outcome of Hepatitis C," *Hepatology* 36, no. 5B (2002): S21–29; D. L. Thomas et al., "Genetic Variation in IL28B and Spontaneous Clearance of Hepatitis C Virus," *Nature* 461 (2009): 798–801.

81. Anwar el Sadat, *In Search of Identity: An Autobiography* (New York: Harper & Row, 1978), 261, 306.

82. G. Alleaume and F. Gad El-Hakk, eds., "Essayons d'en rire: Caricatures publiées dans la presse égyptienne," *Dossiers du CEDEJ* (Cairo) 14, no. 5 (1982).

83. M. Fintz and S. Thierno-Youla, "Les guerres de la grippe aviaire," in *Figures de la santé en Egypte,* ed. M. Fintz, A. M. Moulin, and S. Radi (Cairo: Egypte Monde Arabe, 2007), 4:269–302.

84. S. El-Dâlî, *Al-Fâshlûn* [The Losers] (Cairo: Kitâba misr hayat wa ikhrâj, 2000).

85. Doctors remain at the highest rung of the social ladder, and entrance into medical faculty is very much prized by families.

86. Interview with Sister K, Cairo, July 2011.

87. S. Radi, "L'hépatite C et les défaillances du système de santé publique: Itinéraires thérapeutiques et solutions palliatives," in Fintz, Moulin, and Radi, *Figures de la santé en Egypte,* 4:127–46.

88. A. Regourd, "Deux coupes magico-thérapeutiques," in *Coran et talismans: Textes et pratiques magiques en milieu musulman,* ed. Constant Hames (Paris: Karthala, 2007), 309–46.

89. See A. Amin, *Qâmûs al-ʿadât wa-l-taqalîd wa–l-taʾâbîr al-misriyya* (Cairo: Lajnat al-taʾlîf wa-l-tarjama wa-l-nachr, 1953).

90. See K. Fahmi, *All the Pasha's Men ; A. Mikhail, Nature and Empire in Ottoman Egypt: An Environmental History* (New Haven:Yale University Press, 2011).

91. S. Deuffic-Burban et al., "Expected Increase in Hepatitis C-Related Mortality in Egypt due to Pre-2000 Infections," *Journal of Hepatology* 44, no. 3 (2006): 455–61; M. M. El Gaafary et al., "Surveillance of Acute Hepatitis C in Cairo, Egypt," *Journal of Medical Virology* 76 (2005): 520–25; A. Munier et al., "Frequent Transient Hepatitis C Viremia without Seroconversion among Healthcare Workers in Cairo, Egypt," PLoS ONE 8, no. 2 (2013): e57835. doi: 10.1371/journal.pone.0057835.

92. M. Talaat et al., "Overview of Injections Practices in Two Governorates in Egypt," *Tropical Medicine and International Health* 8, no. 3 (2003): 234–41.

93. Doctors mention tonsillectomy as a potential cause of transmission of hepatitis C, explaining some infections in children. See interview with Dr. Tewhida Yassin Abdel Ghaffar, Liver Center, Cairo, April 2011.

94. V.-K. Nguyen, *The Republic of Therapy: Triage and Sovereignty in West Africa's Time of AIDS* (Durham, NC: Duke University Press, 2010).

95. During the French Revolution, some speakers advocated medical transparency and called for clinical observations occurring under the gaze of informed citizens. This suggestion was consonant at the time with the ephemeral proposal of suppressing medical faculties as conservatories for elitist, secret knowledge out of the public purview. P. Pinel, "Rapport fait à l'École de médecine de Paris, sur la clinique d'inoculation, le 29 fructidor, an VII (1799)," document published in *La France médicale*, no. 357 (1901).

96. S. Radi and A. M. Moulin, "La société égyptienne au risque de la grippe aviaire: Une pandémie au quotidien," in "Islams et santé," ed. Laurence Kotobi and Anne Marie Moulin, special issue, *Revue sociologie santé*, no. 31 (March 2010): 115–37.

97. D. McNeeley et al., "Changes in Antischisosomal Drug Usage Patterns in Rural Qalubiya, Egypt," *American Journal of Tropical Medicine and Hygiene* 42, no. 2 (1990): 158.

98. A. M. Moulin, "La santé est aussi un enjeu politique: Les révolutions arabes," *L'histoire* 52 (2011): 84.

7 "SNAKE IN THE BELLY"

Africa's Unhappy Experience with Cholera during the Seventh Pandemic, 1971 to the Present

MYRON ECHENBERG

One of the most feared maladies of the nineteenth century, modern cholera is a severe diarrheal disease.[1] Its bacterium, *Vibrio cholerae,* is spread mainly by water contaminated with the fecal discharges of cholera patients. Once the pathogen is ingested, an incubation period as short as twelve hours can ensue, often with frightening symptoms; these include an explosive dehydration from both watery diarrhea and vomiting, to darkened skin and thickened blood, and finally to circulatory or kidney failure and death. Untreated with oral rehydration therapy (ORT), a previously healthy person can be dead in hours.

Cholera's Global Reach

A frightening and repugnant disease, cholera was responsible for millions of deaths as it spread from its reservoir in the Ganges delta of the Bay of Bengal in a series of six pandemics beginning in 1816.[2] Higher urban densities and crowded meeting places provided fertile ground. Millions of Muslim pilgrims at Mecca and Hindu pilgrims at Hardwar, India, succumbed, as did city dwellers in such far-flung locations as London, Paris, Hamburg, St. Petersburg, Montreal, New York, and Rio de Janeiro. Especially dramatic were losses in Russia between 1892 and 1894, when more than 800,000 deaths occurred. In Africa, Zanzibar city alone lost 70,000 to cholera in 1869–70.

The modern history of cholera turns on two paradoxes. First, the growth of science and technology actually abetted the spread of cholera before medical and public health advances began to catch up with technological change. Expanding global trade and improving land and sea transport after 1830 enabled *Vibrio cholerae* to spread more rapidly and reach human hosts in every corner of the globe. Initially, poor understanding of cholera's etiology caused physicians to prescribe remedies that did more harm than good. By the late nineteenth century, however, cholera became more sporadic and less destructive of human life as advances in public health and sanitation enabled more people to have access to clean sources of drinking water and effective disposal of sewage.

The second paradox, which forms the main problematic of this chapter, is that, as cholera has become a nuisance rather than a killer, the disease now constitutes a major health problem in Africa. Indeed, with over 95 percent of the world's cases since 1995, cholera is now an African disease. Why a disease now well understood scientifically, and for which an inexpensive and effective rehydration treatment exists, should have become more widespread and lethal, not less, requires an explanation based on variables rooted in both biological and social science. The increased severity of risk conditions in Africa is a product both of the changing physical environment and the deteriorating political and economic conditions most sub-Saharan Africans have endured after the mid-1970s.

Cholera's Changing Environment

Vibrio cholerae bacteria rely on water to live and propagate. Modern scientific efforts to understand and control cholera have turned on this obvious relationship between the bacteria and water. Several natural events can transform water into a danger. Floods can cause an overflow of wastewater treatment plants, failure of septic systems, or combined sewer overflows that contaminate surface waters or wells. During droughts, contaminants may be concentrated in available water sources, and multiple use for cleaning and bathing and drinking increases risk.

Classic *Vibrio cholerae,* probably responsible for all six of the nineteenth-century pandemics, gave way to *Vibrio cholerae o1* El Tor during the seventh pandemic beginning in 1961. The early 1990s witnessed the emergence of a new strain of toxigenic cholera called *Vibrio cholerae o139,* or "Bengal" serotype, but its ability to launch an eighth cholera pandemic has not materialized.[3]

For almost a century, scientific dogma held that the only reservoir of cholera was located in the human intestinal tract. Highly host adapted, the bacteria were believed incapable of surviving longer than a few hours or days outside the human body. Today it has been established by leading scholars such as the American Rita Colwell and her South Asian associate Dilip Mahalanabis that toxigenic *Vibrio cholerae o1* El Tor has acquired the ability to stand without a human host and survive in an aquatic milieu.[4] Attaching to shells of shrimps, and in the guts of clams, mussels and oysters, these bacteria are able to survive long periods of starvation by moving into dormancy.

The researchers also investigated the microflora that served as cholera's nutrients in its aquatic environment. They determined the key variables to be temperature and salinity, adherence to surfaces, and colonization of macro-biota with zooplankton blooms, and copepods. The implications for the spread of cholera are enormous. Cholera vibrios are able to survive in association with such common aquatic vegetation as water hyacinths and the blue-green bacterium *Anabena,* as well as other zooplankton and shellfish in the aquatic environment. Cholera outbreaks therefore lack a common source and have a broad distribution as a result of tidal ebb and flow and seasonal flooding. As ocean currents sweep coastal areas, they are able to transport plankton and their bacterial passengers, which have attached to them.[5]

Human agency helps significantly in this proliferation of oceanic algae blooms. The destruction of wetlands, poor erosion control, excessive use of fertilizers, and coastal sewage dumping are some of the factors.[6] Adverse climate changes producing irregular rainfall patterns contribute to cholera's threat, as was the case in 2005 in Senegambia.[7]

Vibrio cholerae have been detected in estuarine and coastal water along the Pacific, Atlantic, and Gulf coasts of the United States. The bacteria have also been isolated in Australia, the island nations of the South Pacific, southeast Asia, Europe, and Africa.[8] Cholera, in brief, no longer has to be imported by a human carrier traveling from a single South Asian reservoir, which typically had been the Bay of Bengal. In several locales in Africa, freestanding cholera is present year round in aquatic settings, and can trigger human outbreaks through the consumption of water containing the vibrio. The major locales are Lake Chad in West Africa and Lakes Kivu, Tanganyika, and Malawi (Nyasa) in East Africa. The estuaries of several rivers in Mozambique are likely reservoirs, and possibly also other Great Lakes of East Africa, though no scientific confirmation has yet occurred.

The standard treatment for cholera patients is oral rehydration therapy (ORT). It is an inexpensive and effective therapy developed by multinational teams in Calcutta and Dhaka in the mid-1960s, needing only sugar and salt, ingredients available throughout the world, and capable of being administered by immediate family caregivers. The most spectacular breakthrough in oral rehydration was led by Dilip Mahalanabis during the Bangladesh War of Independence in 1971. He and his teams proved that ORT in an emergency could save lives otherwise bound to be lost.[9] The procedure is based on the physiological observation by scientists from the 1950s that glucose enhanced the absorption of sodium in the mammalian gut.

The transfer of this basic insight to the clinical practice of medicine occurred within less than a decade, and was, according to a *Lancet* editorial on 5 August 1978, a momentous scientific breakthrough:

> The discovery that sodium transport and glucose transport are coupled in the small intestine, so that glucose accelerates absorption of solute and water, was potentially the most important medical advance this century.

More expensive therapies have not been as successful. Antibiotics have not been effective in altering the course of cholera epidemics. The resistance of *V. cholerae* 01 El Tor to tetracycline, once the drug of choice, together with higher costs that create a false sense of community protection and take resources away from more effective ORT measures, have prompted the World Health Organization (WHO) to "strongly advise health authorities not to employ this measure."[10]

Another option in clinical management of cholera is the use of oral cholera vaccines (OCVs). The older vaccines had never been considered satisfactory for general public health use because of their low protective efficacy. The WHO argues that priority in acute phases of a cholera emergency should be given to basic relief activities rather than to mass immunization.[11]

The Cholera Crisis in Africa

Nyoka, or *manyoka,* translated as "snake in the belly," is a common metaphor in Bantu-speaking East and Central Africa for diarrhea.[12] Gastrointestinal infections, especially among children, have long been a major source of disability and death in the region.[13]

Local culture expressed its preoccupation by assigning no less than eight terms for various kinds of diarrhea, whereas elsewhere in Africa a couple of labels might be the norm. Diarrhea's etiology, as understood locally, is complex. Among infants, contaminated food or water could be causative, but so too could be improper sexual behavior of the father or mother. The snake in question is the symbolic guardian of bodily purity, and needs to be kept calm. Violations of the body that cause it disturbance, whether attributed to diet, environment, social relations, taboo violation, death in the family, miscarriage, or new pregnancy, require purification through the expulsion of impurities.

Mozambique experienced a major cholera outbreak in 1870, but no details have survived.[14] When cholera next appeared a century later during the seventh pandemic, its extensive vomiting and diarrhea were immediately understood as an extreme form of *manyoka.* Central Mozambicans tried familiar treatments for other diarrheas such as the boiling of roots to produce a drinkable liquid. It was not, therefore, a great leap to adapt to modern medicine's ORT.[15]

The recent outbreaks in Mozambique are part of a continuing cholera crisis in Africa, even though the disease has long ceased to be a dreaded affliction in the rest of the world, as figure 7.1 indicates.

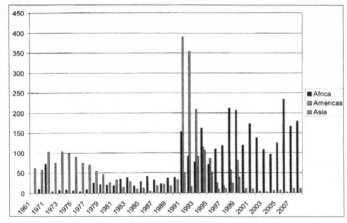

FIGURE 7.1. Seventh cholera pandemic cholera, cases in thousands reported to WHO, 1961–2001.

Source: WHO, *Weekly Epidemiological Record,* annual reports on cholera, 1961–2008.

Since 2000, Africa's cholera cases account for 90 percent or more of the world's totals. Worse, the number of cases is rising. Africa's worst year in 2006 saw it register 234,000 cases, 99 percent of the global number. The latest figures, for 2008, show only a small decline to 179,000 African cases, representing 94 percent of the global total of 190,000.

Not only does Africa have the most cases, it also suffers from the highest case fatality rates, or CFRs (see figure 7.2).

FIGURE 7.2. Seventh cholera pandemic, case fatality rate reported to WHO, 1961–2007

Source: WHO, *Weekly Epidemiological Record,* annual reports on cholera, 1961–2007.

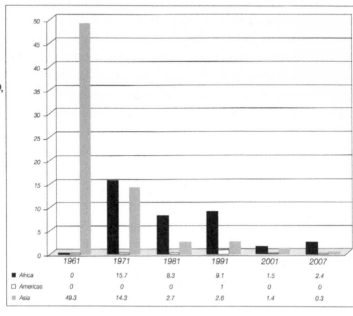

	1961	1971	1981	1991	2001	2007
■ Africa	0	15.7	8.3	9.1	1.5	2.4
□ Americas	0	0	0	1	0	0
▣ Asia	49.3	14.3	2.7	2.6	1.4	0.3

In the early years of the seventh pandemic, CFRs were high everywhere, but with the spread of effective oral rehydration therapy, the rates declined dramatically, enabling the World Health Organization to establish a bench mark of 1 percent as the maximum a sound public health system should tolerate. Only very recently have some African countries fallen below this benchmark. For example, in 2007, the African CFR stood at 2.4 percent, representing 3,994 cholera deaths among 166,000 cases. By contrast the Asian CFR was only 0.3 percent, or 37 deaths from 11,000 cases.

Table 7.1 shows incidences of African cholera outbreaks from 1991 to 2007. Cholera is endemic in at least twenty-one African countries, that is, they have reported cases at least ten times since 1991. Outbreaks have varied in size, but table 7.2 indicates that the attack rates per 100,000 population in the most severe outbreaks have been devastating throughout the regions of Africa. It can also be seen that many countries have experienced their worst cholera epidemics since 2005. Except for a rare handful of imported cases, five countries have been cholera-free (the Central African Republic [CAR], Gabon, Botswana, Namibia, and Lesotho). Among those countries with low rates of incidence, questions with regard to Sudan and Ethiopia arise, because they have usually chosen to describe and report their intestinal infections as "acute watery diarrhea," or AWD.

This anomaly draws attention to the issue of the quality of the statistical data compiled by WHO and used widely in cholera epidemiology. Our main source since the seventh pandemic began are the data published regularly on cholera outbreaks globally, and compiled annually in August or September for the previous year's totals, by the WHO in their weekly publication, The *Weekly Epidemiological Record (WER)*. These aggregate data have been supplied officially by member states of the WHO since 1968, in keeping with their mandatory obligation under the WHO's International Health Regulations (IHR). In 2005, after thirty-seven years, WHO Member States adopted revised IHRs, entering into force on 15 June 2007. No longer would it be compulsory for states to report cases of cholera, or yellow fever or bubonic plague, three once notifiable infectious diseases. Instead, countries would be required to inform the WHO of "public health events of international concern." Despite this vague language, it is unclear what logic lay behind the WHO's public expression of confidence that, with the compulsion removed, countries would feel freer to report accurately.[16]

Over the years, the WHO has issued several caveats concerning the quality of cholera reporting. In 1993, the WHO attributed uneven data to "reporting

TABLE 7.1. Country incidence of cholera, 1991–2007 (17 years)

WEST AFRICA

High (13–17 years)		Medium (7–12 years)		Low (0–6 years)	
Nigeria	17	Guinea	12	Mali	6
Ghana	17	Chad	11	Mauritania	4
Cameroon	16	Guinea-Bissau	10	Gambia	1
Liberia	15	Cote d'Ivoire	10		
Benin	14	Burkina Faso	8		
Togo	14				
Niger	13				

HORN OF AFRICA

High (13–17 years)		Medium (7–12 years)		Low (0–6 years)	
		Somalia	12	Ethiopia	2
		Djibouti	7	Sudan	2
				Eritrea	1

CENTRAL AND EAST AFRICA

High (13–17 years)		Medium (7–12 years)		Low (0–6 years)	
DRC	17	Angola	7	Congo-Brazzaville	4
Tanzania	17			Sao Tome	3
Burundi	16			Equatorial Guinea	2
Uganda	16			Central African Republic	1
Kenya	14			Gabon	1
Rwanda	13				

SOUTHERN AFRICA

High (13–17 years)		Medium (7–12 years)		Low (0–6 years)	
Mozambique	15	Zimbabwe	12	Swaziland	6
Malawi	15	South Africa	8	Namibia	1
Zambia	14			Botswana	0
				Lesotho	0

INDIAN OCEAN

High (13–17 years)		Medium (7–12 years)		Low (0–6 years)	
				Comoros	6
				Madagascar	2

Source: WHO, Weekly Epidemiological Record, annual reports on cholera, 1991–2007.

*Incidence when 50 or more cases occur.

TABLE 7.2. Attack rates in worst outbreak of cholera

WEST AFRICA

Country	Year	Cases	Population (in millions)	Attack rate (per 100,000)
Guinea Bissau	2005	25,111	1.4	1,894
Liberia	2003	34,740	2.8	1,241
Guinea	1994	31,415	7.2	436
Senegal	2005	31,719	12.0	264
Chad	1991	13,915	6.0	232
Benin	1991	7,474	4.9	153
Ghana	1991	13,172	15.8	83
Togo	1998	3,217	4.6	70
Nigeria	1991	59,478	99.0	60
Cameroon	2004	8,005	16.9	47
Niger	1991	3,238	8.0	40

HORN OF AFRICA

Country	Year	Cases	Population (in millions)	Attack rate (per 100,000)
Djibouti	1995	10,055	0.5	2,011
Somalia	2007	41,643	9.3	448
Sudan	2006	30,662	38.5	80
Ethiopia	2006	54,070	77.4	70

CENTRAL AND EAST AFRICA

Country	Year	Cases	Population (in millions)	Attack rate (per 100,000)
Angola	2006	67,257	12.0	560
Uganda	1998	49,514	22.5	220
Tanzania	1997	40,249	31.0	130
DRC	1994	58,057	44.5	130
Kenya	1998	22,432	29.1	77

SOUTHERN AFRICA

Country	Year	Cases	Population (in millions)	Attack rate (per 100,000)
Zimbabwe	2008–09	95,000	11.4	833
South Africa	2001–02	125,000	45.6	274
Malawi	2002	32,618	12.5	261
Mozambique	1999	44,329	17.7	250
Zambia	1991	13,154	8.2	160

INDIAN OCEAN

Country	Year	Cases	Population (in millions)	Attack rate (per 100,000)
Comoros	2000	3,297	0.6	550
Madagascar	2000	29,083	15.7	185

artifacts," but gave no indication of what these were.[17] For the year 1997, the WHO acknowledged that cholera reporting was "far from complete," because member states had powerful disincentives against full disclosure.[18] First were the risks of severe economic repercussions ranging from tourism losses to restrictions on trade exports of foodstuffs. Second was the loss of face African politicians faced in admitting implicitly that their water supply was contaminated by feces. Third were surveillance difficulties, especially in more remote rural areas.

Definitions of cholera and the lack of a standard vocabulary also make the data problematic. WHO cholera data do not include cases defined as AWD, and some member states opted to report only laboratory-confirmed cases. Sudan and Ethiopia have been inclined to report their cases of intestinal disease as AWD; both only began reporting what they called cholera to the WHO in 2006. For years, the WHO reported AWD cases without commentary, but the 2008 report conceded that there were an estimated 500,000–700,000 such cases in "vast areas of Central and South-East Asia and in some African countries." They added that the number of global cholera cases was "much higher."[19]

Can researchers have much confidence in official global cholera data? No is the obvious answer. One study estimates the annual global burden of cholera in the millions rather than one or two hundred thousand. The authors claim that cholera accounts for 0.6 percent of all diarrhea cases, or 11 million cases annually.[20] Fortunately, epidemiologists and cholera specialists have had access to superior data since the mid-1990s. Since then, the Program for Monitoring Emerging Diseases (ProMED), supplies a free online forum for infectious disease specialists, microbiologists, public health officials, and the general public; it has been administered since 1999 through the International Society for Infectious Diseases.[21] It goes without saying that the statistics in this essay represent guidelines and trends, but cannot be considered definitive.

First Risk Condition: Landscapes of Risk

Changing ecological conditions in Lakes Chad, Tanganyika, and Malawi (Nyasa) have enabled cholera to become freestanding, and thus endemic to thousands of people living in these large lake basins.[22]

The Lake Chad basin is essential to the lives of over 20 million people in the four countries touching its shores: Chad, Cameroun, Nigeria, and Niger. Located in the heart of the West African sahel, Lake Chad receives over 90 percent of its water from the Chari River, originating to the south in the tropical forest of the Central African Republic (CAR).[23]

The region's first encounter with the seventh cholera pandemic began in May of 1971, resulting in several thousand cases and a CFR of 15 percent.[24] A well-attended circumcision ceremony for the son of an important Muslim shaykh brought an estimated 20,000 people from Nigeria, Cameroun, Chad, and Niger to the town of Goulfrey in northern Cameroun. A cholera outbreak struck the day after, and in May alone, Goulfrey recorded 801 cases and 121 deaths (a CFR of 15 percent). Medical authorities rushed in to chlorinate drinking water and disinfect all latrines, but the infection spread throughout the Lake Chad basin. Some isolated Camerounian villages endured CFRs of over 50 percent. Fifty kilometers across the border in Chad, the capital of N'Djamena experienced 176 cases and 33 deaths (CFR of 18.8 percent) between May and July, despite a massive vaccination campaign, which administered 189,000 inoculations in three days. A French medical observer described the cholera outbreak in the Lake Chad basin as a "scene of desolation and horror."[25]

Cholera outbreaks in the Lake Chad basin were mild and sporadic for the next twenty years. But, beginning in 1991, and continuing to the present, WHO cholera statistics suggest that the Lake Chad basin has suffered from a continuing endemic presence. Rarely a year passed without significant outbreaks in the Chad basin. Persistently high CFRs, among the worst in Africa, suggested that little treatment of patients occurred.

Of the four countries involved, Niger's poverty, and the remoteness of Lake Chad from the capital of Niamey are no doubt factors in that country's poor performance in controlling cholera. In the case of Chad, even though its capital of N'Djamena is close to the Lake Chad basin, it has been subject to warlord rule since the early 1990s and has not taken care of its basic public health duties. But even though Cameroun and Nigeria have the financial resources available to keep cholera under control, they have failed to do so. Remoteness of the region and its marginal participation in the national economies of the two states only partially explain their poor public health records in containing cholera.

A second endemic focus of cholera is the shore area of Lake Tanganyika, implicating populations of southeastern Democratic Republic of the Congo (DRC), Burundi, western Tanzania, and Zambia. Over 100,000 people are directly involved in the fisheries at roughly 800 sites in the four countries touching on the lake. Conditions in the lake make it hospitable to freestanding *V. cholerae;* its average surface temperature is 25 degrees C, and plankton abound.[26]

The Kaputa district in the northern province of Zambia illustrates the problems posed by cholera to fishing communities in the Lake Tanganyika basin.[27]

This remote area incorporates a population of roughly 50,000, many of whom engage in seasonal fishing to supplement subsistence. Each rainy season sees the opening of temporary, and unsanitary, fishing camps and a cholera season corresponding with the rains between November and February. The presence of traders from neighboring Tanzania and the DRC runs the risk of importing cholera from these countries as well. The worst cholera year in Kaputa district was 1991, when 573 cases and 63 deaths brought the CFR to the alarming level of 11 percent.

Zambian health authorities did attempt control measures. They established eleven cholera treatment centers, but the limited public transport and the remoteness of the region led to shortages of rehydration fluids and staff. Because the Zambian economy suffered in the 1980s and early '90s as the price of copper, its main export, plummeted, the government felt obliged to keep the fishing camps open during the cholera season. Simple educational admonitions to "boil water, wash hands" foundered, meanwhile, because firewood was scarce, charcoal was expensive, and soap not readily available.[28]

Over the seventeen years after 1991, endemic cholera remained an annual health problem for the peoples of the Lake Tanganyika basin. Although CFRs have fallen recently, in 2006, for example, the basin experienced approximately 19,000 cases.[29]

Lake Malawi, also known as Lake Nyasa, is the third largest lake in Africa.[30] Conditions in Lake Malawi would support a hypothesis, as yet unconfirmed, that freestanding *Vibrio cholerae* are present. Annual cholera data for seventeen years starting in 1991 show that both Malawi and Mozambique have reported cholera fifteen times.

The peoples of the Lake Malawi basin have been tied to a long history of labor migration in the direction of South Africa. Population movements, both voluntary and involuntary, have triggered cholera outbreaks in the rest of Mozambique, Zimbabwe, and the northern provinces of South Africa.

Second Risk Condition: Armed Conflict and the Risk to Refugees

Throughout the seventh pandemic, overcrowded refugee camps globally have exposed vulnerable civilians to cholera. Cholera among refugees was a feature of the war of independence of Bangladesh in 1971.[31] The terrible Ethiopian famine of 1985 drove an estimated half million starving civilians from the Ethiopian regions of Tigray, Wollo, and Eritrea into neighboring Sudan, where they contracted cholera.[32] Four years later, refugees from conflict in Liberia and Sierra Leone brought cholera with them when they took shelter in

Guinea. In this instance, the United Nations High Commission for Refugees (UNHCR) complied with the Guinean government's wish to settle the refugees amid existing border villages and towns rather than in camps.[33] Elsewhere, unfortunately, challenged health workers have struggled to provide basic services such as latrines, sufficient quantities of safe water, appropriate rehydration fluids, and enough soap and food for distribution.

The worst cholera disaster of the seventh pandemic struck at Goma, North Kivu, in the DRC (then called Zaire) in July 1994, following quickly after the Rwandan genocide.[34] Medical statistics in the Goma region were estimates, especially in the first few weeks. The toll was terrible, not only from cholera, but from dysentery and meningococcal meningitis as well. In the three weeks following 20 July, OXFAM estimated cholera deaths on some days at 3,000. By mid-August, the death count reached 13,000, and the WHO reported a decline in the CFR from 22 percent in the first days to 3 percent, following the massive response of the international community.[35] Fatalities were higher still for untreated people in the streets of Goma.

The Rwandan genocide provides political context.[36] Between 14 and 17 July 1994, large numbers of ethnic Hutu civilians, together with defeated members of the genocidal former Rwandan regime, ex-FAR (Forces armées rwandaises) soldiers, and the Interahamwe, or Hutu militias, fled west in panic, arriving in the Goma area of the DRC. Initial estimates of the refugees were as high as 1.2 million people, arriving at a rate of 25,000 a day. The first refugees were installed in Goma itself, but four additional camps nearby were soon opened.

The exodus of so many hundreds of thousands of civilians was orchestrated by the ideologues of the genocide, called *génocidaires,* and their armed supporters. They demanded sexual favors from mothers desperate to care for their children, gave themselves priority in the distribution of food, water, and medicine, and sold the extra rations. Adding insult to injury, the *génocidaires* perpetuated ethnic stereotyping and hatred by encouraging the belief that Tutsis caused the cholera by poisoning the water.[37]

Refugee assistance was in the hands of several United Nations agencies, French military forces, and NGOs such as CARE, OXFAM, and Médecins sans Frontières (Doctors without Borders). The UNHCR coordinated efforts, but was overwhelmed by the enormous number of refugees appearing in such a short time. Hunger, disease, and death stalked the camps from the outset, and news agencies reported the catastrophe globally. Media coverage of Goma's cholera disaster was dramatic; "Hell on Earth" was the headline in Newsweek on 1 August, and it seemed not to be hyperbole.[38]

What was absent from news coverage was the moral ambiguity involved in alleviating the suffering of perpetrators of genocide. The French government used humanitarianism as a cover, while protecting the Rwandan *génocidaires*, whom they had supported throughout the crisis. The UN and the NGOs treated these armed camps strictly as refugee settlements, and saw their actions as humane and charitable, turning a blind eye to political coercion exercised in the refugee camps, just as they had failed to help stop the original genocide from unfolding. Mahmood Mamdani makes a persuasive case for judging the international emergency health relief efforts at Goma as a moral failure, whatever the various claims to have brought cholera under control.[39]

Armed conflicts and the dispersal of internal and external refugee populations also played a central role in the recent history of cholera in Mozambique. The ugly and protracted wars that plagued Mozambique for two decades following its independence in 1975 enabled cholera to thrive on malnutrition, the destruction of treatment centers, and especially on the untreated water that millions of people were forced to consume.

Armed rebels opposed to the Mozambique government deliberately targeted public health personnel and infrastructure.[40]

Mozambique's sanitary inheritance from Portugal also contributed to health issues. At independence in 1975, some resentful departing Portuguese settlers spitefully poured cement into drainpipes. Impoverished urban Africans who occupied abandoned houses and apartments later added to the problem by selling items of value such as copper and lead piping. By the 1990s, high-rise buildings had no piped water, and people purchased water by the bucket in markets.[41]

Conflict has placed a heavy disease burden on Mozambicans, but the complex ecology of the region has constituted a second set of conditions for cholera. To the northwest, endemic cholera originating in Lake Malawi has made *Vibrio cholerae* present throughout Mozambique almost annually since 1991. To the east, low-lying estuarine environments such as Mozambique's Indian Ocean coast are vulnerable to the threat of rising sea levels.

Cholera in Mozambique has benefited from both drought and flooding. A widespread drought throughout southern Africa in 1992 made Beira's urban groundwater source on the Pungwe River too saline to drink. In Quelimane, artificial lagoons alongside the River Licuar, from which the city water was pumped, dried up entirely.[42]

By contrast, a devastating flood struck Mozambique in February and March 2000. Five weeks of heavy rains all over the eastern parts of southern Africa left

Cholera during the Seventh Pandemic

Mozambique with at least 800 dead, many more homeless, 20,000 head of cattle lost, and 1,400 square kilometers of arable land spoiled. The capital of Maputo was devastated, and the road to Beira was closed. In the Limpopo Valley as river banks burst, over 45,000 people were rescued from trees and rooftops, including Sofia Pedro, who gave birth in a tree to her daughter Rositha. International responses took up to three weeks. The Beira Central Hospital, second largest in country, and another forty-two health units, were ruined. The floods overwhelmed aging colonial water systems and contaminated drinking water.[43]

Mozambique has long endured endemic cholera in both rural and urban settings. Between the seventeen years from 1991 through 2007, only two, 1995 and 1996, were cholera-free. Given the numerous conditions of risk that the country has faced it is not surprising that it has averaged annually 16,715 cases and 359 deaths, with a relatively low CFR of 2.1 percent. Since the beginning of the twenty-first century, however, Mozambique's local public health officials, with the aid of WHO, have succeeded in driving down the CFR below 1 percent.[44]

Third Risk Condition: Water and Sanitation

Cholera risk is also a function of public health policy choices, especially those involving water and sanitation. On the South Atlantic coast of West Africa, the region of Senegambia has been vulnerable to extreme weather, and thus to cholera. Several times since 1985 extensive flooding following heavy rains has wrecked havoc from Mauritania through to Guiné Bissau. In 1985, when floods struck Dakar, the capital of Senegal, it took its heaviest toll in the poor and low-lying neighborhoods of Médina, Gueule-Tapée, Reubeuss, and Cité Cap-Verdienne, where the piped water supply was defective and open air sewers were often clogged. Only 36 percent of the district buildings were connected to the sewer network, and over 60 percent employed poorly built latrines.[45]

Two decades later, floods in the summer of 2005 contributed to Senegal's alarming national total of 31,719 officially notified cholera cases and 458 deaths (a CFR of 1.4 percent). Once again, several of the same impoverished slums in Dakar became uninhabitable, this time leaving at least 20,000 people homeless.[46]

Although its environment has not been cooperative, the government of Senegal has exacerbated the risk of cholera through poor policy decisions. A functioning African democracy with a strong civil society and a well-developed public health system, Senegal has become the darling of international health agencies. It has a positive public health image as a result of its remarkable success in dealing with Africa's HIV/AIDs crisis.[47] Unfortunately, the country's record is weak in addressing the cholera risk resulting from its exposure to extreme weather and its aging sanitary infrastructure.

In the aftermath of the 2005 cholera crisis, the elected president, Abdulaye Wade, announced an ambitious but poorly executed emergency plan costing $104 million to build 4,000 cement homes with electricity and running water for people displaced by floods. Wade called the plan *Jaxaay*, or "eagle" in Wolof, a symbol of pride.[48] A year later, however, on the site where the houses were to be built, only empty fields stood, and thousands of flood victims still lived in temporary tent camps. Some new housing has been constructed, but the project remained seriously behind schedule. When the rains returned in 2006, the tents sheltering most displaced persons leaked. At one camp called Ganar, 500 people shared six showers and toilets, garbage was never collected, and the infirmary has reported numerous cases of malaria and dysentery since 2005.

A second cholera threat to Senegal, which combines environmental and political risk, is the annual Muslim pilgrimage. Each March, over a million of the faithful congregate at the holy city of Touba, where the shrine of the venerated founder of the Murid brotherhood is located. This festival, called the Grand Magal, is emulated by other Muslim groups in the same general region of Diourbel, 150 kilometers to the northeast of Dakar. As was the case with cholera in the nineteenth century with Hindu pilgrimages at Hardwar in India and Muslim pilgrimages at Mecca, the congested temporary facilities for millions of people enabled cholera to spread rapidly among pilgrims arriving at, and especially leaving, such large gatherings. In Senegal in 2005, health authorities tried to control cholera by installing additional health stations and increasing the amount of chlorinated water for pilgrims, but these measures failed to prevent both an explosion of cholera, and the diffusion of the infection by pilgrims returning to their homes throughout the country. Cholera associated with the Touba pilgrimage peaked on 2 April 2005, when 785 new cases were registered in a single day, after which cases declined from over 3,000 a week to about 500 by June.[49]

To be fair, neither Wade nor his predecessors have dared challenge the autonomy of powerful religious authorities so as not to be perceived as interfering with sacred religious practices. Yet it must be said that no visible efforts to reason with the public have been attempted. Instead, Wade's government has continued policies of accommodation toward the Muslim elite and especially toward the international economic elites. Beginning in the late 1980s, in exchange for renegotiated loans, Senegal, like most indebted countries of the Third World, adopted the so-called Structural Adjustment Programs, or SAPs, which required them to sell off public enterprises and utilities, and to privatize education, health care, electricity, and transportation. Specific to cholera, the World Bank, the IMF, and key regional banks such as the African Development Bank, all encouraged poor countries to permit large European water corporations to run their water systems for profit.[50] In 1995, the national water service provider of Senegal, the Société nationale d'exploitation des eaux du Sénégal (SONES), was split into the state-owned SONES and a private operator, La sénégalaise des eaux (SDE). Water prices to consumers have risen since, although SDE insists that the quality of the service has improved.[51] Many cholera victims in Senegal have continued to remain outside the water system.

Although South Africans have confronted such terrible scourges as tuberculosis and HIV/AIDs, their current exposure to cholera also presents a serious health threat. During the 1990s, while cholera registered only a handful of deaths on two occasions, it was never far from South Africa's borders. Endemic cholera in Malawi and Mozambique posed a danger throughout the region as political power shifted away from white to majority rule.

Suddenly, in mid-August of 2000, a cholera epidemic of dramatic proportions struck the Empangeni/Madlebe region of KwaZulu-Natal, some 160 kilometers north of Durban. Soon the epidemic engulfed most of KwaZulu-Natal, and then spread to the Eastern Cape, Mpumalanga, and other provinces of South Africa. Combined official cholera statistics for the 2000–2001 epidemic reveal a total of 125,818 cases, roughly 60 percent of the world total for the two years, and far and away the most ever recorded for a modern African epidemic. Remarkably, however, the CFR for this cholera explosion was only one-quarter of one percent, or 264 deaths, the lowest reported anywhere in the world.[52]

This success was attributed to rapid mobilization of medical and military personnel. Hospitals erected temporary nursing stations to cope with the epidemic. The Ministry of Health launched a public information campaign using radio, television, and pamphlets to warn against unsafe sources, and they sponsored demonstrations of how to treat water both by boiling and the application of freely provided chlorine bleach.[53] They also sponsored awareness programs through road shows featuring popular presenters and musicians. In addition, they deployed 125 health workers from other provinces to KwaZulu-Natal to boost local capacity.[54]

Equally extraordinary was the intensive mobilization of the then formidable resources of the South African Defence Force (SADF). The military bolstered the water tankers provided by municipalities to distribute safe water in rural KwaZulu-Natal. The army medical corps mobilized helicopters and ambulances to evacuate acute cases from some seventy temporary rehydration tents, set up in convenient sites such as playing fields and schools. There, medical teams treated more than 1,000 patients a day and roughly 100,000 overall.[55]

What was lost amid the almost universal acclaim was the role government policy had played in causing such an enormous cholera explosion. Beginning in 1995, just after majority rule began, the Mbeki-led ANC government adopted a neoliberal development program called Operation Masakhane, "let's build together," which claimed to launch South Africa on a path to sustainable development, but which involved "cost-recovery" for new water installations. The World Bank's water expert on Lesotho and South Africa, John Roome, advised Kader Asmal, then South Africa's Minister of Water Affairs, to introduce a "credible threat of cutting service" to nonpaying customers.[56]

The close correlation between neoliberal cost-recovery policy and the cholera explosion is best illustrated by the impact of water policy where the terrible outbreak began. The KwaZulu-Natal region of Madlebe is a semirural community of poor black South Africans living close to the formerly white town and industrial area of Empangeni.[57] Interviews at nine communal taps in the community by Deedat and Cottle showed that a registration fee for connection to the water supply was unaffordable for most Africans and drove them to use unpurified river water a few months before the cholera outbreak.[58] Even for those who sacrificed to subscribe, the frequent breakdown of the entire system left customers without water for up to three weeks at a time. Clearly, cost recovery represented a terrible threat to the health of the poor.

As the KwaZulu-Natal epidemic was unfolding, the Mbeki government responded with a "Free Basic Water policy," to be implemented by Department of Water Affairs and Forestry (DWAF) Minister Ronnie Kasrils.[59] All South African households would be guaranteed 6,000 liters of free water per month, based on estimates of eight persons per household and consumption of at least twenty-five liters per person per day. As critics pointed out, however, this quantity did not significantly exceed the minimum of four liters a day an individual requires to replenish the body's liquids.[60] Kasrils promised "basic supplies" of water and electricity for all South Africans by 2008.

Kasrils's fine words promised much more than he or the ANC could deliver. Since 2001, progress in extending access to free water has been slow, especially in semi-urban and rural areas, the very places where cholera has been prominent. In addition, inadequate management of water has led to frequent interruptions and cutoffs, burst pipes, slow repairs, and poor general maintenance so that water delivery in urban as well as rural locales could be interrupted for weeks. As late as 2005, only half of the 170 water service providers met water quality standards.[61] In rural areas, only 2 percent of blacks had indoor plumbing.[62] In cities, the fundamental unfairness of water policy in a racially divided society persists, which was not supposed to happen in the new South Africa. All-white suburbs of Johannesburg are given discounted bulk rates, and a household can fill its swimming pool and water its garden at less than half the cost per liter faced by a black family in Alexandra township, for example.[63]

Resistance to cost recovery in the provision of basic services is widespread and ongoing, as is the threat from cholera. From 2002 to 2008, South Africa has experienced an average of 3,500 cholera cases annually. Among the most militant opponents is the South African Municipal Workers' Union (SAMWU). They view privatization as a threat to their jobs and to services for the poor. SAMWU argues that South Africa's cholera problem is clearly linked to the delivery system of clean water, and a new policy must "entail recognition of water-cutoffs as unconstitutional and the principled scrapping of cost-recovery as a determinant of water delivery."[64]

Angola provides a third case study of how public policy can enhance the risk of cholera. The country has experienced cholera at various times since 1973 but reported outbreaks were not worrisome until 2006. A massive epidemic began in February 2006, and ended in the spring of 2007.[65] Cholera infected sixteen of eighteen provinces, including urban slums in the two largest cities, the capital of Luanda, and Benguela. These two largely urban provinces recorded over 50 percent of Angola's total for 2006–7 of 85,679 cases and 3,235 deaths (a high CFR of 3.8 percent). In nine rural provinces, devastating CFRs ranging from 5 and 15 percent were reported, a measure of poor or nonexistent treatment.

To date, no cholera research beyond the rudimentary and politically correct reports of the WHO are available for the Angola outbreak. But careful reporting by the journalist Stephanie Nolen offers some hints, although she does not mention cholera specifically.[66] Nolen shows how a property and construction boom has been occurring in Luanda over the past few years based on extensive oil and diamond exports. The Angolan economy has been growing at 20 percent per annum, and prime real estate space has become so scarce as to be limited to a little patch of seafront land. Three-quarters of the city's 4 million inhabitants, many of them new urban migrants working in the construction boom, live in appalling conditions. Their shacks have no water services or sanitation, and few schools for their children. People pay a dollar a bucket for water from tanker trucks. Those who cannot afford such exorbitant prices must scrounge for water, and expose themselves and their families to illnesses.

Cholera in Luanda, which exposes the whole country to risk, is a function of government choices. Enjoying such windfall wealth from its oil revenues, the government might have chosen to provide a modicum of services for its labor force, rather than having to pay the terrible price in lives and resources needed to control or eliminate cholera. Instead, the Angolan government has opted for a scheme designed to benefit the affluent. Its policy has been to evict people, especially those on prime seafront land, and relocate them some 30 kilometers away from the city. From 2002 to 2006, the government has conducted eighteen mass evictions, displaced 20,000 people, and destroyed 3,000 slum dwellings.

The story of cholera in Africa has revealed how complacency and narrow self-interest have combined to help the cholera pathogen secure its niche in tropical Africa. Comfortable urban Africans, together with tourists and expatriates, too often have paid cholera little thought as they drink bottled water and live sheltered lives.

Yet cholera has long ceased to be a dreaded affliction in most of the globe, with the painful exception of Africa. Despite the risk conditions this paper has outlined, effective control of cholera in Africa can be achieved. The disease is well understood, and oral rehydration therapy is inexpensive and effective. What is required is that governments in Africa and in the West act out of enlightened self-interest.

Angola represents a good example of how cholera thrives because of its government's cynical choices, though the country is by no means alone. Measures to improve public awareness and provide potable water are in the interest of all Angolans. Angola's substantial fiscal assets, together with the availability of international financing and partnerships, could turn back cholera in only a few years if its leaders are willing.

The reluctance of African governments to take the political decisions required is part of the cholera tragedy. But blame also rests with the West, which is ready to intervene in African medical emergencies, but reluctant, for example, to allow fair trade in African export products.[67] Only when there are improvements in their economies will enough African states invest in the affordable public health measures required to end the lethality of this historically dreaded disease, as have developing countries in Asia and Latin America.

Notes

1. There have been four modern edited compilations dealing with cholera science. In chronological order, they are Dhiman Barua and William Burrows, eds., *Cholera* (Philadelphia: W. B. Saunders, 1974); a revised edition by Dhiman Barua and William B. Greenough III, eds., *Cholera* (New York: Plenum, 1992); I. Kaye Wachsmuth, Paul A. Blake, and Orjan Olsvik, eds., *Vibrio Cholerae and Cholera: Molecular to Global Perspectives* (Washington, DC: American Society for Microbiology, 1994); and B. S. Drasar and B. D. Forrest, eds., *Cholera and the Ecology of Vibrio Cholerae* (London: Chapman & Hall, 1996). The latest published overview that is valuable for researchers and lay readers alike is Paul Shears, "Recent Developments in Cholera," *Current Opinion in Infectious Diseases* 14 (2001): 553–58.

2. For a fine new overview of cholera's history and a guide to its voluminous bibliography, see Christopher Hamlin, *Cholera: The Biography* (Oxford: Oxford University Press, 2009).

3. WHO, *Weekly Epidemiological Record* 72 (1997): 235. Hereafter *WER*.

4. Rita Colwell's germinal research in cholera's ecology was conducted in the Bay of Bengal, and later in Chesapeake Bay. She was associated initially with the Centre for Diarrhoeal Disease Research in Dhaka, Bangladesh, where she eventually became its chair, and now she is with the Maryland Biotechnology Institute at College Park, Maryland. Among the many publications, see Rita R. Colwell and William M. Spira, "The Ecology of Vibrio Cholerae," in *Cholera,* ed. Dhiman Barua and William B. Greenough III (New York, Plenum, 1992), 101–27.

5. Paul R. Epstein, "Cholera and the Environment," *Lancet* 339 (1992): 1167–68.

6. J. Patz et al., "Global Climate Change and Emerging Infectious Diseases," *Journal of the American Medical Association* 275 (1996): 220.

7. Rosa R. Mouriño-Pérez, "Oceanography and the Seventh Cholera Pandemic," *Epidemiology* 9 (1998): 355–57.

8. A. Huq et al., "Detection of Vibrio cholerae 01 in the Aquatic Environment by Fluorescent-Monoclonal Antibody and Culture Methods," *Applied and Environmental Microbiology* 56 (1990): 2370–73.

9. D. Mahalanabis et al., "Oral Fluid Therapy of Cholera among Bangladesh Refugees," *Johns Hopkins Medical Journal* 132 (1973): 197–205; and Dilip Mahalanabis, A. M. Molla, and David A. Sack, "Clinical Management of Cholera," in Barua and Greenough III, *Cholera, 253.*

10. *WER* 67 (1992): 260.

11. Roger Glass et al., "Cholera in Africa: Lessons on Transmission and Control for Latin America," *Lancet* 338 (28 September 1991): 793.

12. Edward C. Green, Annemarie Jurg, and Armando Djedje, "The Snake in the Stomach: Child Diarrhea in Central Mozambique," *Medical Anthropology Quarterly* 8 (1994): 4–24.

13. For Southern and Central African medical beliefs see John Janzen, "Health, Religion, and Medicine in Central and Southern African Traditions," in *Caring and Curing: Health and Medicine in World Religious Traditions,* ed. L. Sullivan (New York: Macmillan, 1989), 225–54; and Harriet Ngubane, *Body and Mind in Zulu Medicine* (London:

Academic Press, 1977). For efforts to control gastrointestinal disease, see Julie Cliff, Felicity Cutts, and Ronald Waldman, "Using Surveys in Mozambique for Evaluation of Diarrhoeal Disease Control," *Health Policy and Planning* 5 (1990): 219–25.

14. James Christie, *Cholera Epidemics in East Africa* (London: Macmillan, 1876; reprinted, USA: Kessinger Publishing, 2008).

15. Green et al., "Snake," 16.

16. WHO, "Cholera, 2006," *WER* 82 (2007): 280.

17. *WER* 68 (1993): 155.

18. WHO, "Cholera in 1997," *WER* 73 (1998): 207.

19. WHO, "Cholera: Global Surveillance Summary," *WER* 84 (2009): 309.

20. C. F. Lanata, W. Mendoza, and R. E. Black, *Improving Diarrhea Estimates* (Geneva: WHO Child and Adolescent Health Development Monitoring and Evaluation Team, 2002).

21. ProMED's data are too scattered to be aggregated. Nevertheless, the data and discussions, though by no means definitive, are open to all with Internet access, and are a boon to over 30,000 subscribers in 180 countries.

See www.promedmail.org, and L. C. Madoff and J. P. Woodall, "The Internet and the Global Monitoring of Emerging Diseases: Lessons from the First 10 Years of ProMED Mail," *Archives of Medical Research* 36 (2005): 724–30.

22. This arbitrary grouping of cases does not deny the diversity of local experiences with cholera in Africa. It is reductionist in that multiple risk conditions often operate. For example, cholera outbreaks in Senegal can be assigned three fundamental causes, though it is impossible to determine which is primary. One condition, clearly, is environmental change; a second is the failure of the state to address the public health issues surrounding crumbling water and sewage infrastructure; a third is the exposure of huge gatherings of pilgrims at religious shrines, a common risk condition in the nineteenth century.

23. A major source of water and of fish, Lake Chad has experienced dramatic environmental cycles of expansion and contraction over the past thirteen millennia. Recently, its diminution has accelerated, from an area of 26,000 square kilometers in 1960 to less than 1,500 square kilometers in 2000, with an exceptionally shallow average depth of only 1.5 meters. Experts attribute this shrinkage to combined factors: cyclical patterns of reduced rainfall in what is an arid part of Africa, greatly increased amounts of irrigation water drawn from the Chari River system, and population growth that has dramatically increased water demand in the past half century. It is not surprising that water rights in the Lake Chad basin have produced political and social tensions, mitigated somewhat by a World Bank–funded effort to enable member countries of the Lake Chad Basin Commission to develop a project to divert water from the Ubangi River into the Lake. See Graham Chapman and Kathleen M. Baker, *The Changing Geography of Africa and the Middle East* (London: Routledge, 1992); Michael T. Coe and Jonathan A. Foley, "Human and Natural Impacts on the Water Resources of the Lake Chad Basin," *Journal of Geophysical Research* 106 (2001): 3349–56; "Africa at a Watershed (Ubangi-Lake Chad Inter-Basin Transfer," *New Scientist,* 23 March 1991, 34; "Vanishing Lake Chad—A Water Crisis in Central Africa," *Circle of Blue,* 24 June 2008, 1–2, www .circleofblue.org/waternews/world/vanishing-lake-chad (accessed 19 March 2013).

24. H. Félix, "Le choléra africain," *Médecine tropicale* 31 (1971): 619–28.

25. Ibid., 624.

26. "Data summary: Lake Tanganyika," www.ilec.or.jp/database/afr/dafr06.html. Accessed 19 March 2013.

27. J. E. A. M. van Bergen, "Epidemiology and Health Policy—A World of Difference? A Case-Study of a Cholera Outbreak in Kaputa District, Zambia," *Social Science and Medicine* 43 (1996): 94–95.

28. Ibid., 97.

29. *WER* 82 (2007): 274.

30. World Lakes Database, International Lake Environment Committee Foundation, accessed 19 March 2013, www.ilec.or.jp/database/afr/afr-13.html.

31. Dhiman Barua and Michael H. Merson, "Prevention and Control of Cholera," in Barua and Greenough III, *Cholera,* 345–46.

32. Kim Mulholland, "Cholera in Sudan: An Account of an Epidemic in Eastern Sudan, May–June, 1985," *Disasters* 9 (1985): 247–58.

33. The UNHCR paid a fee to the Guinean health service, and foreign donors made supplementary payments. Small epidemics of cholera, measles, and meningitis did occur, but most refugees living in Guinea enjoyed a high degree of autonomy and avoided the squalor and acute illness typical of camps. William Van Damme, "Do Refugees Belong in Camps? Experiences from Goma and Guinea," *Lancet* 345 (1995): 260–64.

34. Paul Epstein, "Climate, Ecology, and Human Health," in *Plagues and Politics: Infectious Disease and International Policy,* ed. Andrew T. Price-Smith (New York: Palgrave, 2001), 43.

35. *WER* 70 (1995), 201–8.

36. For medical data, see Goma Epidemiology Group, "Public Health Impact of Rwanda Refugee Crisis: What Happened in Goma, Zaire, in July, 1994," *Lancet* 345 (1995): 339–44; for the political story, see Mahmood Mamdani, *When Victims Become Killers: Colonialism, Nativism, and the Genocide in Rwanda* (Princeton: Princeton University Press, 2001), and Gérard Prunier, *The Rwanda Crisis: History of a Genocide* (New York: Columbia University Press, 1995).

37. Prunier, *Rwanda Crisis,* 314; for poisoning rumor, see Liisa Malkki, "Speechless Emissaries: Refugees, Humanitarianism, and Dehistoricization," *Cultural Anthropology* 11 (1996): 395. For the continuing politicization of the camps, see Sarah Kenyon Lischer, *Dangerous Sanctuaries: Refugee Camps, Civil War, and the Dilemmas of Humanitarian Aid* (Ithaca, NY: Cornell University Press, 2005), and Kate Halvorsen, "Protection and Humanitarian Assistance in the Refugee Camps in Zaire: The Problem of Security," in *The Path of Genocide: The Rwanda Crisis from Uganda to Zaire,* ed. Howard Adelman and Astri Suhrke (New Brunswick, NJ: Transaction Press, 1999), 307–20.

38. For a graphic account of how French military engineers used bulldozers to bury corpses in mass graves, see Thomas P. Odom, *Journey into Darkness: Genocide in Rwanda* (College Station: Texas A&M University Press, 2005), 106.

39. Mamdani, *When Victims,* 254–55.

40. For case studies of cholera, see Andrew E. Collins, *Environment, Health and Population Displacement: Development and Change in Mozambique's Diarrhoeal Disease Ecology*

(Aldershot: Ashgate, 1998). For politics, see J. Hanlon, *Mozambique: Who Calls the Shots* (London: James Curry, 1991), and John Saul, ed., *A Difficult Road: The Transition to Socialism in Mozambique* (New York: Monthly Review Press, 1985). For public health, see G. Walt and A. Melamed, eds., *Mozambique: Towards a People's Health Service* (London: Zed Books, 1984).

41. David A. McDonald and Greg Ruiters, eds., *The Age of Commodity: Water Privatization in Southern Africa* (London: Earthscan, 2005), 46.

42. Collins, *Environment*, 228–29.

43. "Born above the Floodwaters," *BBC News*, 2 March 2000, in BBC News Africa, http://news.bbc.co.uk/2/hi/Africa/662472.stm; "Mozambique Flood: The Threat of Disease," *BBC News*, 28 February 2000, in BBC News Africa, http://news .bbc.co.uk/2/hi/health/medical_notes/e-f/659684.stm.

44. See, for example, *WER* 82 (2007): 274, and 83 (2008): 270.

45. P. S. Sow et al., "L'épidémie de choléra de 1995–1996 à Dakar," *Médecine et maladies infectieuses* 29 (1999): 105–9.

46. *WER* 81 (2006): 300–302.

47. John Iliffe, *The African AIDS Epidemic: A History* (Oxford: James Currey, 2006), 57.

48. "Utopian Plan Belies Dismal Reality for Flood Victims," news item, 19 December 2006, posted on http://www.irinnews.org/printreport.aspx?reportid=62800.

49. "Senegal: Lingering Cholera Epidemic Gains New Strength," Integrated Regional Information Networks, 23 June 2005.

50. For background on water politics in Africa, see Maude Barlow, *Blue Covenant: The Global Water Crisis and the Coming Battle for the Right to Water* (Toronto: McClelland & Stewart, 2007), 35–43; Ann-Christin Sjolander Holland, *The Water Business: Corporations versus People* (New York: Zed Books, 2005); and Kate Bayliss and Terry McKinley, *Privatizing Basic Utilities in Sub-Saharan Africa: The Millennium Development Goal Impact* (for the UNDP International Poverty Centre (January 2007).

51. "Water for Life," accessed 19 March 2013, www.un.org/waterforlifedecade /factsheet.html.

52. *WER* 76 (2001): 233–40, and 77 (2002): 257–68.

53. Hameda Deedat and Eddie Cottle, "Cost Recovery and Prepaid Water Meters and the Cholera Outbreak in KwaZulu-Natal: A Case Study in Madlebe," in *Cost Recovery and the Crisis of Service Delivery in South Africa,* ed. David A. MacDonald and John Pape (Cape Town: Human Sciences Research Council Publishers, 2002), 94.

54. David Hemson, "Still Paying the Price: Revisiting the Cholera Epidemic of 2000–2001 in South Africa," Occasional Papers Series, No. 10, Municipal Services Project, David A. McDonald and Greg Ruiters, series editors (Grahamstown: Grocott's Publishers, 2006), 17–18.

55. Ian Crowther, "Saluting the South African Medical Health Service's Involvement in Cholera Prevention and Treatment in KwaZulu-Natal," *Milmed* 17 (2001): 18–19.

56. Jacques Pauw, "Metered to Death: How a Water Experiment Caused Riots and a Cholera Epidemic," *Global Policy Forum* (5 February 2003): 6.

57. The two sources for the Madlebe case study are Deedat and Cottle, "Cost Recovery," and Hemson, "Still Paying."

58. Deedat and Cottle, "Cost Recovery," 11.

59. A prominent member of Prime Minister Thabo Mbeki's Cabinet, Ronnie Kasrils had been a senior member of the ANC, a founding member and commander of its armed wing, Umkhonto we Sizwe, and a prominent figure in the South African Communist Party during the struggle against apartheid. He was appointed Deputy Minister of Defense from 1994 to 1999, Minister of Water Affairs and Forestry from 1999 to 2004, and since then, Minister for Intelligence Services. As head of the DWAF he proved to be an artful dodger of criticism directed toward the ANC government, and a loyal supporter of President Mbeki.

60. "Dead in the Water," CBC, The Fifth Estate, broadcast of 31 March 2004, www.cbc.ca/fifth/deadinthewater/.

61. Hemson, "Still Paying," 37.

62. Pauw, "Metered," 5.

63. John Jeter, "South Africa's Driest Season," *Mother Jones*, November/December 2002, 4.

64. "Joint SAMWU-RDSN (Rural Development Services Network) World Water Day Press Statement," 22 March 2006, www.worldwaterday.org.

65. *WER* 82 (2007): 273–75, and 83 (2008): 270.

66. Stephanie Nolen, "Land of the State, Home of the Poor," *Toronto Globe and Mail*, 9 September 2008.

67. In his history of malaria, Randall Packard has made a similar argument about bringing malaria under control. Although malaria's grip on humans is more tenacious and destructive, cholera can also be tamed when social, political, and economic changes in its disease ecology occur. See Randall M. Packard, *The Making of a Tropical Disease: A Short History of Malaria* (Baltimore: Johns Hopkins University Press, 2007).

PART III

❖

The Past in the Future

8

MALE CIRCUMCISION AND HIV CONTROL IN AFRICA

*Questioning Scientific Evidence
and the Decision-Making Process*

MICHEL GARENNE, ALAIN GIAMI, AND CHRISTOPHE PERREY

The HIV/AIDS epidemic expanded rapidly in sub-Saharan Africa in the 1980s and 1990s, with major health and demographic implications. According to the Joint United Nations Program on HIV/AIDS (UNAIDS), more than 50 million persons have been infected with the virus since 1976. By 2009, 35 million persons were living with HIV, and another 2 million were dying every year, mostly in Africa.[1] Most HIV transmission in Africa occurs through adult heterosexual relations and through maternal-child contact during pregnancy, delivery, and breastfeeding. Early in the epidemic, other modes of transmission also took place, including iatrogenic transmission through unsafe blood transfusion and possibly unsafe injections.[2] The sudden emergence and expansion of this epidemic has been an enormous shock for African populations and has had major demographic, economic, and social consequences. The epidemic has also inflicted considerable strain on African health systems, requiring new forms of diagnosis, treatment, and care delivery, and new sources of financing.

In response to this epidemic, national and international agencies have developed several strategies to reduce the virus's transmission and, later, to lower mortality. These efforts first began by securing blood supplies when a diagnostic test to screen for the virus became available (1984–85). By the late 1980s and early 1990s, the focus shifted to reducing the risk of heterosexual transmission through the "ABC" strategies ("Abstinence," "Be faithful," "Condom use"). When well implemented, these strategies could curb the course of the epidemic within a few years, as exemplified in Uganda.[3] A few years later, health policymakers sought to limit mother-to-child transmission by promoting caesarean section delivery, providing antiviral drugs to mothers, and offering advice about breastfeeding. In the mid-2000s, low-cost HAART (highly active antiretroviral therapy) drugs became available and more widely used, thus significantly reducing mortality and limiting HIV transmission.

Another recommended protective measure has been "medical male circumcision" (MMC). Following the World Health Organization's March 2007 recommendation, some African health services began to offer MMC to young men as an additional means of preventing female to male transmission. This recommendation inspired wide-ranging reactions about the ethical and practical questions involved in MMC, notably from anticircumcision activists and from biomedical scientists, especially epidemiologists and demographers.

This chapter investigates the rationale (or lack thereof) of the MMC strategy for HIV control. The first section briefly reviews the social anthropology and history of male circumcision in past and contemporary African societies. The second section investigates the nature of scientific evidence mobilized to support official recommendations that MMC be included in programs to control HIV transmission. The third section analyzes the decision-making process that led to the WHO recommendation.

The literature on "circumcision" and on "circumcision and HIV" is vast, with thousands of titles covering scientific, historical, sociopolitical, and religious issues. In this overview, we cannot do justice to all publications. Instead, our citations refer readers to existing bibliographies and synthetic works. This literature is often conflicting and controversial, so we occasionally mention some of these debates.[4]

Social Anthropology and a Brief History of Male Circumcision
MALE CIRCUMCISION IN EARLY AND PRECOLONIAL AFRICAN SOCIETIES

Male circumcision seems to be very ancient in Africa, particularly throughout the Sahelian belt from Senegal to Somalia.[5] The first evidence of this practice appeared over five thousand years ago, although some interpretations of rock paintings and engravings depicting circumcision have been questioned.[6] The practice may have originated among societies of ancient Nubia (present-day Sudan and Ethiopia), a locus of early agriculture and animal domestication. Descendants of early practitioners of male circumcision continued this practice well after their conversion to Islam or Christianity. Various forms of female genital cutting, including excision, were also widely practiced, although not universally.

The symbolic justification for both practices is similar: removing the female parts from the males, and removing the male parts from the females. In both cases, circumcision and excision were practiced on adolescents, as part as a highly celebrated ritual, as a *rite de passage* to adulthood. From some sociopolitical standpoints, this practice can be considered as a form of power abuse from elder generations on younger ones, and Margaret Mead has contended that it also expressed elder fears of sexual competition and anxieties about aging.[7]

Bantu-speaking peoples, whose beginnings linguists now trace to southeastern Nigeria and western Cameroon, probably learned circumcision from northern groups, but do not currently practice it routinely. Bantu speakers carried their language, ironworking techniques, agricultural practices, and ritual practices like circumcision through waves of migration and interaction with indigenous groups through central, eastern, and southern Africa; as a result, circumcision seems to have spread sporadically in eastern and southern Africa, but was never universal, and it currently remains a marginal practice among most Bantu-speaking groups. Note also that these dynamics are complex and probably evolved over time.[8] A good example is that of the Zulu, an ethnic group living in South Africa. The Zulus seem to have practiced male circumcision until the eighteenth century, but dropped it in the early nineteenth century during the *mfecane,* or Zulu wars, primarily because it was seen as incompatible with the military training required by their leader, Shaka Zulu (1787–1828).

The map of male circumcision in Africa is particularly complex because, outside of North Africa and the Sahelian band where it remains universal, male circumcision is mostly ethnic specific, and part of ethnic identity. Within a single country, certain ethnic groups practice male circumcision as a defining feature of their identities, whereas others refuse it for the same reasons. Elsewhere, certain social groups practice—or refuse to practice—male circumcision for other reasons; new syncretic Christian churches, for instance, recommend that adherents also practice male circumcision because Jesus Christ was circumcised, and some African Initiated Churches require the practice as a condition of membership within the church community.

CIRCUMCISION AMONG PEOPLE OF MONOTHEIST RELIGIONS

Male circumcision probably expanded in Egypt and in Arabia a long time ago. In ancient Egypt, the earliest document depicting the practice is a bas-relief on the wall of a temple of the sixth dynasty (2325 to 2155 B.C.E.), the Ankhmahor Mastaba in Saqqara. Egyptians were in close contact with Nubian cultures and may have learned the practice from them. Male circumcision seems to have been a compulsory ritual for those seeking admission to the temple community and to the priesthood. The Greek historian Herodotus explains that Mediterranean people practicing male circumcision in Antiquity (Phoenicians, Philistines) learned it from the Egyptians, the only known people to practice it, along with Ethiopian populations and Colchis of the southern Caucasus of present-day Georgia, also of Egyptian origin.[9] The practice seems to have receded in Egypt under the influence of the Romans and the Greeks, who opposed any form of bodily mutilation; male circumcision then became generalized after the Arab invasion.

Captive Jews in Egypt seem to have learned the practice from the Egyptians. Some of them were initiated in Egyptian temples, and likely had to undergo the ritual like the other priests (around 1600 B.C.E.). The obligation to circumcise newborn babies, a major change from previous practices, seems to have occurred later, around 1500 B.C.E. At this time, Jewish priests dramatically expanded their political power and required newborn male circumcision as a necessary condition for membership in the Jewish faith. This obligation, symbolizing the Jews' covenant with God, is clearly stated in the Bible.[10] Since then, male circumcision at the seventh day of life has remained a strict obligation for all observant Jews. Only recently have some Jewish families begun to reject this practice, shifting from the traditional *Brit Milah* to the modern *Brit Shalom* without circumcision, although this movement had its beginnings in nineteenth-century Germany.[11]

Muslims follow similar practices. The Qu'ran does not explicitly require male circumcision, but it is nevertheless part of Muslim tradition (*sunnah*). A virtually universal practice among Muslims, male circumcision is considered a necessary prerequisite for the pilgrimage to Mecca. Primarily a symbol of cleanliness, circumcision usually occurs sometime between birth and adolescence, and often between seven and ten years of age throughout the Muslim world, from Maghreb to Central Asia, and in Muslim India and Indonesia.[12]

NINETEENTH- AND TWENTIETH-CENTURY BRITISH AND NORTH AMERICAN PRACTICES

A later wave of circumcision took place in nineteenth-century England, its sociopolitical dynamics well documented by contemporary historians.[13] Briefly, the medical establishment encouraged male circumcision as a prophylactic measure to prevent onanism and sexually transmitted diseases. Medical authorities observed that Jewish men had fewer sexually transmitted infections (STIs) and perceived the Jewish family as a model for others, contending that it embraced laudable work ethics and sexual behaviors. The late nineteenth-century medical profession's authority (which coincided with developments in hygiene and biology) led to a large proportion of British male infants being circumcised for the next century. Medical practitioners and parents progressively abandoned the practice after 1945, when they realized that it had few of its anticipated effects.

Meanwhile, other English-speaking countries such as the United States, anglophone Canada, Australia, and New Zealand adopted male circumcision. In the United States, male circumcision became prevalent in the early twentieth century, and increasingly widespread after 1945 when private health insurance companies began to reimburse costs of the operation on the grounds that it maintained cleanliness and prevented STIs, particularly syphilis. In any case, male circumcision soon became good business for obstetricians and gynecologists, and nearly two-thirds of American families circumcised their male newborn children. But since 1990, under increasing pressure from human rights and other groups opposing such practices, some Americans have abandoned male circumcision. In response to legal claims filed by men seeking compensation for the loss of their foreskin, certain private insurance companies now refuse to reimburse the costs of the operation. And in 2011, major political fights erupted over the outlawing of newborn male circumcision.[14] For many years, the American Academy of Pediatrics (AAP) was reluctant to tolerate MMC or any form of genital cutting. It has, however, altered its recommendations recently. In April 2010, the AAP published a controversial policy statement mentioning that some physicians supported a "ritual nick" in lieu of female genital cutting. The AAP statement indicated that this procedure was "not physically harmful" and "much less extensive than routine male genital cutting."[15] Although the organization fell short of explicitly recommending this "ritual nick," subsequent outrage among obstetricians and activists forced it to state categorically that it did not endorse this procedure. But in August 2012, it allowed medical male circumcision, as an answer to the pressure from pro-circumcision scientists. This recommendation provoked an expression of outrage from anticircumcision activists, and intense debates are now under way.

EXPORTING CIRCUMCISION TO REGIONS UNDER AMERICAN INFLUENCE

After World War II, male circumcision became fashionable in countries under American control, particularly in South Korea, and to a lesser extent, Japan. The recent promotion of male circumcision in Africa may be interpreted as an expansion of this policy. Male circumcision never disappeared—and perhaps never even declined from previous levels—in Africa. Before contemporary campaigns of MMC, about two-thirds of African males were circumcised. A meta-analysis of Demographic and Health Surveys (DHS) conducted in twenty countries covering about 56 percent of the total populations of sub-Saharan Africa concluded that 71 percent of adult men between fifteen and fifty-nine were circumcised.[16] Most men were circumcised at adolescence, mostly by traditional practitioners, although African families are increasingly seeking physicians and nurses to conduct the procedure in order to avoid serious secondary effects (e.g., mutilation, infection, or, rarely, death).

ETHICAL AND LEGAL ISSUES IN CONTEMPORARY SOCIETIES

Male circumcision on infants, children, or adolescents has raised many questions for contemporary societies. Although widely accepted in some societies, many groups now perceive it as unacceptable for several reasons: it imposes severe psychological and physical pain on the patient, and it violates the first principle of medical ethics, "First, do no harm." From an ethical standpoint, male circumcision could be considered acceptable if it proved to be strongly effective protection from infection. But the reduction of susceptibility to several pathogens is negligible or nil, and as we shall see below, this is particularly true for HIV/AIDS.

Scientific Evidence about the Relationship between Male Circumcision and HIV Incidence and Prevalence

Here we evaluate the scientific evidence that led the WHO to recommend MMC as a measure of protection from HIV transmission.

CLINICAL OBSERVATIONS

The debate began with clinical observations conducted in the United States during the early years of the HIV epidemic. These observations, published as two short letters in the prestigious *New England Journal of Medicine,* found that circumcised patients were less infected by syphilis and herpes, an observation that could apply to HIV as well.[17] Similar clinical observations had precipitated the very same debate in western Europe during the early nineteenth century.[18] These debates continued into the early 1990s in South Africa, when the HIV epidemic exploded. One author of the present chapter (MG) spoke at the time with physicians working in Tintswalo hospital of the present-day Mpumalanga province (formerly Eastern Transvaal), who observed the opposite phenomenon: circumcised patients were *more* infected with HIV than others. Of course, this type of observation is only circumstantial and may be influenced by observer bias or numerous selection biases.

MICHEL GARENNE, ALAIN GIAMI, AND CHRISTOPHE PERREY

A second type of evidence introduced in the late 1980s was the geographical correlation between circumcision and HIV. In Africa, populations in which more men were circumcised (e.g., Sahelian West Africa) had fewer HIV infections than those populations with fewer circumcised men (e.g., Eastern Africa). John Bongaarts first presented a paper at the 1988 International Union for the Scientific Study of Population meeting on African Demography in Dakar, Senegal, subsequently publishing the piece in the journal *AIDS*.[19] His paper addressed both HIV1 and HIV2 infections and focused on populations in cities where data had recently become available. Stephen Moses followed with a similar paper.[20] Both studies had several weaknesses. In the late 1980s, data on male circumcision came only from ethnographic studies, conducted by anthropologists studying ethnic groups in the early twentieth century, but these studies covered only a small proportion of the more than two thousand ethnic groups in Africa. Neither Bongaarts nor Moses accounted for possible variations within ethnic groups, particularly among urbanized populations. Furthermore, these studies were conducted in the first years of the HIV epidemic, when much of southern Africa was still free of HIV. Fifteen years later, southern African countries ranked the most heavily infected.

Several selection biases could have influenced the studies' conclusions. The most important seems to have been a correlation between age at marriage and sexual permissiveness. Men living in countries in the Sahelian belt are universally circumcised, but both men and women within these predominantly Muslim societies have a much lower age at marriage and much lower tolerance for premarital and extramarital intercourse. Southern African populations, however, have a very high age at marriage, a high proportion of women who never marry, and a high tolerance for premarital and extramarital intercourse, which enables a person to have more partners from the age of first intercourse until his or her first marriage. Southern African countries also have experienced rapid social change: industrialization, urbanization, and apartheid policies have all had devastating effects on southern African families. In contemporary times, a higher median age at marriage can be a strong indicator of social disruption. Premarital fertility (birth of a child before first marriage) is a function of age at marriage, of permissiveness of premarital intercourse, and of premarital contraceptive use. Levels of premarital fertility thus bring together all risks associated with premarital intercourse. Subsequently, researchers recognized this correlation between HIV prevalence and age at first marriage, and even more strongly with premarital fertility. The map of high HIV seroprevalence in Africa coincides with those regions where populations marry later, and even more so where populations have high levels of premarital fertility.[21]

Furthermore, these findings are more than simple correlations: mathematical models demonstrate the effects of age at marriage and sexual behavior on the course of the epidemic. Microsimulation models of HIV epidemics based on age at marriage reproduced the large differences in HIV prevalence noted between southern Africa and Sahelian Africa.[22] In contrast, microsimulation models based solely on male circumcision explained only a tiny fraction of the differences in HIV prevalence observed between southern and Sahelian Africa.[23] Note that most epidemiological models developed in the 1980s and 1990s, whether compartmental or microsimulation models, ignored marriage entirely; in demographic models, however, marriage appears as the most important variable of the dynamics of the African HIV epidemic. This conclusion is easy to understand: women who marry late, who have unprotected intercourse before first marriage and with several partners are more likely to become pregnant and contract STIs. Demographic evidence shows that most large HIV epidemics are associated with high HIV prevalence among young women, especially in the fifteen- to twenty-four-year-old cohort, and high HIV prevalence is in turn highly correlated with premarital fertility. Subsequent analyses of geographical patterns in HIV prevalence repeated these same weaknesses, including religion as a confounding variable.[24] These analyses suffered from the same biases: they did not account for age at marriage, sexual permissiveness, and condom use.

ECOLOGICAL STUDIES

Several case/control studies followed, investigating whether observations about circumcision and HIV could be confirmed. Case/control studies are classic epidemiological methods that evaluate the relationship between a risk factor and a particular health outcome and measure this relationship with an odds ratio. A case/control study compares an outcome (in this case, HIV seroprevalence) according to a risk factor (in this case, male circumcision); it calculates an odds ratio—the ratio of the risk of being HIV-infected if circumcised compared with that if not circumcised. The method can be extended to multivariate analysis to control for confounding factors. Some studies were based on selected groups, including "high-risk groups" such as truck drivers or hospital patients, whereas others were population-based, thus labeled "cross-sectional" studies. One influential study was conducted in four African cities, two with low HIV prevalence (Cotonou, Benin, and Yaoundé, Cameroon) and two with

MICHEL GARENNE, ALAIN GIAMI, AND CHRISTOPHE PERREY

high HIV prevalence (Kisumu, Kenya, and Ndola, Zambia).[25] This study did not elucidate reasons for the difference in HIV prevalence between the groups but found only two significant risk factors: male circumcision and co-infection with the herpes virus (HSV).

Cohort studies were also conducted in Africa. Another method of epidemiological investigation, cohort studies investigate prospectively the risk of becoming infected over time, and compare this risk between circumcised and uncircumcised men. Cohort studies compute the relative risk of becoming infected (and not only the odds ratio as in case/control studies), and can conduct multivariate analysis to control for cofactors. The results of these cohort studies often concluded that a lower risk of HIV was associated with male circumcision, but not always.

Comprehensive meta-analysis was first conducted on twenty-two studies, and then on twenty-seven studies (twenty cross-sectional, four case/control, two cohort, and one partner study), finding a risk ratio of 0.52, reduced to 0.42 in multivariate analysis.[26] The results, however, were far from homogeneous, since eight studies showed a risk ratio $\geq$ 1, and most were large-scale population-based studies. Another meta-analysis of thirty-five case/control studies in Africa found precisely the opposite: an excess risk of HIV infection associated with male circumcision.[27] A more rigorous Cochrane meta-analysis of similar studies concluded that the findings were quite heterogeneous and thus produced no firm conclusion.[28] Green et al. have summarized the debates generated by the evidence and analyses.[29]

Long-term cohort studies on other STIs were conducted in the United States, England, Australia, and New Zealand, where STI prevalence and incidence among male adults was compared according to circumcision status. For instance, in Dunedin, New Zealand, STI incidence was found to be identical in the two groups by age thirty-two.[30] Other studies with larger sample sizes reached similar conclusions in the United States, England, and Australia.[31] Whatever the transmission mode of STIs (heterosexual or homosexual), these studies clearly indicate that male circumcision does not protect against transmission.

RANDOMIZED CONTROLLED TRIALS

In epidemiology, the formal proof of an effect is usually provided by randomized controlled trials (RCT). This is a technique developed for testing the effect of new drugs or new vaccines. It consists of randomly allocating volunteers into two groups, sometimes three or more groups when several strategies are simultaneously compared. The first group receives the treatment under investigation, and the second does not; the investigation then compares the outcome (infection, disease, death, etc.) after a given duration of observation (a few weeks, months, or years). The role of randomization is to control for any potential bias associated with socioeconomic factors or behavior that could interact with the outcome. Considered in epidemiology to be the "gold standard," the methodology is well known, well accepted, and well standardized, and it has been used in numerous studies throughout the world. The main limitation of RCTs is sample size, and results are always given with a confidence interval around the mean effect. When several trials are available, they can be combined into a meta-analysis, leading to a more precise estimate of the effect and smaller confidence intervals.

Three randomized controlled trials were conducted to investigate the effect of male circumcision on HIV infection, in South Africa, Kenya, and Uganda, three countries heavily affected by HIV.[32] The three trials were similar in their design: uncircumcised young men between the ages of eighteen and twenty-four or more were asked to participate and were allocated into two groups: one underwent circumcision, and the other remained uncircumcised. Sample size was large enough to ensure statistical significance (3,274, 2,784, and 4,996 men, respectively). Results were unambiguous: in all three trials, male circumcision at time (t) reduced the risk of acquiring HIV within eighteen or twenty-four months by about half, confirming the findings from many case/control and cohort studies. These positive and consistent results from three different trials were the main justification for the 2007 WHO recommendation.

But these three trials had several limitations that were not properly considered. First, the incidence (number of new cases per person per year) remained very high, even in the circumcised groups. The order of magnitude was 1 percent per year (0.9, 1.1, and 0.7 new infections per year, respectively), which would lead to some 40 percent of infected men between, say, ages twenty and fifty-nine, assuming constant incidence. An incidence of 1 percent per year is very high, and shows that circumcision cannot be considered "protective" against HIV. Second, the studies calculated HIV incidence within a relatively short time period (e.g., eighteen months), but they should have discounted both the healing period after circumcision (about six to eight weeks) during which intercourse is rare, and the time to observe seroconversion (time between primo-infection and the measurable rise of antibodies), also a period of several weeks. Third, and most important, this observation did not match demographic evidence. Note that when a new drug is tested, its long-term

MICHEL GARENNE, ALAIN GIAMI, AND CHRISTOPHE PERREY

demographic impact is unknown. The purpose of RCTs is to document a biological effect, in the hopes that this biological effect will translate into a demographic impact. But only long-term surveillance provides a full-scale estimation of demographic impact. This is particularly true for vaccines because of herd immunity, and also for drugs, because possible side effects are not visible in the short run. The demographic impact of a new health program (drug, vaccine, etc.) is usually assessed in what is called "phase IV" trials, not in "phase III" trials such as the classic RCTs. But this was not the case for male circumcision: male circumcision was not a new program, and demographic evidence of long-term impact was available, to the extent that many scientists did not even consider RCTs to be necessary.

DEMOGRAPHIC EVIDENCE

Two types of demographic evidence became available in the early 2000s, at the same time as the RCTs were conducted. The first type was provided by Demographic and Health Surveys (DHS).[33] These are large-scale, high-quality demographic surveys, based on representative samples of national populations, and they include special modules for men ages fifteen to fifty-nine, for women ages fifteen to forty-nine, for children ages zero to four, and various other sociodemographic information. In some countries, the module for men includes a question on male circumcision and a blood sample for HIV screening. By 2007, some nineteen African surveys with information on circumcision and HIV were available, and a few more have since been added. For each country survey, one could compute the risk ratio of being infected with HIV depending on circumcision status, which gives a measure of the risk of being infected at given exposure, that is, given the level of infection in the population. Later, one could merge all the surveys to conduct a meta-analysis and obtain stable results.

Results were unambiguous: the standardized risk ratio was 1.00 (95 percent CI = 0.95–1.05), meaning that there was no difference in HIV prevalence by circumcision status throughout Africa in the long run, that is, about thirty years after the epidemic's beginning.[34] Only two countries, Kenya and Uganda, had an HIV prevalence that was significantly lower among circumcised groups than among uncircumcised groups, but three other countries (Lesotho, Malawi, and Tanzania) showed the precisely opposite pattern—a higher level of infection among circumcised groups than among uncircumcised groups. These data were based on very large representative samples, together evaluating more than 80,000 men. Although such results do not exclude a biological effect of circumcision, because of the many potential biases involved, they clearly

Male Circumcision and HIV Control

demonstrate a lack of demographic impact. This demographic impact is very clear with other interventions. Comparing two groups of vaccinated and unvaccinated children, for instance (e.g., for measles, whooping cough, or tetanus) will yield a huge difference with respect to the response variable in general populations (incidence of the disease), often in the range of 1 to 100. Similarly, comparing two groups of women using and not using efficient contraception (e.g., pill, IUD, injectable) will yield a huge difference in fertility rates, thus confirming the demographic impact of contraception. In the case of HIV prevalence and male circumcision, a standardized relative risk of 1.00 demonstrates just the opposite.

Proponents of male circumcision to control HIV also proposed that large-scale male circumcision would affect the dynamics of the epidemic by reducing female to male transmission. Yet the opposite could be demonstrated in South Africa, the only country with a routine, high-quality surveillance system of HIV infection among pregnant women attending antenatal clinics. In the ten provinces studied, the dynamics of the epidemic were very much the same between 1990 and 2008, regardless of whether the dominant ethnic group was circumcised or not. There were some minor differences in the timing of the epidemic; some provincial populations were infected earlier, but the dynamics remained similar, with the exception of the Western Cape that has a different ethnic composition. For instance, the increase in seroprevalence between 1994 and 2006 in the North-West Province, populated by Tswana peoples who are not circumcised, was basically the same as that of the Eastern Cape, populated by Xhosa peoples who are all circumcised (HIV prevalence of 29 percent and 29 percent respectively in 2006). Again, this analysis demonstrates no demographic impact of male circumcision on the dynamics of the epidemic. Further analysis of a large-scale population-based survey in South Africa also found no effect of male circumcision on HIV prevalence.[35]

BIOLOGICAL EFFECT VERSUS DEMOGRAPHIC IMPACT

In debates over MMC's putative effects on HIV incidence and prevalence, it is important to distinguish between clinical efficacy found in RCTs, the effects measured in case/control and cohort studies, and the population impact or effectiveness. This is not a new issue, and the epidemiological literature contains many examples of differences between clinical efficacy and population effectiveness. Two classic examples include the cholera vaccine and the rhythm method for contraception. The cholera vaccine, developed in the 1980s and tested in Bangladesh, was found to have a 50 percent efficacy in clinical trials,

MICHEL GARENNE, ALAIN GIAMI, AND CHRISTOPHE PERREY

but nevertheless demonstrated a very small population impact and did not change the course of cholera epidemics; even vaccinated groups had a high incidence of cholera.[36] The cholera vaccine is thus not recommended for general use, since there exist many other ways of controlling cholera (basic hygiene in treatment of water, food, and hands will suffice) and of reducing cholera mortality (rehydration and antibiotics) (see Echenberg, this volume). Likewise, the rhythm method is based on solid biological evidence and induces a 50 percent reduction in fecundability (monthly probability of becoming pregnant if exposed), but it has virtually no long-term effect on protection: under repeated exposure, most women using the rhythm method eventually become pregnant. These two classic examples demonstrate important commonalities with circumcision and HIV: about 50 percent reduction in short-term HIV incidence in trials, but no long-term impact on prevalence under intense, repeated exposure. These two observations are, in fact, compatible. A further commonality with these classic examples of cholera vaccination and the rhythm method is that more effective alternative strategies exist.

The arguments for and against MMC to control HIV can be summarized as follows. In favor of the practice, MMC is a single, definitive procedure that somewhat reduces the risk of infection for men. Avoiding or delaying a few infections could be seen as an achievement, particularly in the context of very high levels of infection. And while MMC programs are costly, international aid can cover some of those costs.

But MMC as a strategy to control HIV transmission also has many significant shortcomings. First, it will not have any major population impact, nor will it curb the course of HIV epidemics, as many studies cited in this chapter demonstrate. Second, it diverts human and financial resources into a single strategy that could be better used in other more effective strategies. Most African countries, for instance, lack physicians and nurses who are so badly needed to provide HAART treatments and other kinds of care; these countries also lack finances for their health care systems. In such a context, using scarce resources for a strategy that is unlikely to have a major population-level impact is questionable. Third, because circumcision has deep social, cultural, and emotional implications, MMC cannot be imposed on men; individuals must freely choose circumcision, so that population coverage will likely be low. Fourth, MMC on a large scale may have deleterious unintended consequences, ranging from infection to mild or moderate mutilation; these consequences are often disregarded in cost/benefit analyses. Fifth, MMC as an HIV control strategy may encourage more dangerous practices: if circumcised men feel more protected, they may engage in riskier practices, such as using condoms less frequently. Currently, there is no evidence for such practices, but they may only become visible over the longer term, perhaps in another ten or twenty years. In such a case, the overall effect of MMC would be negative, opening up the possibility for those who were circumcised and subsequently infected with HIV to claim compensation.

In order for MMC to have the full impact of reducing HIV transmission, it should be proposed to boys before the age of first intercourse, yet many parents and observers would consider such an intervention a violation of children's rights. One author of this chapter (MG) observed that in a Durban, South Africa, clinic in 1999–2000, half of the men seeking voluntary MMC (mean age = twenty-five years) were already infected with HIV. None of these considerations have been seriously considered by proponents of MMC, nor have they addressed the lack of demographic impact of this intervention. The history of public health has repeatedly demonstrated that hiding the negative findings of an intervention is the worst possible strategy, one that can lead to many undesirable consequences. Recommending MMC under current conditions in southern Africa appears to be more of a "minefield" than a "magic bullet."

In any case, even the fiercest proponents of MMC still advise men to use a condom in any casual encounter or in case of intercourse with infected people, whether circumcised or not. But if condom use suffices for individual protection, and if large-scale condom use can control HIV transmission in a population, why would circumcision be necessary?

Anatomy of the WHO/UNAIDS
Decision-Making Process to Recommend Male Circumcision

> The partial protective effect of male circumcision is remarkably consistent across the observational studies (ecological, cross-sectional and cohort) and the three randomized controlled trials conducted in diverse settings. . . . The efficacy of male circumcision in reducing female to male transmission of HIV has been proven beyond reasonable doubt. This is an important landmark in the history of HIV prevention.

This extract comes from the conclusions and recommendations of the WHO/UNAIDS technical consultation, held on 6–7 March 2007 in Montreux, Switzerland.[37] The report recognized male circumcision as a new means of preventing female to male transmission of HIV during sexual relations, and its recommendations targeted primarily southern African countries.[38]

This recommendation, however, simultaneously raised ethical and scientific concerns, not to mention questions about MMC implementation in different socioeconomic and cultural contexts, about its long-term effects among populations, and about its psychological, physiological consequences, particularly because of deep religious and symbolic connotations of circumcision.[39] Moreover, even the most ardent proponents of MMC questioned the capacity of health systems to implement this measure under sufficiently safe, hygienic conditions.[40] In light of these questions, the following analysis reviews the factors that shaped the Montreux decision-making process.

CONTEXT OF THE HIV EPIDEMIC AND PREVENTION SCHEMES

The broad epidemiological context certainly facilitated the decision at Montreux. At that time, the annual number of new HIV infections remained very high, and the year 2006 alone saw an estimated 4.3 million new infections, close to the peak of incidences since 1980. Despite notable successes in HIV prevention in such countries as Cambodia, Brazil, Haiti, and India, most preventive measures were limited in their impact. One UN report showed that most people had no access at all to preventive measures.[41] Since then, international organizations have responded by intensifying available strategies and proposing new ones. Without such efforts, they risked being accused of inefficacy and of not doing enough.

Some officials expressed doubt about the sustainability of prevention programs, and about the promise of new control strategies. Some prevention programs that sought to change behavior (condom use, reducing number of partners, abstinence, etc.) were demonstrably effective, as in Uganda and Tanzania,[42] but they nevertheless appeared unsustainable over the long run. Peter Piot and Kevin O'Reilly, for instance, argued that despite localized results, these educational efforts had not had a large effect.[43] Moreover, although interest in biomedical interventions was increasing, particularly under the influence of such funding agencies as the Gates Foundation,[44] there was grim news on several fronts. In 2007, a failed Phase II microbicide trial was stopped, and other clinical trials similarly offered little promise of success.[45] The three randomized control trials on male circumcision thus offered a ray of hope in an otherwise dismal context.

OBSERVATIONAL EPIDEMIOLOGICAL STUDIES: TIME FOR DEBATE

The results of geographical and ecological studies produced divergent interpretations and recommendations. From 1999, some researchers argued for the official integration of male circumcision into HIV control programs. In 1999, Daniel Halperin and Robert Bailey's comprehensive literature review in the

Lancet urged international public health organizations to implement programs that incorporated male circumcision as a new preventive method:

> In the face of such compelling evidence, we would expect the international health community to at least consider some form of action. However, the association between lack of male circumcision and HIV transmission has met with fierce resistance, cautious skepticism, or, more typically, utter silence, which is evidenced by a dearth of public-health information on the issue.[46]

A subsequent paragraph entitled "time to action" continued, "The hour has passed for the international health community to recognize the compelling evidence that show a significant association between lack of male circumcision and HIV infection."[47]

For Michel Caraël, an anthropologist and then chief of prevention of UNAIDS, the multi-site study conducted in four African cities had produced sufficient evidence to support male circumcision as a preventive measure.[48] When interviewed, he recalled:

> At that time I was head of the prevention unit at UNAIDS, and I had a team of about fifteen persons. I met with Peter Piot. I was giving seminars; I was meeting with WHO colleagues. Everywhere I tried to propagate the idea that it was necessary to use male circumcision for preventing HIV.[49]

An informal meeting at the 13th International AIDS Conference (2000) in Durban discussed the results of this study. According to one WHO official,

> Some people felt the data were strong enough; others felt that it was unlikely to be sufficiently convincing unless there were randomized trial data, and in 2000, I convened a small consultation in the Durban AIDS conference, which brought together the people who had been working in the field. And here again we reviewed the data, and the recommendation there was that some randomized control trials should be launched, and in fact three randomized trials were launched as you know.[50]

Researchers thus sought to resolve four problems (confounding factors; the measure's efficacy on newly circumcised persons; delay to decreasing incidence; and global level of efficacy) that had dogged previous studies by conducting randomized controlled trial (RCTs). But simultaneously, several anticircumcision organizations actively protested, including to the UNAIDS director.[51]

The first results of the Orange Farms trial in South Africa were presented in the summer of 2005 at the International AIDS Society conference by the physician-epidemiologist Bertran Auvert.[52] These results precipitated several meetings aimed at implementing circumcision in target countries. By August 2005, an interagency task team coordinated by UNAIDS had taken up the question. Composed of international and regional representatives from WHO, UNICEF, UNFPA, and the World Bank, the team sought to gather necessary information to recommend and implement the policy. It conducted consultations and meetings, assessed countries' reactions, and developed guidelines for safe implementation. In 2006, it issued precise recommendations to target priority populations and to develop communication kits and implementation strategies.[53]

Results of the American clinical trials[54] confirmed Auvert's results, showing a decline of 51 percent and 59 percent, respectively, of HIV incidence among circumcised men compared with intact men. Thus three randomized controlled trials on some 10,000 men convinced WHO and UNAIDS decision makers.

Simultaneously, several mathematical models sought to evaluate the potential impact of the measure, concluding that male circumcision programs could induce a 30 percent reduction of HIV incidence among males (by direct effect) and a 15 percent reduction among females (by indirect effect). HIV prevalence could drop 20 to 30 percent within two years.[55] The cost/benefit ratio was seen as excellent.[56] Authors concluded that the measure had an acceptable level of efficacy and was relatively cheap (40 dollars per person). Even before the clinical trial, epidemiologists conducted acceptability studies of large-scale circumcision and a literature review, concluding that there existed a widespread positive perception of MMC.[57] Frequently conducted in response to intense advocacy, these studies focused on the potential benefits, not the risks associated with circumcision. Quite likely they measured primarily the pervasive efficacy of information sessions concerning circumcision, presented and perceived as a prophylactic measure that improved hygiene.

Public health planners and researchers did consult social scientists who were well placed to offer insight into such questions. But they only consulted social scientists to facilitate the measure's implementation at the country level. A January 2007 colloquium in Durban sought to determine the future research priorities about MMC, and charged the group SAHARA (Social Aspects for HIV/AIDS Research Alliance) to coordinate forthcoming studies.[58]

Nevertheless, WHO and UNAIDS officials did not wait for the study results to make their recommendation, for several epidemiologists and WHO/UN-AIDS task force members formed a strong coalition favoring the measure. These researchers (B. Auvert, R. Bailey, R. Gray, S. Moses, and D. Halperin) had undertaken the clinical trials, impact studies, cost/effectiveness studies, and acceptability studies of MMC. As faculty members of prestigious universities or research centers, they had published widely in well-regarded biomedical journals and had long been convinced of circumcision's efficacy. As such, they did not consider M. Garenne's demographic arguments about the lack of population impact, which he had presented to the WHO working group in Geneva.[59]

Opponents of MMC, however, were more heterogeneous and included clinicians, epidemiologists, demographers, and sociologists, HIV/AIDS advocacy group representatives (divided on this issue), and activists from anti–genital mutilation organizations.

Nevertheless, the clinical trials offered the WHO/UNAIDS working group the ethical grounds on which to make their decision. Not to act would have been morally indefensible. The working group publicly presented the results and made an official recommendation for the integration of male circumcision as a new measure to reduce the risk of HIV transmission.

MONTREUX:
CONSTRUCTING THE LEGITIMACY OF THE RECOMMENDATION

The Montreux technical consultation was more a formality to present justifications for MMC to a larger audience of political authorities and association representatives, and less an opportunity for open debate about its rationale and predicted consequences. Taking place a month after the publication of the Gray and Bailey trials, the working group had clearly already decided to recommend the measure.[60] The precise content of the recommendation, its implementation, the target countries, and the measure's value for HIV seropositive people remained to be decided. One expert who organized the meeting recalled: "We knew already the important themes ... the topics on which we wanted a recommendation, but the precise sentences were not yet written, the words were not there, and we worked a lot during the meeting to find the words." The meeting's chairs, participants, speakers, themes, and timing were all chosen so as not to cast doubt on the measure, but rather to focus on the recommendation's specific contents.

Eighty participants attended, including academic researchers, members of international health organizations, gender relations specialists, representatives of UN funding agencies (World Bank, UNICEF, UN Population Fund) and of other public and private institutions (Global Fund, ANRS, Bill and Melinda Gates Foundation), political representatives of target countries, association members, youth organization members, human rights and women's health activists, and the editor of a scientific journal.[61] Organizers clearly saw the meeting's heterogeneous nature—its multi-occupational, multidisciplinary, and international character—as a sign of a healthy democratic process.

Meeting participants included many medical scientists, but very few social scientists and lawyers.[62] Epidemiologists gave most of the presentations, dominating discussions of meta-analyses, observational studies, clinical trials, cost/effectiveness analysis, and models of the potential impact. Yet known and published critics of the measure, including urologists, sexologists, and demographers, were not invited to the meeting.[63] The sole critic of MMC who was invited was the sociologist Gary Dowsett, but the meeting's organization seriously impeded his ability to voice any critical remarks.

The meeting program focused discussion on the measure's medical, scientific, and technical aspects through presentations and round tables. It devoted two hours to ethical issues (human rights) and to the Durban social sciences meeting about male circumcision. Catherine Hankins, a physician and scientific adviser to UNAIDS, and not Gary Dowsett or another social scientist, delivered this presentation. The meeting devoted one day to implementation strategies.

THE FINAL TEXT

Members of the WHO/UNAIDS wrote the final text, presenting it as eleven conclusive points with recommendations. The document underscored the efficacy of circumcision in reducing female-to-male HIV transmission, a new and important tool for HIV prevention. It acknowledged that male circumcision was not fully protective and should be considered a supplementary tool to existing measures.[64] It stressed that effective communication and community participation were important, as were respecting international ethical codes, including informed consent, confidentiality, and nondiscrimination. Guidelines published two months after Montreux addressed the measure's ethical dimensions.[65] It also mentioned the need to undertake circumcision under good sanitary conditions, but never specified the means to be devoted for doing so.

The report presented target countries and groups for these programs and studies needed for monitoring the measure. Such studies would assess the impact on female-male relations and on perceptions of the measure and on individual and community behavior. It would evaluate service delivery, as well as the effects of circumcision for homosexual or heterosexual anal sexual intercourse.

Two weeks after Montreux, Kevin de Cock (director of the HIV/AIDS department at WHO), Catherine Hankins (associate director, strategic information and chief scientific adviser to UNAIDS), and Jean-François Delfraissy (the director of ANRS, the French Agence nationale de recherches sur le sida et les hépatites virales) presented the official press release at a press conference in Paris. The measure is now being implemented in target countries.

❖

The French philosopher Michel Foucault described in his books and lectures what he called the emergence of "biopower" in the eighteenth and nineteenth centuries.[66] Foucault saw biopower as a new form of sociopolitical power, mobilized to function as a "government of populations," and differing from previous, classical forms of power, including military and economic. The "government of populations" created some positive consequences for modern societies, including the organization of public health in the nineteenth century, which led to dramatic changes in the ecological balance between germs and human populations, to major improvements in morbidity and mortality and to an extraordinary increase in life expectancy at birth. The development of tools for measurement and especially of statistical tools to evaluate and monitor progress made this government of populations possible. But this new paradigm also negatively affected human populations, particularly because it put into place diverse forms of repression (on sexual behavior and on those with mental disorders), and it culminated with the eugenics movement in the late nineteenth century.

Although medical male circumcision does not present the dire consequences that eugenics did, Foucault's concept of biopower is nevertheless useful in illuminating what is at stake in debates over MMC and its potentially repressive features. Male circumcision has long entailed the exercise of elder power over younger generations, and indeed, we would argue that it constitutes an abuse of power. Is medical male circumcision, then, a new avatar in the male circumcision saga—a new form of power abuse, exercised by an informal alliance of international organizations, funding agencies, and various lobbies of scientists and political activists? Proponents have supported this measure of "prophylaxis," justifying it with "scientific evidence" presented as absolute proof produced by the "gold standard." But they disregarded crucial scientific evidence showing that the measure has no effect on the population level.

Most surprising has been the silence of much of the press in the face of these debates over MMC. Newspapers intensively covered the findings of the clinical trials, but hardly addressed any counterevidence and discordant voices, even with the availability of publications and the plethora of international conferences on the topic, including those addressing genital integrity and human rights. But questions remain about why the press remained silent, and why WHO/UNAIDS working groups so systematically ignored counterevidence and critical perspectives on male circumcision.

Acknowledgments

Michel Garenne wrote the first two sections, introduction, and conclusion; Alain Giami and Christophe Perrey wrote the third section. All authors read and approved the final text.

Notes

1. World Health Organization/UNAIDS Report, 2007, accessed online at http://data.unaids.org/pub/Report/2007/mc_recommendations_en.pdf; UNAIDS report, 2009.

2. Some authors have even argued that iatrogenic transmission is an important factor in the African HIV epidemic, but this argument remains controversial. D. Gisselquist et al., "Let It Be Sexual: How Health Care Transmission of AIDS in Africa was Ignored," *International Journal of STD and AIDS* 14, no. 3 (2003): 148–61; M. Garenne, R. Micol, and A. Fontanet, "Unsafe Health Care and Sexual Transmission of HIV: Demographic Evidence," *International Journal of STD and AIDS* 15, no. 1 (2004): 65–66.

3. D. Mulder et al., "Decreasing HIV-1 Seroprevalence in Young Adults in a Rural Ugandan Cohort," *British Medical Journal* 311, no. 7009 (1995): 833–36; G. Asiimwe-Okiror et al., "Change in Sexual Behaviour and Decline in HIV Infection among Young Pregnant Women in Urban Uganda," *AIDS* 11, no. 14 (1997): 1757–63; D. Low-Beer, "HIV Incidence and Prevalence Trends in Uganda," *Lancet* 360, no. 9347 (2002): 1788; D. Low-Beer and R. L. Stoneburner, "Behaviour and Communication Change in Reducing HIV: Is Uganda Unique?" *African Journal of AIDS Research* 2, no. 1 (2003): 9–21.

4. See, for instance, R. Darby, *A Surgical Temptation: The Demonization of the Foreskin and the Rise of Circumcision in Britain* (Chicago: University of Chicago Press, 2005); P. Lafargue, "La circoncision, sa signification sociale et religieuse," *Bulletins de la Société d'anthropologie* (Session of 16 June 1887). See also Robert Darby's site, www.historyofcircumcision.net (accessed 21 March 2013).

5. Male circumcision has long been practiced around the world, likely abandoned and reinvented several times.

6. H. Lhote, "L'abbé Breuil et le Sahara," *Journal de la Société des africanistes* 32, no. 1 (1962): 63–74; F. Soleilhavout. "Images sexuelles dans l'art rupestre du Sahara," *Sahara* 14, no. 1 (2003): 31–48.

7. More than sixty years ago, Margaret Mead observed, "In South America, in Africa and in the South Seas, there are tribes in which the old men's antagonism to the springing sexuality of the young induces fears that are later reduced in pantomime, cruel initiatory rites in which the young men are circumcised, their teeth knocked out, and, in various ways they are reduced and modified and humbled, and then permitted to be men." Margaret Mead, *Male and Female* (New York: Harper, 1949), 84.

8. J. Mark, "Aspects of Male Circumcision in Sub-Equatorial African Culture History," *Health Transition Review* 7, Suppl. (1997): 337–59.

9. Herodotus, Liber II, Euterpe §104.

10. Genesis 17:10–12.

11. See, for instance, www.jewsagainstcircumcision.org, and www.tikkun.org /nextgen/circumcision-identity-gender-and-power?pr (both accessed 21 March 2013).

12. See http://www.circumstitions.com/Islam.html and http://www.missionislam .com/health/circumcisionislam.html (both accessed 21 March 2013).

13. Darby, *Surgical Temptation*.

14. See, for instance, the websites of Doctors Opposing Circumcision, http:// www.doctorsopposingcircumcision.org, NORM-UK www.norm-uk.org, International Coalition for Genital Integrity, www.icgi.org (all accessed 21 March 2013).

15. Committee on Bioethics, "Policy Statement—Ritual Genital Cutting of Female Minors," *Pediatrics* 125, no. 5 (2010): 1092.

16. See Demographic and Health Surveys (DHS), accessed 21 March 2013, at www.measuredhs.com.

17. A. Fink, "A Possible Explanation for Heterosexual Male Infection with AIDS," *New England Journal of Medicine* 315, no. 8 (1986): 1167; A. Fink, "Circumcision and Heterosexual Transmission of HIV Infection to Men," *New England Journal of Medicine* 316, no. 24 (1987): 1546–47.

18. Claude-François Lallemand, a French physician who taught medicine at University of Montpellier, claimed that circumcision prevented "night pollution," masturbation, and numerous disorders associated with penile diseases. The French Academy of Medicine and academies in Germany, Spain, and other European countries refuted the claim. The claim, however, stuck in England. See C. F. Lallemand, *Des pertes séminales involontaires,* 2 vols. (Paris: Béchet-Jeune, 1839); Darby, *Surgical Temptation*.

19. J. Bongaarts et al., "The Relationship between Male Circumcision and HIV Infection in African Populations," *AIDS* 3, no. 6 (1989): 373–77.

20. S. Moses et al., "Geographical Patterns of Male Circumcision Practices in Africa," *International Journal of Epidemiology* 19, no. 3 (1990): 693–97.

21. J. Bongaarts, "Late Marriage and the HIV Epidemic in Sub-Saharan Africa," *Population Studies* 61, no. 1 (2007): 73–83; M. Garenne and J. Zwang, "Premarital Fertility and HIV/AIDS in Africa," *African Journal of Reproductive Health* 12, no. 1 (2008): 64–74.

22. P. Leclerc, A. Matthews, and M. Garenne, "Fitting the HIV/AIDS Epidemic in Zambia: A Two-Sex Micro-Simulation Model," *PLoS One* 4, no. 5 (2009): e5439.

MICHEL GARENNE, ALAIN GIAMI, AND CHRISTOPHE PERREY

23. S. Clark, "Male Circumcision Could Help Protect against HIV Infection," *Lancet* 356, no. 9225 (2000): 225.

24. P. K. Drain et al., "Male Circumcision, Religion, and Infectious Diseases: An Ecologic Analysis of 118 Developing Countries," *BioMed Central Infectious Diseases* 6 (2006): 172–81.

25. B. Auvert, A. Buvé, E. Lagarde, M. Kahindo, J. Chege, N. Rutenberg, R. Musonda, M. Laourou, E. Akam, and H. A. Weiss, for the study group on the heterogeneity of HIV epidemics in African cities, "Male Circumcision and HIV Infection in Four Cities In Sub-Saharan Africa," *AIDS* 15, Suppl. 4 (2001): S31–S40.

26. S. Moses et al., "The Association between Lack of Male Circumcision and Risk for HIV Infection," *Sexually Transmitted Diseases* 21, no. 4 (1994): 201–10; H. A. Weiss, M. A. Quigley, and R. K. Hayes, "Male Circumcision and Risk of HIV Infection in Sub-Saharan Africa: A Systematic Review and Meta-Analysis," *AIDS* 14, no. 15 (2000): 2361–70.

27. R. S. Van Howe, "Circumcision and HIV Infection: Review of the Literature and Meta-Analysis," *International Journal of STD and AIDS* 10, no. 1 (1999): 8–16; R. S. Van Howe, "Does Circumcision Influence Sexually Transmitted Diseases? A Literature Review," *British Journal of Urology International* 83, Suppl. 1 (1999): 52–62.

28. N. O'Farrell, M. Egger, "Circumcision in Men and the Prevention of HIV Infection: A Meta-Analysis Revisited," *International Journal of STD and AIDS* 11, no. 3 (2000): 137–42; N. Siegfried et al., "Male Circumcision for Prevention of Heterosexual Acquisition of HIV in Men," *Cochrane Database of Systematic Reviews* 3 (2003), CD003362. Revised in 2007.

29. L. W. Green et al., "Male Circumcision and HIV Prevention: Insufficient Evidence and Neglected External Validity," *American Journal of Preventive Medicine* 39, no. 5 (2010): 479–82.

30. N. P. Dickson et al., "Circumcision and Risk of Sexually Transmitted Infections in a Birth Cohort," *Journal of Pediatrics* 152, no. 3 (2008): 383–87.

31. E. O. Laumann, C. M. Masi, and E. W. Zuckerman, "Circumcision in the United States: Prevalence, Prophylactic Effects, and Sexual Practice," *JAMA* 277, no. 13 (1997): 1052–27; S. S. Dave et al., "Male Circumcision in Britain: Findings from a National Probability Sample Survey," *Sexually Transmitted Infections* 79, no. 6 (2003): 499–500; J. Richters et al., "Circumcision in Australia: Prevalence and Effects on Sexual Health," *International Journal of STD and AIDS* 17, no. 8 (2006): 547–54.

32. B. Auvert et al., "Randomized, Controlled Intervention Trial of Male Circumcision for Reduction of HIV Infection Risk: The ANRS 1265 Trial," *PLoS Medicine* 2, no. 11, e298 (2005): 1–111; R. C. Bailey et al., "Male Circumcision for HIV Prevention in Young Men in Kisumu, Kenya: A Randomised Controlled Trial," *Lancet* 369, no. 9562 (2007): 643–56; R. H. Gray et al., "Male Circumcision for HIV Prevention in Men in Rakai, Uganda: A Randomised Controlled Trial," *Lancet* 369, no. 9562 (2007): 657–66.

33. See the DHS website for details: www.measuredhs.com.

34. M. Garenne, "Male Circumcision and HIV Control in Africa," *PLoS Medicine* 3, no. 1 (2006): e78; M. Garenne, "Long-Term Population Effect of Male Circumcision in Generalized HIV Epidemics in Sub-Saharan Africa," *African Journal of AIDS*

Research 7, no. 1 (2008): 1–8; M. Garenne, "Mass Campaigns of Male Circumcision for HIV Control in Africa: Clinical Efficacy, Population Effectiveness, Political Issues," in *Genital Autonomy. Protecting Personal Choice,* ed. G. C. Denniston, F. M. Hodges, and M. F. Milos (Dordrecht: Springer Science+Business Media B.V., 2010), 49–60.

35. C. Connolly et al., "Male Circumcision and Its Relationship to HIV Infection In South Africa: Results of a National Survey in 2002," *South African Medical Journal* 98, no. 10 (2008): 789–94.

36. M. Ali et al., "Herd Immunity Conferred by Killed Oral Cholera Vaccines in Bangladesh: A Reanalysis," *Lancet* 366, no. 9479 (2005): 44–49; J. D. Clemens et al., "Field Trial of Oral Cholera Vaccines in Bangladesh: Results from Three-Year Follow-Up," *Lancet* 335, no. 8684 (1990): 270–73.

37. WHO/UNAIDS, *New Data on Male Circumcision and HIV Prevention: Policy and Programme Implications: WHO/UNAIDS Technical Consultation on Male Circumcision and HIV Prevention: Research Implications for Policy and Programming: Conclusion and Recommendation* (Montreux: WHO/UNAIDS, 2007).

38. The recommendation pertains to countries with generalized epidemics (HIV prevalence in the general population above 15 percent), with hyperendemic prevalence (between 3 and 15 percent), where heterosexual contact is the main mode of transmission, and where most men (more than 80 percent) are uncircumcised. Mostly southern African countries were thus targeted: Botswana, Burundi, Central African Republic, Kenya (Nyanza province), Lesotho, Liberia, Malawi, Mozambique, Namibia, Rwanda, South Africa, Swaziland, Tanzania, Uganda, Zambia, and Zimbabwe.

39. D. L. Gollaher, *A History of the World's Most Controversial Surgery* (New York: Basic Book, 2000); E. O. Laumann, C. M. Masi, and E. W. Zuckerman, "Circumcision in the United States: Prevalence, Prophylactic Effects, and Sexual Practice," *JAMA* 277, no. 13 (1997): 1052–57; J. Richters et al., "Circumcision in Australia: Prevalence And Effects on Sexual Health," *International Journal of STD and AIDS* 17, no. 8 (2006): 547–54; B. Bettelheim, *Les blessures symboliques* (1954; Paris: Gallimard, 1971).

40. R. C. Bailey, O. Egesah, and S. Rosenberg, "Male Circumcision for HIV Prevention: A Prospective Study of Complications in Clinical and Traditional Settings in Bungoma, Kenya," *Bulletin of the World Health Organization* 86, no. 9 (2008): 669–77.

41. Condom use protected only 9 percent of high-risk sexual contact, and global need for condoms far outstripped condom availability. In sub-Saharan African countries, the most hard-hit by HIV, only 12 percent of men and 10 percent of women know their serological status. Only 11 percent of HIV-infected pregnant women in countries with medium and low income benefited from antiretroviral therapy. Likewise, prevention services reached only 9 percent of men who had sex with men, 8 percent of intravenous drug users, and less than 20 percent of commercial sex workers. UNICEF, WHO, UNAIDS, "Towards Universal Access: Scaling Up Priority HIV/ AIDS Interventions in the Health Sector: Progress Report," April 2007.

42. G. Slutkin et al., "How Uganda Reversed Its HIV Epidemic," *AIDS and Behavior* 10, no. 4 (2006): 351–60; U. Vogel, *Towards Universal Access to Prevention, Treatment and Care: Experiences and Challenges from the Mbeya Region in Tanzania—A Case Study* (Geneva, 2007).

MICHEL GARENNE, ALAIN GIAMI, AND CHRISTOPHE PERREY

43. Peter Piot was the executive director of UNAIDS from 1995 to 2008. K. R. O'Reilly and P. Piot, "International Perspectives on Individual and Community Approaches to the Prevention of Sexually Transmitted Disease and Human Immunodeficiency Virus Infection," *Journal of Infectious Diseases* 174, Suppl. 2 (1996): S214–22.

44. These biomedical measures included screening, postexposure prophylaxis, antiretroviral treatment of seropositive mothers and newborns, microbicides, and vaccines. On the influence of the Bill and Melinda Gates Foundation on these technological approaches to malaria control, see Randall Packard, *The Making of a Tropical Disease: A Short History of Malaria* (Baltimore: Johns Hopkins University Press, 2007); T. J. Coates, L. Richter, and C. Caceres, "Behavioural Strategies to Reduce HIV Transmission: How to Make Them Work Better," *Lancet* 372, no. 9639 (2008): 669–84.

45. G. Ramjee et al., "South Africa's Experience of the Closure of the Cellulose Sulphate Microbicide Trial," *PLoS Medicine* 4, no. 7 (2007): e235.

46. D. T. Halperin and R. C. Bailey, "Male Circumcision and HIV Infection: 10 Years and Counting," *Lancet* 354, no. 9192 (1999): 1814.

47. Ibid.

48. Many epidemiologists cosigned the article. B. Auvert et al., "Ecological and Individual Level Analysis of Risk Factors for HIV Infection in Four Urban Populations in Sub-Saharan Africa with Different Levels of HIV Infection," *AIDS* 15, Suppl. 4 (2001): S15–30; Auvert et al., "Male Circumcision and HIV Infection."

49. Telephone interview with Michel Caraël, conducted in 2011.

50. Telephone interview with official in charge of prevention at WHO, conducted in 2011.

51. These associations include the National Organization to Halt the Abuse and Routine Mutilation of Males (NOHARMM), the National Organization of Circumcision Information Resource Centers (NOCIRC), Brothers United for Future Foreskin (BUFF), Recovery of a Penis (RECAP), and Doctors Opposing Circumcision (DOC).

52. Auvert et al., "Randomized, Controlled Intervention," e298.

53. WHO, *Strategies and Approaches for Male Circumcision Programming* (Geneva: WHO, 2006).

54. Bailey et al., "Male Circumcision"; Gray et al., "Male Circumcision for HIV."

55. R. H. Gray et al., "The Impact of Male Circumcision on HIV Incidence and Cost per Infection Prevented: A Stochastic Simulation Model from Rakai, Uganda," *AIDS* 21, no. 7 (2007): 845–50; N. J. Nagelkerke et al., "Modelling the Public Health Impact of Male Circumcision for HIV Prevention in High Prevalence Areas in Africa," *BioMed Central Infectious Diseases* 7 (2007): 16; "Making Decisions on Male Circumcision for HIV Risk Reduction: Modeling the Impact and Costs. Report from a UNAIDS/WHO/SACEMA Consultation, Stellenbosch, South Africa" (15–16 November 2007).

56. J. G. Kahn, E. Marseille, and B. Auvert, "Cost Effectiveness of Male Circumcision For HIV Prevention in a South African Setting," *PLoS Medicine* 3, no. 12 (2006): e517.

57. P. Kebaabetswe et al., "Male Circumcision: An Acceptable Strategy for HIV Prevention in Botswana," *Sexually Transmitted Infections* 79, no. 3 (2003): 214–19;

N. Westercamp and R. C. Bailey, "Acceptability of Male Circumcision for Prevention of HIV/AIDS in Sub-Saharan Africa: A Review," *AIDS and Behavior* 11, no. 3 (2007): 341–55.

58. WHO/UNAIDS, *New Data on Male Circumcision and HIV Prevention.*

59. Garenne, "Male Circumcision," e76.

60. Presumably the organizers knew of the impending publications in *The Lancet.*

61. Attending researchers included key members of the circumcision random controlled study teams. The WHO/UNAIDS Male Circumcision Working Group, an informal group composed of two prominent organizations in medical circumcision and HIV, also attended.

62. Some 52.5 percent had a medical doctorate or equivalent, and 75 percent had biomedical training. Only five attendees (6.3 percent) had social sciences training, and just one had a law degree.

63. These critics included sexologist/urologist J. N. Krieger, epidemiologists M. W. Tyndall, C. L. Mattson, and J. G. Kahn, demographer M. Garenne, social scientist D. Peltzer, and representatives of major associations critical of mutilations Dean Ferris, national co-coordinator of the National Organization of Circumcision Information Resource Centers and Michael Bahinyoza from Uganda.

64. The cited measures include delaying the age of first sexual encounter, engaging in sex without penetration, decreasing number of sexual partners, promoting and using correctly and regularly male and female condoms, counseling and testing for HIV, and providing services for sexually transmitted disease treatment.

65. WHO/UNAIDS, *New Data.*

66. M. Foucault, *Surveiller et punir, naissance de la prison* (Paris: Gallimard, 1975); M. Foucault, *Naissance de la biopolitique, Cours au collège de France, 1978–79* (1979; Paris: Editions EHESS, 2004).

MICHEL GARENNE, ALAIN GIAMI, AND CHRISTOPHE PERREY

9

HEROIN USE, TRAFFICKING, AND INTERVENTION APPROACHES IN SUB-SAHARAN AFRICA
Local and Global Contexts

SHERYL MCCURDY AND HARUKA MARUYAMA

Heroin use in Africa is a startling phenomenon. Since the 1980s, repackaging and transshipment locations on the African continent have proliferated, and growing numbers of Africans from all regions have been buying and using heroin. During the early 1990s, some African governments began mobilizing legal resources to monitor and prosecute trafficking practices in response to local and international demands to monitor, reduce, and ultimately eradicate the heroin trade. Heroin dependence expanded in the 1990s and 2000s, and heroin flows continued unabated, even as African countries implemented their local versions of the US-led "War on Drugs."

In the late 1990s, East African heroin users, who previously had smoked or inhaled the drug, began injecting it. For the first time, injection drug use had been introduced into a region with an entrenched HIV/AIDS epidemic. A chill swept through public health networks. Practitioners, researchers, and government leaders feared that injection drug use threatened public health advances to contain the HIV/AIDS epidemic. They struggled to develop new ways to control heroin use.

Harm reduction was an alternative approach, helping users, families, communities, and states work together to reduce the individual and social harms of drug use. The guiding principle—reducing harm—has as its goal assisting users in becoming autonomous, healthy, and contributing members of society. It offers strategies to reduce infectious disease transmission and helps people who use drugs not to transmit diseases to others. Such interventions are successful, however, only when the political will exists to create national policies that support their implementation. Many African governments were unwilling or unable to manage the movement of illicit substances; their inaction mirrored their reluctance to recognize and respond to the problem of local heroin consumption.

In this chapter, we examine the evolution and characteristics of heroin trafficking and use in sub-Saharan African countries, as well as the myriad responses to heroin use on the continent. We discuss the causes and consequences of two different responses to the heroin epidemic: a foreign-led, top-down drug control approach, and a public health– and human rights–focused harm-reduction approach. In the first section we examine the historical and political context for heroin trafficking in Africa and discuss interventions to control drug trafficking. In the second section we examine the extent and characteristics of recent heroin use in Africa, focusing especially on the shift to injecting. We show how these developments led certain African states to embrace a harm-reduction approach, and we highlight the experiences of Tanzania. By examining how the heroin situation unfolded in Africa, we demonstrate the importance of understanding historical, economic, political, and social contexts of drug use to develop timely and effective responses to an emerging, rapidly changing public health problem.

The Context of Heroin Use and Trafficking in Africa from the Antitrafficking Intervention Perspective

THE FOUNDATIONS FOR TRAFFICKING IN AFRICA IN THE POST-INDEPENDENCE ERA

The postcolonial political and economic climates of many sub-Saharan African countries set the stage for the emergence of narcotics trafficking. Following decolonization, African states had to cope with the limited resources and minimal infrastructures that they had inherited. Many were beset by political instability, and few possessed effective legal and law enforcement systems. During the mid-1980s, these states struggled with financial crises, brought on by global economic recession as well as International Monetary Fund (IMF) and the World Bank structural adjustment policies and loan programs. Illicit drugs flowed across porous borders. By the late 1980s in Eastern and Southern Africa, as the AIDS crisis began to dominate national and international concerns, debates, and initiatives, few policymakers recognized illicit drug trafficking as a problem, and even fewer were aware of its local impacts.

IMF–World Bank structural adjustment policies facilitated the further integration of African countries into the market-based, capitalist system of the world economy. Owing to technological advances in transportation and communications, larger volumes of goods traveled faster and accelerated the development of the free-market system. Some low-resource countries in Africa also expanded tourism opportunities in an attempt to bring in wealth.

SHERYL MCCURDY AND HARUKA MARUMAYA

Meanwhile, globalization brought images, music, and ideas about other ways of living to people everywhere, and increasingly, migration promised better opportunities and lives. Many youth in low-income countries were influenced by the youth-focused popular culture embedded in the music, clothing, language, and practices of high-income countries, and many sought to participate in the global economy, escape desperate circumstances, and have meaningful lives that could be facilitated by a cash income. Many young Africans had very few options for finding meaningful, licit work. IMF structural adjustment conditions (including the privatization of nationally held companies and loss of access to free education) had contributed to the creation of an unskilled, unemployed labor force. A massive cohort of discontented youth had been bypassed by the new opportunities enjoyed by a small middle class at home. A few motivated, well-connected individuals participated in the drug trade, as did the poor and unemployed who faced coercive, desperate circumstances. The drug trade promised lucrative financial opportunities, depending on one's position in its organization.

Alcohol and tobacco consumption also increased during this period, a consequence of the international distribution of these products, improvements in advertising, and local tobacco production, processing, and distribution. Adolescents, in particular, had easier access to substances such as alcohol, cannabis, and tobacco. Yahya Affinnih refers to "the climate of experimentation" in the 1980s, when many drugs became available for misuse, including cannabis, amphetamines, Mandrax (Methaqualone), barbiturates, Valium (diazepam), and Librium (chlordiazepoxide).[1] Cocaine traffickers in West Africa and heroin traffickers in East Africa expanded their operations.

In essence, African countries offered traffickers a unique opportunity. First, reduced border controls after the mid-1980s allowed for increased movement and exchange of people, ideas, money, and objects. Some Africans went abroad and returned with new connections, knowledge, and ideas, and some foreigners entered African markets to exploit opportunities. Local markets served as transit locations for processing and repackaging drugs. Second, high unemployment and poverty rates meant that local people could be lured into working in the lucrative drug-trafficking business. Poor security and policing infrastructure made African countries compelling sites for illicit trade. Finally, Africa's lengthy coastlines with many international ports lay between the main narcotics producers in Asia and Latin America and the main consumers in North America and Europe.

In the 1960s, 80 percent of the heroin in the United States originated in Turkey, one of the few countries authorized to produce opium for pain-relief medications. Illicit opium production increased significantly in the 1960s in the Golden Triangle (Burma/Myanmar, Lao People's Democratic Republic, and Thailand); by the 1970s and 1980s, this area produced most of the world's opium.[2]

The demand for drugs in Europe and North America grew by the 1980s, but increased security on flights to Europe and North America forced transporters to find new routes to transport illicit narcotics. Some traffickers began to move their products through African countries, where they could take advantage of political instability, weak infrastructure, corrupt officials, and poorly regulated borders.[3] Some brought cocaine from South America to West and Southern Africa en route to Europe. Others brought heroin from Burma and Afghanistan to East Africa, where the drug was repackaged and sent to Europe and North America.[4]

In West Africa during the early 1980s, Nigerian and Ghanaian cannabis traffickers added cocaine and heroin to their portfolios.[5] Nigerians began to import heroin from Pakistan and repackage it for shipment to the United States. Nigerians came to dominate the trade, and Nigeria became a prominent hub in this traffic.[6] The trade expanded to Ghana in the late 1980s, when the Nigerian government tightened drug-trafficking controls.[7] West Africans also acted as intermediaries and couriers for transshipment of heroin and cocaine en route to North America and Europe.

By the mid-1980s, East Africa became part of a second drug-networking system on the continent. Nigerians also dominated this trade, and Mozambicans and Tanzanians increasingly participated in it.[8] Local informants link the appearance and expansion of heroin use on the Swahili coast to the arrival of Italians in the early 1980s and the subsequent growth of the tourist industry,[9] although East African seamen who first used heroin learned of it in foreign ports.[10]

Outsiders, however, did not single-handedly expand the heroin trade in East Africa: several factors within the region facilitated this development. Coastal East Africa's strategic position and its geographical and cultural proximity to the Arabian Peninsula and South Asia made it a prime site for drug trafficking. Additionally, the landlocked countries of Burundi, Rwanda, Uganda, and the eastern portion of the Democratic Republic of Congo depend on the Dar es Salaam and Zanzibar ports in Tanzania for their imported goods. Criminal groups based in Dar es Salaam appeared to be linked to associates in Kenya, Zambia, and South Africa who participated in this expanding trade.[11] Drug consignments from Pakistan, Afghanistan, and other sites that arrived in Dar es Salaam and other East and Southern African ports were repackaged and then routed to the United States and Europe.[12] At the same time, African youth migrated to Europe and South Asia for work; the drug-trafficking networks expanded and intermingled, as they recruited new young African participants. In West and Southern Africa, similar activities took place and the movement of cocaine from South America further enlarged their volume of trade.

During the 1990s, Nigerian traffickers continued to facilitate an African and global heroin trade. They effectively developed and superimposed a bulk heroin trade (transported via large air and sea containers) over an existing courier trade system. This massive trade was first detected during 1993 when Nigerian authorities arrested a Nigerian for transporting 250 kg from Thailand.[13] By the decade's end, Nigerian crime syndicates dominated the Moscow retail market and controlled 80 percent of the North American heroin trade coming from Southeast Asia.[14]

Across the continent, some participants in the drug trade became users and brought their habits home.[15] Others who were entrenched in local drug transit sites' tasting, repackaging, and distribution networks also became users. Still others learned new drug-using practices from friends and family. Combined with the rapid social and economic changes, the accessibility and availability of drugs, and the lack of effective control efforts, drugs easily filtered into an ordinary citizen's life. By 1987, the Division of Narcotic Drugs of the UN Secretariat reported opiate abuse across Africa.[16]

While heroin became entrenched in the trafficking routes through Africa, opium production escalated in Afghanistan toward the end of the 1980s. It rose from 200 metric tons of opium base at the time of the Russian invasion in 1980 to 1,600 metric tons at their departure in 1990. Production steadily increased to an estimated 3,300 tons by 2001, when the Taliban outlawed it. Production subsequently fell to the 1980 level. With a three-year supply of opium in reserve, however, this lost year of production did not affect opium prices or supplies in subsequent years. Following the US invasion of Afghanistan in 2002, opium production soared. Afghanistan, the "Golden Crescent," dominated global opium production.[17] By 2007, Afghanistan produced an estimated 8,000 tons—90 percent of the world's opium supply. Global opium production had also massively escalated, from around 1,040 tons in 1980 to 8,870 tons in 2007.[18]

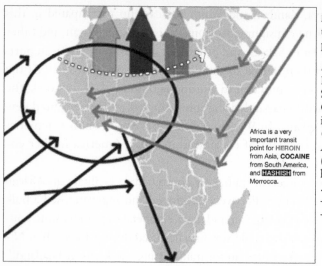

MAP 9.1. Global drug trafficking: Africa's expanding role (2009)

Source: Woodrow Wilson International Center for Scholars Africa Program, Conference Proceedings from 28 May 2009, *Global Drug Trafficking: Africa's Expanding Role* (2009). Retrieved from http://www.wilsoncenter.org/publication/global-drug-trafficking-africas-expanding-role.

Africa is a very important transit point for HEROIN from Asia, COCAINE from South America, and HASHISH from Morrocca.

RESPONSES TO DRUG TRAFFICKING—INTERVENTIONS FROM A DRUG-CONTROL PERSPECTIVE

As opium production and trafficking escalated, nation-states and international agencies sought to disrupt and reduce the supply. This top-down approach employs treaties, legislation, and police functions to implement antitrafficking measures. These measures include: (1) prosecuting members of criminal organizations, drug barons, and their employees, (2) monitoring and limiting the supply of illicit drugs through drug seizures, and (3) promoting the reduction of poppy production. Within this framework, individual countries have little latitude to develop their own responses. The African countries that harbored drug transit sites submitted to drug-trafficking rules and regulations that affected both the economic and political livelihoods of their people as well as their national stability and security.

The three UN conventions designed to regulate international drug control require signatory states to take action to criminalize drug-related activities. These treaties are the 1961 Single Convention on Narcotic Drugs, the 1971 Convention on Psychotropic Substances, and the 1988 Convention against Illegal Traffic in Narcotic Drugs and Psychotropic Substances. The UN Commission on Narcotic Drugs (CND), the United Nations Office on Drugs and Crime (UNODC), and the International Narcotics Control Board (INCB) provide oversight. Fifty-three UN member states populate the CND, the central policy-making body on drug control. The UNODC focuses on member states' national struggles against illicit drugs, crime, and terrorism. The INCB consists of thirteen individuals and describes itself as the "independent and quasi-judicial monitoring body for the implementation of the United Nations international drug control conventions."[19]

The 1961 Single Convention on Narcotic Drugs required UN member signatory states to establish measures to criminalize the drug-related uses of controlled substances that were not slated for medical or scientific purposes. The treaty did not succeed at containing illicit heroin production or use. In the United States alone, during the first decade of the 1961 Convention, the number of heroin users increased tenfold, from 50,000 in 1960 to approximately 500,000 in 1970.[20] The conventions focus on criminalization and penalties for drug-related activities, but, as Elliott et al. note, they also contain important qualifications that can, "if interpreted and implemented courageously by policy-makers, make some space for harm-reduction initiatives, even if this 'room for maneuver' is limited."[21] Elliot et al. observe that the 1961 and 1971 treaties allow states to follow a harm-reduction approach to address drug users' needs through treatment, rehabilitation, and social reintegration. These offerings can provide alternatives to or can accompany criminal penalties. Elliot et al. further argue that although the 1988 convention "requires each state to criminalize possession of a controlled substance even if only for personal consumption," it also acknowledges that this obligation is "subject to the constitutional principles and the basic concepts of its legal system."[22] Thus states can provide different harm-reduction measures if they choose to interpret the treaty from a health-promoting perspective, although many countries such as the United States have not.

The US response to the treaties was to intensify efforts to punish and ostracize nations implicated in drug production and trafficking. In 1986, the United States introduced a drug certification process sanctioning states designated as drug-producing or drug-transit.[23] Each year, the US president had to submit an International Narcotics Control Strategy Report to the House of Representatives and the Senate Committee on Foreign Relations, detailing evidence about cultivation, manufacture, and trafficking of illicit drugs in drug-producing and trafficking countries, information about their antitrafficking efforts and their attempts to address drug-related government corruption. The president certified to Congress whether or not each country on the list was working to comply fully with the 1988 Convention goals and objectives. Any listed country certified as a drug-producing or trafficking nation would find 50 percent of US bilateral assistance withheld. The United States could also oppose multilateral development assistance from six international development banks and could cut off security assistance.

US certification profoundly affected listed African countries. From 1994 to 1998, for instance, foreign investment and overseas borrowings dwindled in Nigeria, which consequently experienced financial hardship. The United States denied Nigeria aid for health and education, military training, and sales of arms and equipment. Nigerians faced difficulties in undertaking international travel, and relations with the United States became strained.[24]

The United States subsequently took limited steps to respond to both internal and external complaints about the deleterious effects of certification. In 2003, the US government enacted the Foreign Relations Authorization Act for Fiscal Year 2003 (FRAA) (H.R. 1646/P.L. 107–228). Under the FRAA, a listed country did not suffer any consequences for the first twelve months of this designation. After that year, they would lose only US aid, and would not be subject to other multilateral aid and trade sanctions.[25] Nevertheless, the United States effectively exported the War on Drugs to other nations by using economic threats and sanctions, and many African countries suffered as a result. Although the FRAA act tamed earlier legislation and limited US influence, the United States developed other strategies that intensified the War on Drugs and offered assistance to African countries to increase military and antitrafficking efforts.

Since the 1990s, the US annual federal budgets for drug-law enforcement have exceeded US$15 billion. By the mid-2000s, an estimated $65 billion was spent on drugs in the United States, and the Drug Enforcement Administration's (DEA) efforts to stop trafficking increased.[26] The US Department of Defense (DOD) also has provided funds to train, equip, and improve counternarcotics capacities in select countries. During fiscal year 2009, Congress authorized the DOD and US Africa Command (AFRICOM) to work in Africa and offer counternarcotics assistance to African countries.[27] Since then, AFRICOM has provided approximately $20 million a year in African counternarcotic assistance.[28] In 2011 alone, AFRICOM conducted 71 counter-trafficking training events related to weapons, narcotics, and human beings with twenty-four African partner nations.[29]

Despite such intense efforts to contain illicit trafficking in Africa and elsewhere, drug production and markets boomed. Earnings from the drug trade skyrocketed, and antitrafficking efforts stopped only some 20 percent of the global traffic. The UNODC has estimated that 375 tons (80 percent) of the 2009 global heroin traffic reached consumers.[30] The "War on Drugs" is failing.

Within Africa, the criminalization of individual drug use has led to numerous human rights abuses against drug users, including police brutality, unequal access to treatment for HIV/AIDS, and denial of necessary interventions.[31]

This punitive approach to drug use has forced drug users to engage in risky behaviors that facilitate HIV transmission.[32] In sum, forcing African countries to import the "War on Drugs" did not succeed in resolving the drug-related crises. It escalated them.

Injecting Drug Use and the Harm-Reduction Approach
DRUG-USE PATTERNS IN THE GLOBAL CONTEXT

As the production of opium and other drugs expanded, so did drug consumption levels worldwide. Between 2005 and 2010, illicit global drug use averaged between 3.4 and 6.6 percent of the adult (fifteen to sixty-four years) population.[33] According to the UNODC in 2012, illicit drug use is largely a youth phenomenon, with prevalence rates peaking as users reached their early twenties. The mortality consequences of drug use are significant: illicit drug use resulted in 0.5 to 1.3 percent of deaths (99,000 to 153,000) of drug users between fifteen and sixty-four in 2010,[34] and the average age for drug-related deaths is often in the mid-thirties.[35] Of the approximately 153 to 300 million illicit drug users worldwide, 10 to 13 percent are problem users with drug dependence and/or drug-use disorders. Of these, a small percentage receive treatment services (12 to 30 percent in 2009); some 11 to 33.5 million problem drug users go without treatment.[36]

Every year, according to the UNODC, illicit drug use causes between 23.1 and 58.7 deaths per million for ages fifteen to sixty-four.[37] Drug dependency itself is a major health problem: the UNODC estimates that 50 percent of heroin users develop drug dependency and become problem users.[38] Some drug users inject substances, and sharing injecting equipment, needles, and syringes is one of the most efficient ways to transmit HIV, hepatitis B virus (HBV), hepatitis C virus (HCV), and other blood-borne pathogens; using contaminated injection equipment can be almost six times more efficient in transmitting HIV compared to heterosexual acts.[39] Worldwide, the prevalence of HIV, hepatitis C, and hepatitis B among drug users is estimated at 18.9 percent (3,000,000), 46.7 percent, and 14.6 percent respectively.[40] Of the approximately 1.78 million heroin users, an estimated 534,500 to 3,022,500 injected drugs, among whom approximately 221,000 (range: 26,000–572,000) were HIV positive.[41]

HEROIN-USE PATTERNS IN SUB-SAHARAN AFRICA

The global increase in illicit drug use did not spare Africa. According to the UNODC, some 1.23 million Africans used heroin in 2008 (11 percent of the world's total), and consumed approximately 7 percent of the product.[42]

Drug-related deaths account for 1 in 150 deaths in Africa.[43] In addition, the physical, social, cultural, political, and economic harms of drug trafficking, use, and associated diseases lead to both short- and long-term consequences at every level of society. Users' fear of the pain of withdrawal symptoms drives them to find their next dose and experience stigma for their drug-associated activities. Family relationships sometimes disintegrate. Users and drug-affected communities often experience chaos, declining economic productivity, and decreased political, economic, and social stability. Drug-related practices threaten both individual and community safety, increasing crime and resulting in wide-ranging harms, including overdoses and improperly discarded drug paraphernalia.

Changes in drug consumption practices accompanied the rise in heroin use across Africa. Until the late 1990s, most heroin consumed in East Africa was adulterated "brown" heroin, which users primarily smoked, inhaled, or snorted.[44] In Tanzania, most users smoked heroin via "joints" (tobacco) or "cocktails" (laced with cannabis and tobacco). Over time, some graduated to snorting, which they could do for about six months before developing nosebleeds or losing their sense of smell. They would then switch to inhaling through a pipe, known as "chasing," or "chasing the dragon" as it is known in Asia.

After 1999, when white heroin from Afghanistan began to dominate world markets, East Africa became a primary transshipment hub for heroin from Southwest Asia, and illicit drug use on the African continent increased.[45] The post-1999 glut of Afghan heroin, trafficked through East Africa, dramatically altered patterns of heroin use. Injecting drug use (IDU) became more commonplace. During the earlier "brown" heroin era, users shifting to injections would purify the heroin by mixing it with water and lime in an upturned gin bottle cap and heating it with a candle or a lighter. This process was laborious and time-consuming.[46] But the white heroin from Afghanistan, called "White Crest"[47] in Kenya and "white" and "cocaine" in Tanzania, was more refined than brown heroin from the Golden Triangle of Burma/Myanmar; it was so pure that it did not require cooking before injecting.[48] Injection was also a more efficient and cost-effective way to consume heroin because it went directly into the bloodstream.[49] This water-soluble, easily injectable form of heroin gained popularity in the coastal towns of East Africa.[50]

Accurately measuring the national or regional prevalence of People Who Inject Drugs (PWIDs) across sub-Saharan Africa is difficult, and the data collection methods highlight several problems. Most studies conducted are cross-sectional, and although this "snapshot" type of data can be useful, it does little to measure long-term trends. Many are also hospital-based, so only people

SHERYL MCCURDY AND HARUKA MARUMAYA

who seek or receive treatment for substance abuse or related comorbidities are counted. Users who cannot or do not want treatment are not captured by these studies, and thus estimates likely underestimate numbers of PWIDs. It remains difficult to capture a representative sample of users in a locale; PWIDs experience stigma, fear criminalization, migrate, and suffer high mortality rates. Many countries lack monitoring systems to measure prevalence.

Several studies have attempted to estimate IDU levels in Africa. A 2004 review by Aceijas et al. found nine countries with reports of IDU: Cote d'Ivoire, Ghana, Guinea, Mauritius, Niger, Nigeria, Somalia, South Africa, and Zambia, totaling an estimated 9000 PWIDs.[51] In 2008, Mathers et al. conducted a systematic review, reporting injecting drug use in thirteen out of forty-seven sub-Saharan African countries.[52] Only some countries produced mean prevalence estimates of PWIDs aged fifteen to sixty-four: Kenya (0.73 percent, or an estimated 130,748 persons), Mauritius (2.07 percent, or 17,500 persons), and South Africa (0.87 percent, or 262,975 persons).[53] A subsequent review by Mathers et al. in 2010 expanded this list of IDU reporting countries to include Sierra Leone, Swaziland, and Togo.[54]

Although many sub-Saharan African countries do not produce national prevalence rates, there are abundant smaller-scale studies of injecting drug use.[55] A rapid assessment conducted in Mombasa, Kenya, in March 2004 included 496 heroin users, among whom 15 percent had "ever injected" heroin and 7 percent were currently injecting heroin, although the authors acknowledged that their results were likely an underestimation.[56] A 2009 study in Tanzania produced estimates of 15,000 PWIDs in Dar es Salaam and another 25,000 across the country.[57] Despite most countries' lack of funding and political will to conduct national-level surveillance drug studies, local-level research indicates that injecting drug use occurs in every region of the continent.

The shift to injecting drug use had numerous negative consequences on users' health. Heroin dependence from injecting can be more severe than from noninjecting methods of consumption.[58] A study comparing chasers and injectors in Switzerland showed that the severity of dependence (measured by the addiction severity index) was significantly worse for the injectors.[59] Additionally, longitudinal studies have shown a significant difference between the mortality of chasers and injectors, with higher rates for the latter.[60] Injectors typically have a higher risk of overdose than noninjectors because injecting puts a large amount of heroin in the bloodstream quickly.[61]

Injectors using unsafe injection practices also risk transmitting infectious diseases. Unsafe injection practices include intentional or accidental sharing of needles and syringes tainted with pathogen-containing blood. This drug-related harm is heightened in sub-Saharan Africa where resource-poor nations struggling with poverty, hunger, and social, political, and economic inequities are also challenged by HIV, HBV, and HCV epidemics. A 2004 study in South Africa found that 89 percent of heroin users who acknowledged injecting heroin in the last month reported that they had shared a needle at least once during that time.[62] In addition to sharing practices, other high-risk practices developed in different contexts. For example, in 2005 in Tanzania, a practice known as *flashblood* emerged among female heroin users in Dar es Salaam; it spread to male heroin users in Zanzibar by 2006 and subsequently north along the Swahili Coast to Kenya.[63] *Flashblood* began as an altruistic practice, in which injectors tried to help one another stave off withdrawal symptoms. One injector would draw back a syringe full of their blood immediately after injecting heroin and pass it to another user to inject.[64] Practices like *flashblood* thus compounded the risks of injecting drug use.

Available research findings from different African countries support the conclusion that PWIDs are disproportionally affected by HIV and other infectious diseases. Mathers et al. estimated HIV positive prevalence rates among PWIDs of 42.9 percent in Kenya and 12.4 percent in South Africa.[65] A multinational, retrospective analysis study of HIV and HCV coinfection found that the method of exposure of HIV was a significant predictor, with 92.7 percent of injecting drug use cases being positive for both.[66] A study of heroin users in Nairobi, Kenya, revealed that HIV and HCV prevalence among 146 PWIDs was 36.3 percent and 42.2 percent, respectively—staggeringly high when compared to prevalence among those who never injected (13.51 percent and 3.24 percent, respectively).[67] Furthermore, the numbers of HIV cases in Kenya attributable to drug use have been increasing, constituting 4.8 percent of new infections in 2005.[68] By 2006 in Mauritius, where there were an estimated 17,000 to 18,000 PWIDs and needle sharing was estimated at 25–50 percent, injection drug use surpassed heterosexual contact as the main mode of HIV transmission.[69] In Tanzania, where the adult (fifteen to forty-nine years old) prevalence rate of HIV is just under 6 percent, one study found that among a sample of PWIDs, 28 percent of men and 64 percent of women tested positive for HIV.[70] A study in Zanzibar found that the prevalence of infectious disease among PWIDs was significantly higher when compared to those who did not inject (HIV: 30 percent versus 12 percent and hepatitis C: 22 percent versus 15 percent, respectively).[71]

Although the literature and data on PWIDs and HIV is limited in many African countries, the available research warrants concern. Heterosexual transmission remains the main mode of transmission in sub-Saharan Africa,[72] but HIV seroprevalence rates among PWIDs are extremely high, and in many cases, rising. While numbers of heroin users have increased in several African countries, governments and public health systems have largely ignored their plight: only an estimated 5 percent of drug users in Africa received treatment services during 2009. Most demands for treatment in Africa as a whole come from cannabis users (64 percent), but in certain countries, opiate users are the predominant group seeking treatment: 81 percent of those treated in Mauritius, 55 percent in Mozambique, 45 percent in Seychelles and 33 percent in Tanzania. Among the few countries reporting mortality data for substance groups, drug-related deaths were most often found among opiate users.[73]

Injection drug use, in the context of existing HIV and hepatitis B and C epidemics, threatened to introduce a new wave of infections just when several of the most-affected African countries had lowered HIV seroprevalence rates. These challenges necessitated a new approach. Not until 2011 did the political will at the international level coalesce around efforts to eliminate new HIV infections among PWIDs worldwide. In June of that year, states attending the UN High Level Meeting on AIDS signed the *Political Declaration on HIV and AIDS: Intensifying Our Efforts to Eliminate HIV and AIDS,* explicitly identifying the WHO/UNAIDS/UNODC comprehensive harm-reduction package and concrete measures to reduce HIV among PWIDs by 50 percent by 2015. Countries submitted their first progress reports detailing their progress toward the 2015 goals to UNAIDS in March 2012.[74]

The costs for evidence-based treatment versus indirect costs attributed to untreated drug dependence (law enforcement, crime, prisons, unemployment, and deteriorating health) are estimated to produce a 3:1 savings rate in terms of reduced numbers of crime victims and expenditures for the criminal justice system. A broader calculation of costs associated with crime, health, and social productivity increases this rate of savings to investment to 13:1.[75] Furthermore, the high risk of horizontal transmission of HIV/AIDS and other infectious diseases from injectors to the general population highlighted the need for interventions to reduce the harmful effects of injecting use at the individual and community levels. A public health approach through harm reduction was one answer.

THE PRINCIPLES AND APPLICATION OF HARM REDUCTION

Harm reduction is a public health approach to manage the effects of drug use in the individual and the community.[76] Rather than a specific set of rigid "interventions," the harm-reduction perspective provides a guiding framework for understanding and responding to drug use. As Don Des Jarlais noted, first, we need to accept that drug abuse is here to stay. Wherever trafficking occurs, "nonmedical drug use" is inevitable, as are the individual and social harms that result.[77] Second, the harm-reduction framework recognizes that drug users are also part of a community, and thus protecting community health requires improving the health of the drug users, rather than isolating them. Third, the framework recognizes that the harms of nonmedical drug use on the individual and the wider society are multifaceted. They require different kinds of interventions, and eliminating or reducing drug use may not always be necessary to reduce harm. The harm-reduction perspective, then, lends itself well to utilizing research findings because of its context-driven nature. The specific programming strategies of harm reduction can vary across locales and depend on the context of the local drug use and resource availability. Harm reduction can thus constitute multiple interventions that target individual users, wider communities, and government-level policy changes.

Harm reduction focuses on prevention and treatment to enable drug users to make better choices that will help them reduce their risk-related practices. The goal is to help users to manage their drug dependence and comorbidities with less harm to themselves and others. Harm reduction seeks to help users reduce the possibilities of overdose, infection, or transmission of HIV, HBV, HCV, and sexually transmitted infections (STIs). Interventions can include access to treatment for substance abuse disorders (e.g., opioid substitution and overdose medication such as Naloxone), condoms, clean needles and syringes and other drug paraphernalia, education to avoid abscesses and infections associated with poorly administered injections and treatment for these wounds, the ability to inject without threat of arrest, the provision of antiretrovirals as needed, access to food and shelter, and a support system. In the midst of the HIV epidemic, the three pillars of modern harm reduction for PWIDs are needle and syringe exchange programs (NSPs), medication assisted treatment/opioid substation therapy (MAT/OST), and the provision of antiretroviral therapy (ART). Evidence reveals that when OST or MAT,[78] NSPs, and ART are employed together to 60 percent of a PWID population, they can reduce HIV infection in that population by 40 percent.[79]

HARM-REDUCTION UPTAKE AND BARRIERS IN SUB-SAHARAN AFRICA

The emerging injection drug use epidemic in AIDS-entrenched sub-Saharan Africa led funders in the late 2000s to promote harm reduction. Harm reduction is an approach that began from needle and syringe exchange programs

SHERYL MCCURDY AND HARUKA MARUMAYA

pioneered in western Europe in the mid-1980s to prevent hepatitis B transmission among PWIDs. Such programs spread with the availability of diagnostic tools, which detected in the later 1980s an escalating HIV epidemic among PWIDs in Europe. Methadone maintenance treatment, also a strategy of this harm-reduction approach, had existed in some European countries since the late 1960s, but many countries revitalized and expanded methadone treatment for PWIDs in response to the HIV epidemic in the 1990s.

Although the harm-reduction approach first developed in western Europe, its flexibility permitted its appropriation and adaptation in Africa. Two countries, Mauritius and Tanzania, initiated programs to address the harm of injecting drug use in their communities. In Tanzania, AIDS was already entrenched in the general population when the injecting epidemic occurred. International funders and the Tanzanian government, confronted with the evidence that heroin injection existed and was a threat, feared that high HIV seroprevalence among PWIDs (42 percent) would lead to a new wave of infections among those who did not use drugs.[80] But how to develop appropriate measures, accounting for limited resources and for local governments' willingness and capacities to respond remained a critical challenge. Because PWIDs are a stigmatized community, only extenuating circumstances would allow for them to receive special attention, funds, and programming. What seems to be the most convincing argument is that PWIDs' needs should be addressed to protect the health and security of the general population. This is where harm-reduction policies and programs can effectively intervene.

Although evaluations have shown NSP, MAT, and ART interventions to be effective in reducing HIV/AIDS prevalence in high-income countries, many sub-Saharan African countries face structural challenges that can inhibit long-term change. As early as 1997, Adelekan and Stimson identified some of these challenges: lack of social and economic resources to develop harm-reduction approaches, low prioritization of drug abuse as an important public health issue, criminal justice systems that criminalize drug misuse, and moral perceptions of drug dependence as a crime, not a disease or public health concern, leading to victim-blaming.[81] Lack of political will, weak health care systems, and legislation that prohibits prescriptions of OST medications are also significant barriers.[82]

Perhaps these numerous challenges have slowed the uptake of a harm-reduction approach in sub-Saharan African countries. By 2006, only Mauritius, Tanzania, and Kenya had specifically addressed the prevention of HIV among PWIDs in their national HIV/AIDS strategic plans.[83] OST or MAT is available in a very limited context in a few countries. In South Africa, only six private drug treatment facilities provide buprenorphine; in Kenya, only private clinics offer methadone because current governmental policy bans its use in public health facilities, and in Senegal, buprenorphine is reportedly available for OST, but there is no data on coverage thus far.[84]

Despite these poor responses to PWID needs, Mauritius and Tanzania have pioneered harm reduction on the continent. Mauritius passed legislation in February 2006 to permit the use of methadone in detoxification or maintenance therapy for heroin users.[85] Since then, the program has expanded to reach an estimated 2,000 people receiving methadone maintenance treatment at fourteen sites.[86] Mauritius is also the only country in the region with established NSPs, with the exception of a limited, small-scale NSP independently run by a French organization, Médecins du Monde, in Temeke District of Dar es Salaam, Tanzania. The official program in Mauritius runs thirty-one sites, while nongovernmental organizations (NGOs) run an additional eight sites.[87] The NSPs reach nearly one in three PWIDs in the country.[88]

In Tanzania, several events converged in 2006 and 2007, leading to the introduction of harm-reduction services there.[89] First, the media publicized the heroin epidemic and trafficking situation. Second, research demonstrating that PWIDs existed and that they engaged in behaviors that heightened their risk of blood-borne infections was published in peer-reviewed scientific journals. Third, members of the Tanzanian medical and political establishment mobilized their interest, political will, and commitment, using these research findings to persuade the Tanzanian government that policy and programmatic interventions were needed. Finally, committed international funders offered funding in response to the Tanzanian calls for harm-reduction assistance.

By August 2012, four Tanzanian community-based organizations (CBOs) provided outreach services to PWIDs in Kinondoni District of Dar es Salaam. These services included distribution of health kits (including condoms, bleach kits for cleaning needles and syringes, wound care materials, and education materials) and psychosocial support (including individual counseling, self-support groups, Narcotics Anonymous and Methadone Anonymous meetings, and family group therapy meetings). The CBOs identified and supported individuals by screening and enrolling them in a limited pilot methadone program. By early August 2012, clinicians had enrolled 431 former PWIDs into MAT at the Muhimbili National Hospital in Dar es Salaam.

SHERYL MCCURDY AND HARUKA MARUMAYA

This project will expand to Dar es Salaam's other two districts in 2013. In addition, a small comprehensive project with a drop-in center in Temeke District offers a range of services, including needle and syringe exchange and food and clothing.

In Zanzibar, the recovery-oriented systems of care model focusing on 12-step recovery and sober houses emerged. By May 2012, former heroin users operated eight male sober houses and one female sober house. National agencies and nongovernmental organizations also trained outreach workers to provide HIV prevention information, HIV testing, and linkages to care and treatment as needed. In addition, there are static and mobile HIV testing and counseling, outreach services for STI and tuberculosis screening, and for those who need it, peer escort referrals for HIV care and treatment.

Nevertheless, resource-limited settings encounter specific challenges after the implementation of harm-reduction interventions. Many Dar es Salaam drug users take heroin to escape the harsh realities of life and past traumas, from child abuse to homelessness and unemployment.[90] Even if harm-reduction activities reduce or eliminate heroin dependence, many clients worry about long-term prospects for employment and housing because of their poverty and lack of education or training.[91] Nadine Ezard terms these "vulnerability factors," which "constrain choices and limit agency . . . [and] arise out of and are reinforced by past and present social context and experience."[92] Therefore, unless the state and international community offer broader "vulnerability reduction" efforts[93] to help recovered users reintegrate and pursue functional positions and steady employment in society, harm reduction may only offer short-term benefits. Furthermore, funding and difficulties with sustainability are constant worries in these low-resource settings.

Tanzania and Mauritius are pioneers of harm reduction in sub-Saharan Africa. They overcame numerous ideological and structural barriers to offer services such as medication assisted treatment. These two countries recognized the severity of HIV/AIDS specifically in the PWID population and responded to the problem via specific public health programming. This alone is a monumental achievement given a political atmosphere that favors drug trafficking control and the criminalization of drug use. Most significantly, the uptake of services in these two countries demonstrates that PWIDs accept them and that, although "Western" ideas of harm reduction originally shaped harm-reduction services, the specific aims and projects can expand and change to address the specific local contexts of heroin use. Despite their numerous challenges, Tanzania and Mauritius can serve as positive examples for coordinated public health responses to injecting drug use epidemics in sub-Saharan Africa.

Evidence from sub-Saharan Africa reveals drug supplies are at an all-time high and likely growing. Growing numbers of disaffected youth, create a ready market for this supply. How do we address drug users' needs and contain a potential public health disaster? Recognizing a "potential" threat does not make it inevitable. Attempting to police PWIDs' practices in the absence of drug treatment and harm-reduction interventions will only alienate users who desperately need treatment or risk-reduction services.[94] Narcotics in Africa are here to stay, and control efforts alone are not sufficient to mitigate their negative effects on society and individuals. Some nations have successfully managed simultaneous epidemics of IDU and HIV/AIDS using public health strategies. Harm-reduction initiatives can be effective in many settings in and out of Africa. These initiatives respect drug users and drug-affected communities and recognize them as agents of change by empowering them to manage their drug-related practices. Injecting safely is the key principle of harm reduction, whether in conjunction or not with efforts to reduce drug intake levels. If injectors use clean needles every time they inject, they will not get or spread a blood-borne infection.

An intervention that works in one locale at a particular moment will not necessarily work in another place or time. Context matters. Specific historical and structural factors, including structural adjustment policies and the resulting decline in educational and economic opportunities, rural-to-urban migration, structural violence, and poverty offer contexts in which drug traffickers cultivate their clientele, and in which alienated and dejected youth seek escape through drugs. The interactions between different interventions and control approaches, policing, drug availability, and different stakeholders, as well as the general public's opinions regarding drug use can have a very real impact on heroin users' health and lives. Mixed-methods research employing ethnography can gain an accurate portrayal of heroin users' and their families' and communities' experiences. Translational research with community-based interventions can then address the relevant contexts and be developed as part of a team effort to ensure success and sustainability. As the Tanzanian case highlights, having the essential elements (media coverage, published research results, political will, and funding) and advocates converging at the right moment can transform ideas into action, creating policies and programs to improve the lives of PWIDs and the communities in which they live.

Notes

1. Y. Affinnih, "Revisiting Sub-Saharan African Countries' Drug Problems: Health, Social, Economic Costs, and Drug Control Policy," *Substance Use and Misuse* 37, no. 3 (2002): 276.

2. United Nations Office on Drugs and Crime (UNODC), *A Century of International Drug Control* (Vienna: UNODC, 2008), 65. Retrieved from http://www.unodc .org/unodc/en/drug-trafficking/index.html.

3. E. Akyeampong, "Diaspora and Drug Trafficking in West Africa: A Case Study of Ghana," *African Affairs* 104, no. 416 (2005): 429–47; J. Adelekan, "Substance Use, HIV Infection and the Harm Reduction Approach in Sub-Saharan Africa," *International Journal of Drug Policy* 9, no. 5 (1998): 315–23.

4. The other heroin-producing region is Latin America (Colombia and Mexico). Heroin is manufactured from opium and acetic anhydride, a substance that refines morphine into heroin. UNODC, *World Drug Report 2010* (United Nations Publication, Sales No. E.10.XI.13) (Vienna: UNODC, 2010), 140.

5. West Africa was a transit site for heroin trafficking as early as the 1950s, when Lebanese smuggled Near East heroin from Beirut through Kano, Nigeria, and Accra, Ghana, to New York City. S. Ellis, "West Africa's International Drug Trade," *African Affairs* 108, no. 431 (2009): 171–96.

6. M. Shaw, "West African Criminal Networks in South and Southern Africa," *African Affairs* 101, no. 404 (2002): 297, citing Drug Enforcement Administration, Intelligence Division, Drug Intelligence Brief, *The Price Dynamic of Southeast Asian Heroin* (Washington, DC: DEA, February 2001).

7. Akyeampong, "Diaspora."

8. UNODC, *Organised Crime and Trafficking in Eastern Africa: A Discussion Paper,* for the regional ministerial meeting on promoting the rule of law and human security in Eastern Africa, Nairobi, Kenya, 23–24 November 2009 (Vienna: UNODC, 2010), 29. Retrieved from http://www.unodc.org/documents/easternafrica/regional -ministerial-meeting/Organised_Crime_and_Trafficking_in_Eastern_Africa _Discussion_Paper.pdf.

9. United Nations Office for Drug Control and Crime Prevention (UNODCCP), *The Drug Nexus in Africa,* issue 1 (Vienna: UNODCCP, 1999), 20, 74; S. Beckerleg, " 'Brown Sugar' or Friday Prayers: Youth Choices and Community Building in Coastal Kenya," *African Affairs* 94, no. 374 (1995): 23–39.

10. S. Beckerleg, M. Telfer, and G. Hundt, "The Rise of Injecting Drug Use in East Africa: A Case Study from Kenya," *Harm Reduction Journal* 2, no. 12 (2005): doi:10.1186/1477-7517-2-12; S. Beckerleg, M. Telfer, and A. Sadiq, "A Rapid Assessment of Heroin Use in Mombasa, Kenya," *Substance Use and Misuse* 41, no. 6–7 (2006): 1029–44.

11. UNODC, "Tanzania: Country Profile" (UNODC, 2002). Retrieved from http://www.unodc.org/.

12. Ibid. UNODCCP, *Organised Crime,* 31; International Narcotics Control Board, *Report of the International Narcotics Control Board for 2001* (United Nations Publication, Sales No. E.02.XI.1), (United Nations, 2001), 41. Retrieved from http://www.incb .org/incb/en/publications/annual-reports/annual-report-2001.html.

13. Ellis, "West Africa," 190.

14. By 1993, Nigerians had joined Chinese traffickers delivering the bulk of Southeast Asian heroin into the United States. Ellis, "West Africa"; Drug Enforcement Administration (DEA), "Drug Enforcement Administration History in Depth, 1990–1994," n.d., retrieved from http://www.justice.gov/dea/about/history.shtml.

15. Beckerleg, "Brown Sugar"; S. A. McCurdy et al., "Heroin and HIV Risk in Dar es Salaam, Tanzania: Youth Hangouts, *Mageto* and Injecting Practices," *AIDS Care* 17, Suppl. 1 (2005): S65–76; S. McCurdy et al., "Harm Reduction in Tanzania: An Urgent Need for Multisectoral Intervention," *International Journal of Drug Policy* 18, no. 3 (2007): 155–59.

16. Division of Narcotic Drugs of the United Nations Secretariat, "Review of Drug Abuse and Measures to Reduce the Illicit Demand for Drugs by Region," *Bulletin on Narcotics* 1 (1987): 3–30.

17. UNODC, *2007 World Drug Report* (United Nations Publication, Sales No. E.07.XI.5) (Slovakia: UNODC, 2007).

18. C. Beyrer, "The Golden Crescent and HIV/AIDS in Central Asia: Deadly Interactions," *Global Public Health* 6, no. 5 (2011): 571.

19. International Narcotics Control Board, "Mandate and Functions," retrieved from http://www.incb.org/incb/en/about/mandate-functions.html (n.d.) and http://www.incb.org/incb/en/about/membership.html.

20. D. Musto. *The American Disease: Origins of Narcotic Control* (Oxford: Oxford University Press, 1999), 248.

21. R. Elliott, et al., "Harm Reduction, HIV/AIDS, and the Human Rights Challenge to Global Drug Control Policy," *Health and Human Rights* 8, no. 2 (2005): 113.

22. Ibid., 114.

23. J. Ayling, "Conscription in the War on Drugs: Recent Reforms to the U.S. drug Certification Process," *International Journal of Drug Policy* 16, no. 6 (2005): 376–83. Between 1986 and 2002, the Foreign Assistance Act of 1961 was used to control funding directed toward countries deemed to need certification of their antitrafficking efforts. The Foreign Relations Authorization Act superseded it in 2003.

24. I. S. Obot, "Assessing Nigeria's Drug Control Policy 1994–2000," *International Journal of Drug Policy* 15, no. 1 (2004): 21.

25. Ayling, "Conscription," 378.

26. DEA, "Drug Enforcement Administration History in Depth, 2003–2008," n.d. Retrieved from http://www.justice.gov/dea/about/history/2003-2008.pdf, 180.

27. During the 2000s, DOD provided counternarcotics training assistance and assisted twenty-two countries in their counternarcotics efforts by providing personnel and navigation equipment, secure and nonsecure communications, radar surveillance, night vision systems, and land, air, and sea vehicles.

28. L. S. Wyler and N. Cook, *Illegal Drug Trade in Africa: Trends and U.S. Policy* (CRS Report No. R40838) (Washington, DC: Congressional Research Service, 2009), 50; N. Dalrymple, "AFRICOM-Funded Projects Assisting African Partners Develop Capacity to Counter Drug Trafficking" (U.S. AFRICOM Public Affairs, 6 January 2012). Retrieved from http://www.africom.mil/getArticle .asp?art=7532&lang=0.

SHERYL MCCURDY AND HARUKA MARUMAYA

29. General Carter F. Ham, USA Commander, U.S. Africa Command (AFRICOM), "Statement to the U.S. House Armed Services Committee" (29 February 2012), 14. Retrieved from http://www.africom.mil/fetchBinary.asp?pdfID=20120301102747.

30. UNODC, *World Drug Report 2011* (United Nations Publication, Sales No. E.11.XI.10) (Vienna: UNODC, 2011), 54.

31. R. Jürgens et al., "People Who Use Drugs, HIV, and Human Rights," *Lancet* 376, no. 9739 (2010): 475–85.

32. J. Cohen and D. Wolfe, "Harm Reduction and Human Rights: Finding Common Cause," *AIDS* 22, Suppl. 2 (2008): S93–S94.

33. UNODC, *World Drug Report 2012* (United Nations Publication, Sales No. E.12.XI.1) (Malta: UNODC, 2012), 1.

34. Ibid., 1, 7.

35. Ibid., 59.

36. UNODC, *World Drug Report 2010*, 131.

37. UNODC, *World Drug Report 2011*, 33.

38. UNODC, *World Drug Report 2010*, 80.

39. UNODC, *World Drug Report 2005* (United Nations Publication, Sales No. E.05.XI) (Vienna: UNODC, 2005).

40. UNODC, *World Drug Report 2012*, 1.

41. C. Beyrer et al., "Time to Act: A Call for Comprehensive Responses to HIV In People Who Use Drugs," *Lancet* 376, no. 9740 (2010): 551–63; UNODC, *World Drug Report 2012*, citing Reference Group to the United Nations on HIV and Injecting Drug Use (2011 estimates), 18.

42. UNODC, *Addiction, Crime and Insurgency: The Transnational Threat of Afghan Opium* (Vienna: UNODC, 2009), 26. Retrieved from http://www.unodc.org/documents/data-and-analysis/Afghanistan/Afghan_Opium_Trade_2009_web.pdf.

43. UNODC, *World Drug Report 2012*, 17. Most African countries do not commonly monitor drug-related deaths, so these estimates are rough predictions.

44. Beckerleg, Telfer, and Sadiq, "Rapid Assessment"; McCurdy et al., "Heroin and HIV Risk."

45. Wyler and Cook, *Illegal Drug Trade*, citing International Narcotics Control Board (INCB), *Report of the International Narcotics Control Board for 2008*, E/INCB/2008/1 (2009), 1; Drug Enforcement Administration, *Drug Enforcement Administration History in Depth, 1999–2003*, n.d., 117. Retrieved from http://www.justice.gov/dea/about/history.shtml.

46. McCurdy et al., "Heroin."

47. Beckerleg, Telfer, and Sadiq, "Rapid Assessment." They hypothesize that white crest probably came from Thailand in the late 1990s.

48. McCurdy et al., "Heroin and HIV Risk."

49. R. H. Needle et al., "Substance Abuse and HIV in Sub-Saharan Africa: Introduction to the Special Issue," *African Journal of Drug and Alcohol Studies* 5, no. 2 (2006): 83–94.

50. Beckerleg, Telfer, and Sadiq, "Rapid Assessment"; McCurdy et al., "Heroin and HIV Risk."

51. C. Aceijas et al., "Global Overview of Injecting Drug Use and HIV Infection among Injecting Drug Users," *AIDS* 18, no. 17 (2004): 2295–2303.

Heroin Use, Trafficking, and Intervention Approaches

52. B. M. Mathers et al., "Global Epidemiology of Injecting Drug Use and HIV among People Who Inject Drugs: A Systematic Review," *Lancet* 372, no. 9651 (2008): 1733–45.

53. Ibid.

54. Ibid.

55. For Tanzania, see sources in this chapter. For Nigeria, see M. L. Adelekan and R. A. Lawal, "Drug Use and HIV Infection in Nigeria: A Review of Recent Findings," *African Journal of Drug and Alcohol Studies* 5, no. 2 (2006): 117–28.

56. Beckerleg, Telfer, and Sadiq, "Rapid Assessment."

57. J. Mbwambo and S. A. McCurdy, "IDU Size Estimates for Dar es Salaam and Tanzania," Presentation at the Centers for Disease Control [Tanzania], October 2009.

58. M. Gossop et al., "Severity of Dependence and Route of Administration of Heroin, Cocaine, and Amphetamines," *British Journal of Addiction* 87, no. 11 (1992): 1527–36.

59. R. Stohler et al., "A Comparison of Heroin Chasers with Heroin Injectors in Switzerland ," *European Addiction Research* 6, no. 3 (2000): 154–59; D. Tashkin, "Airway Effects of Marijuana, Cocaine, and Other Inhaled Illicit Agents," *Current Opinion in Pulmonary Medicine* 7, no. 2 (2001): 43–61.

60. M. Gossop et al., "Changes in Route of Drug Administration among Continuing Heroin Users: Outcomes One Year after Intake to Treatment," *Addictive Behaviors* 29, no. 6 (2004): 1085–94.

61. M. Brugal et al., "Factors Associated with Non-Fatal Heroin Overdose: Assessing the Effect of Frequency and Route of Heroin Administration," *Addiction* 97, no. 3 (2002): 319–27; S. Chiang et al., "Heroin Use among Youths Incarcerated for Illicit Drug Use: Psychosocial Environment, Substance Use History, Psychiatric Comorbidity, and Route of Administration," *American Journal on Addictions* 15, no. 3 (2006): 233–41; G. Harding, "Patterns of Heroin Use: What Do We Know?" *British Journal of Addiction* 83, no. 11 (1988): 1247–54.

62. A. Pluddermann et al., "Heroin Users in Cape Town, South Africa: Injecting Practices, HIV-Related Risk Behaviors, and Other Health Consequences," *Journal of Psychoactive Drugs* 40, no. 3 (2008): 273–79.

63. D. McNeil, Jr., "Desperate Addicts Inject Others' Blood," *New York Times,* 12 July 2010. Retrieved from http://www.nytimes.com/2010/07/13/health/13blood.html.

64. M. Dahoma et al., "HIV and Substance Abuse: The Dual Epidemics Challenging Zanzibar," *African Journal of Drug and Alcohol Studies* 5, no. 2 (2006): 130–39; S. McCurdy et al., "Flashblood: Blood Sharing Among Female Injecting Drug Users in Tanzania," *Addiction* 105, no. 6 (2010): 1062–70. The heroin used in 2005 was white Afgani and reputedly very pure. No one tested the product for us, nor were we able to test the amount of heroin that might have been in the blood-filled syringe that injectors gave their friends. Our outreach worker saw flashblood recipients nod off as if they had taken a dose of heroin. We do not know if the amount of heroin was enough to cause that response, or if it was a placebo effect, purely the power of suggestion. The practice of flashblood is now extremely rare. Our latest survey found only 2 out of 298 had ever injected flashblood. See J. Atkinson et al., "HIV Risk Behaviors, Perceived Severity of Drug Use Problems, and Prior Treatment Experience in a Sample of Young

Heroin Injectors in Dar es Salaam, Tanzania," *African Journal of Drug and Alcohol Studies* 10, no. 1 (2011): 1–9.

65. Mathers et al., "Global Epidemiology."

66. J. J. Amin et al., "HIV and Hepatitis C Coinfection within the CAESAR Study," *HIV Medicine* 5, no. 3 (2004): 174–79.

67. M. Odek-Ogunde et al., "Seroprevalence of HIV, HBC and HCV in Injecting Drug Users in Nairobi, Kenya: World Health Organization Drug Injecting Study Phase II Findings," XV International Conference on AIDS, Bangkok, 2004. Abstract WePeC6001.

68. C. Deveau, B. Levine, and S. Beckerleg, "Heroin Use in Kenya and Findings Form a Community-Based Outreach Programme to Reduce the Spread of HIV/ AIDS," *African Journal of Drug and Alcohol Studies* 5, no. 2 (2006): 95–106.

69. R. Abdool, F. Sulliman, and M. L. Dhannoe, "The Injecting Drug Use and HIV/AIDS Nexus in the Republic of Mauritius," *African Journal of Drug and Alcohol Studies* 5, no. 2 (2006): 107–16.

70. M. L. Williams et al., "HIV Seroprevalence in a Sample of Tanzanian Intravenous Drug Users," *AIDS Education and Prevention* 21, no. 5 (2009): 474–83.

71. Dahoma et al., "HIV and Substance Abuse."

72. United Nations Programme on HIV/AIDS (UNAIDS) and World Health Organization (WHO), *AIDS Epidemic Update* (UNAIDS/09.36E / JC1700E) (Geneva, Switzerland: UNAIDS, 2009).

73. UNODC, *World Drug Report 2011*, 56.

74. C. Stoicescu, *The Global State of Harm Reduction 2012: Towards an Integrated Response* (London: Harm Reduction International, 2012), 12–13.

75. UNODC, *World Drug Report 2010*, 128.

76. T. Rhodes and D. Hedrich, "Harm Reduction and the Mainstream," in *Harm Reduction: Evidence, Impacts, and Challenges,* ed. European Monitoring Centre for Drugs and Drug Addiction (Luxembourg: Publications Office of the European Union, 2010), 19–36. Drug-related harm reduction's longer history includes the prescription of heroin and morphine to opioid dependent persons in the U.K. during the 1920s and the introduction of methadone maintenance in the United States in the 1960s. During the 1970s, the WHO recommended harm-reduction policies to "prevent or reduce the severity of problems associated with the non-medical use of dependence-producing drugs."

77. Unless otherwise noted, this paragraph draws from Des Jarlais's editorial. D. Des Jarlais, "Harm Reduction—A Framework for Incorporating Science into Drug Policy," *American Journal of Public Health* 85, no. 1 (1995): 10–12.

78. OST or MAT is a medically supervised procedure of replacing illicit opioid drugs such as heroin with controlled narcotic substances (typically methadone or buprenorphine, which are the only approved drugs for opioid treatment in the United States) that have less severe side effects. When prescribed a proper dose, a client on methadone or buprenorphine should be able to lead a functional life without using heroin; these drugs are longer-lasting, mitigate withdrawal symptoms, and produce less euphoric effects than heroin.

79. S. A. Strathdee et al., "HIV and Risk Environment for Injecting Drug Users: The Past, Present, and Future," *Lancet* 376, no. 9737 (2010): 268–84.

80. Williams et al., "HIV Seroprevalence."

81. M. L. Adelekan and G. V. Stimson, "Problems and Prospects of Implementing Harm Reduction for HIV and Injecting Drug Use in High Risk Sub-Saharan African Countries," *Journal of Drug Issues* 27, no. 1 (1997): 97–116.

82. C. Cook, ed., *The Global State of Harm Reduction 2010: Key Issues for Broadening the Response* (London: International Harm Reduction Association, 2010).

83. Needle et al., "Substance Abuse."

84. Ibid.; Cook, *Global State.*

85. Abdool, Sulliman, and Dhannoe, "Injecting Drug Use."

86. Cook, *Global State,* citing F. Sulliman, chair of the SAHRN Steering Committee, "Global State of Harm Reduction Information Response" (2010).

87. Cook, *Global State.*

88. Ibid.

89. McCurdy et al., "Harm Reduction."

90. H. Maruyama, Field notes, Summer 2011; S. McCurdy, Field notes, Summer 2011; S. McCurdy, *Vijana Mateja* interviews; S. McCurdy et al., "Young Injecting Drug Users' Needs and Vulnerabilities in Dar es Salaam, Tanzania (Poster)," International Harm Reduction Association 22nd International Conference, Beirut, Lebanon, 2011.

91. H. Maruyama, Field notes, Summer 2011.

92. N. Ezard, "Public Health, Human Rights and the Harm Reduction Paradigm: From Risk Reduction to Vulnerability Reduction," *International Journal of Drug Policy* 12, no. 3 (2001): 213.

93. Ibid.

94. Williams et al., "HIV Seroprevalence."

SHERYL MCCURDY AND HARUKA MARUMAYA

ABOUT THE CONTRIBUTORS

MYRON ECHENBERG is Professor Emeritus of History at McGill University. He is the author of *Plague Ports: The Global Urban Impact of Bubonic Plague, 1894–1901* (New York University Press, 2007); *Black Death, White Medicine: Bubonic Plague and the Politics of Public Health in Colonial Senegal, 1914–1945* (Heinemann, 2002); and *Africa in the Time of Cholera: A History of Pandemics from 1817 to the Present* (Cambridge University Press, 2011).

MICHEL GARENNE, PhD, works on population and health interactions, with emphasis on communicable diseases, their dynamics and their consequences. He is the author of numerous articles on mortality and fertility changes in African countries. He is based at the Epidemiology of Emerging Diseases Unit of the Pasteur Institute in Paris, where he directs a research project on HIV/AIDS epidemics in Africa.

ALAIN GIAMI is a Research Professor at the Institut National de la Santé et de la Recherche Médicale (INSERM). Trained in psychology and the social sciences, he has published numerous books and articles. His research focuses on the sociological, historical, and psychological dimensions of health and sexuality, including HIV prevention, contraception, and sterilization, as well as on the medicalization of sexuality.

TAMARA GILES-VERNICK conducts anthropological and historical research on hepatitis B and C transmission and control, buruli ulcer, and the beginnings of HIV in central Africa. Based at the Epidemiology of Emerging Diseases Unit of the Pasteur Institute in Paris, she has published on public health and environmental history, including *Cutting the Vines of the Past: Environmental Histories of the Central African Rain Forest* (University of Virginia Press, 2002) and (with Susan Craddock) *Influenza and Public Health: Learning from Past Pandemics* (Earthscan/Routledge, 2010).

GUILLAUME LACHENAL is a Lecturer in History of Science at the University of Paris Diderot–Sorbonne Paris Cité and a member of the Institut Universitaire de France. His research is on the history and anthropology of biomedicine in Africa, especially Cameroon. Among other case studies, he has studied the history of sleeping sickness campaigns in the post–World War II period, the history of the decolonization of French medical research institutions in Africa, and the history of AIDS research and emerging viruses research in Central Africa. His current project, "Memorials and Remains of Medical Research in Africa" (MEREAF), is conducted in collaboration with anthropologists and studies how memories of the past shape the contemporary experience of medical research in Africa.

HARUKA MARUYAMA, MPH, graduated from the University of Texas, School of Public Health, with a concentration in Global Health. Her undergraduate background included a self-designed Bachelor of Arts in African Studies and a minor in Global Health Technologies from Rice University in Houston. She spent most of her childhood in Zambia and Kenya and is currently a Research Advisor with the International Center for AIDS Care and Treatment Center in Tanzania.

SHERYL MCCURDY is an Associate Professor at the University of Texas, School of Public Health. During the last ten years her work has focused on HIV prevention and heroin use in Dar es Salaam, Tanzania. Her publications are in public health, medicine, and African Studies journals and books, including (with Dorothy Hodgson) *'Wicked' Women and the Reconfiguration of Gender* (Heinemann, 2001).

ANNE MARIE MOULIN is a Director of Research with the Centre National de la Recherche Scientifique (CNRS) and based in the unit SPHERE (Sciences, Philosophie, Histoire). Trained in medicine and philosophy, she has published numerous books and articles on the history of medicine in Europe, North Africa and the Middle East. Her work has addressed wide-ranging topics, including immunology, vaccination, medical ethics, transplantation, and trachoma. Her most recent books are entitled *Le médecin du prince: Voyage à travers les cultures* (The Prince's physician: A cross-cultural voyage) (Odile Jacob, 2010) and *Islam et revolutions médicales: Le labyrinthe du corps* (Karthala, 2013).

CHRISTOPHE PERREY (PhD, social anthropology) conducts research on the sociology of science and expertise, as well as on research ethics in developing countries. With Guy de Thé, he authored *Le souple et le dur: Les sciences humaines au secours des sciences biomédicales* (The pliable and the hard: Social sciences to the rescue of biomedical sciences) (CNRS Editions, 2009), which focused on the interdisciplinary dialogue between ethnology and epidemiology. He recently published a second monograph, *Un ethnologue chez les chasseurs de virus* (L'Harmattan, 2012) (An ethnologist among the virus hunters), on the social factors shaping the research questions in an epidemiology unit at the Institut Pasteur. He is currently a researcher associated with the unit titled Gender, Sexual, and Reproductive Health, in the Center for Research in Epidemiology and Population Health at the Institut National de la Santé et de la Recherche Médicale (INSERM).

STEPHANIE RUPP is Assistant Professor of Anthropology at the City University of New York, Lehman College. Recent publications include *Forests of Belonging: Identities, Ethnicities, and Stereotypes in the Congo River Basin* (University of Washington Press, 2011), an ethnography based on her research in southeastern Cameroon. She also has published an edited volume with Sarah Strauss and Thomas Love on ethnographies of energy, *Cultures of Energy* (Left Coast Press, 2013). She is the editor of a forthcoming (2013) special issue of *African Studies Review* concerning ethnographic perspectives on China-Africa relations.

JENNIFER TAPPAN is Assistant Professor of African History at Portland State University. She received her doctorate from Columbia University with a focus on East African history and the history of colonial and tropical medicine in Africa. Her research examines the history of nutritional research, therapy, and programming in Uganda. Forthcoming publications include an article in a special edition of the *International Journal of African Historical Studies* on Health and Disease in Africa.

WILLIAM H. SCHNEIDER (PhD, University of Pennsylvania) is Professor of History at Indiana University–Purdue University in Indianapolis. He directs the Medical Humanities and Health Studies Program and also has an adjunct appointment in the Department of Medical and Molecular Genetics in the School of Medicine. His many articles and monographs include a book on the history of eugenics in France, *Quality and Quantity: The Quest for Biological Regeneration in Twentieth-Century France* (Cambridge University Press, 1990); and an edited volume, *Rockefeller Philanthropy and Modern Biomedicine* (Indiana University Press, 2002), on Rockefeller Foundation funding of medical

ABOUT THE CONTRIBUTORS

research around the world. He is currently finishing a monograph on the history of blood transfusion in Africa.

JAMES L. A. WEBB, JR. is a Professor of History at Colby College, where he teaches courses in comparative world history, global health history, and African health history. He is the editor for the Ohio University Press of the series Perspectives on Global Health and the Series in Ecology and History. He is the author of *Humanity's Burden: A Global History of Malaria* (Cambridge, 2009), and he is currently writing a book on the historical epidemiology of African malarial infections and interventions.

ABOUT THE CONTRIBUTORS

INDEX

elephants (*Loxodonta africana*), 122, 123, 129, 135n35
elimination (of disease), 15, 28, 29, 32, 34, 36, 38, 39, 41n28, 62, 70, 71, 84, 177, 223, 224, 227. *See also* eradication
El Katscha, Samiha, 147
el Sadat, Anwar, 149
emerging diseases, 8, 10, 20n39, 25, 117; biomedical research on, 118, 119–21, 130; Program for Monitoring Emerging Diseases (ProMED), 167
environment. *See* ecology
environmental management. *See* drainage; larvicide
epidemics, 16n2, 26, 30, 130–31. *See also* cholera; Ebola voris; hepatitis C; malaria; sleeping sickness; smallpox
epidemiology, 2, 14, 56, 74, 131, 143, 144, 145–46, 164, 192, 193, 194–95; case/control studies, 192–93; cohort studies, 193; historical, 1, 15–16n1; of HIV/AIDS, 191–95; of sexually transmitted infections, 193; randomized controlled trials (RCTs), 193–95, 200. *See also* clinical trials
Equatorial Africa. *See* Central Africa
eradication, 5, 18n18, 25, 27, 32, 38, 39, 42, 43, 52–62, 71, 74, 80, 84. *See also* guinea worm eradication; malaria; polio; smallpox; World Health Organization (WHO)
ethics, 82, 83, 84
Ethiopia, 164, 169; famine of 1985, 169
European colonial powers. *See individual states*
European Union, 9
Expanded Program in Immunization, WHO, 6
Expert Committee on Nutrition (FAO/WHO, 1949), 94–95, 97, 98
Ezard, Nadine, 227

Fahmy, Khaled, 150
Fang, 124
Farley, John, 141
Fenner, Frank, 25, 34, 37–38, 39n4
fertility, 191–92, 196
filariasis, 118
Firestone Tire and Rubber Company, 43, 64n11
First World War. *See* World War I
flashblood, 222. *See also* injection drug use
flooding, 160, 171, 172
Foege, William, 32–33
Food and Agriculture Organization (FAO), 94, 95, 98
Foucault, Michel, 73, 204

France, 9, 171; and colonies, 12, 73, 76; and colonial medicine, 36, 76, 77
French Algeria, 75
French Congo, 29
French Equatorial Africa, 29, 36, 81
French Guinea, 56, 59
French Soudan, 28–29, 35
French West Africa, 29, 31
Fulani, 37

Gabaldón, Arnaldo, 61
Gabon, 29, 122, 123, 125
Garenne, Michel, 202
Garnett, Geoffrey, 72
Gates Foundation. *See* Bill and Melinda Gates Foundation
Gbaya, 123
gender, 147–48
genealogy, 72–73, 74, 83–84
German East Africa, 74, 76
German Kamerun, 76
Germany, 9, 74, 95
Ghaffar, Yasin Abdel, 144
Ghana, 214, 221
Giglioli, M.E.C., 54
Gilks, John, 77
Gillies, M.T., 52
Global Alliance for Vaccines and Immunizations (GAVI), 9
Global Fund to Fight AIDS, Tuberculosis, and Malaria, 9, 203
global health, 1–3, 5–8, 84; biomedical research institutions and, 9; colonial antecedents, 3–4, 26–38, 84; definition, 2–3, 132n2; diplomacy, 16n2; disease-specific interventions, 5, 10–12; funding, 8–10; and security, 8, 117–18; technical approach, 107; vertical approach, 5, 10–11. *See also* eradication; international health; primary health care
globalization, 132n2, 231
Global Polio Eradication Initiative, 8, 9, 10, 39
Gold Coast, 31, 33, 35
gorillas, western lowland (*Gorilla gorilla gorilla*), 119, 120, 121, 122, 123, 124, 125, 126–27, 129, 130
governance, 1, 150–52, 168, 169, 174–77, 204
Granich, Reuben, 70, 71
Gray, R., 202, 204
great apes, 13, 118–37
Great Aswan Dam, 143
Great Britain, 189; and colonies, 9, 31, 44; and colonial medicine, 76, 77, 87n35, 89n66, 141; and colonial science, 21n48